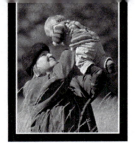

CASE STUDIES

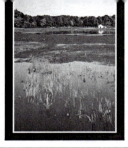

CONTRIBUTORS

Lisa Anderson-Shaw, DrPH, MA, MSN
Director, Clinical Ethics Consultation Service and
  Assistant Clinical Professor, University of Illinois Medical Center

Angeline Bushy, PhD, RN, FAAN
Professor and Bert Fish Endowed Chair,
  University of Central Florida-College of Nursing

Ann Freeman Cook, PhD
Director, National Rural Bioethics Project
Research Professor, Department of Psychology,
  University of Montana-Missoula

Rachel Davis, MD
Faculty, University of Colorado Denver
Denver Health Medical Center Psychiatric Emergency Services

Paul B. Gardent, MBA, CPA
Senior Associate, Center for Leadership and Improvement,
  The Dartmouth Institute for Health Policy & Clinical Practice
Adjunct Professor of Business Administration, Tuck School of Business at
  Dartmouth

Jacqueline J. Glover, PhD
Associate Professor, Department of Pediatrics and the Center for Bioethics
  and Humanities, University of Colorado Denver

Mary Ann Greene, MS
Research Associate, Community and Family Medicine,
  Dartmouth Medical School

Helena Hoas, PhD
Research Professor, Department of Psychology, University of
  Montana-Missoula

Barbara Elliott, PhD
Professor and Director, Clinical Research, Department of Family Medicine
and Community Health Duluth, University of Minnesota Medical School
Duluth
Associate Faculty, Center for Bioethics, University of Minnesota.

David A. Fleming, MD, MA, FACP
Professor of Clinical Medicine, Director, MU Center for Health Ethics,
University of Missouri School of Medicine

William A. Nelson, MDiv, PhD
Director, Rural Ethics Initiatives, Associate Professor Community and Family
Medicine, Dartmouth Medical School
Associate Professor, The Dartmouth Institute for Health Policy &
Clinical Practice

Denise Niemira, MD
Family Physician, Newport, VT

Andrew Pomerantz, MD
Chief, Mental Health and Behavioral Sciences, VA Medical Center,
White River Junction, VT
Associate Professor of Psychiatry, Dartmouth Medical School

Ruth B. Purtilo, PhD
Professor of Ethics, Massachusetts General Hospital, Institute of Health
Professions, Boston, Massachusetts
Marsh Professor-at-Large, University of Vermont

Susan A. Reeves, RN
Vice President, Dartmouth-Hitchcock Medical Center
Chair, Department of Nursing, Colby-Sawyer College

Laura Weiss Roberts, MD, MA
Charles E. Kubly Professor and Chair, Department of Psychiatry and
Behavioral Medicine; and Professor of Bioethics, Department of
Population Health, Medical College of Wisconsin

Karen E. Schifferdecker, PhD
Research Assistant Professor, Director, Office of Community-based
Education and Research, Dartmouth Medical School

Tom Townsend, MD
Professor, Department of Family Medicine and Director, Program in Clinical Ethics, Quillen College of Medicine East Tennessee State University

Aruna Tummala, MD
Fellow in Geriatric Psychiatry at Medical College of Wisconsin Affiliated Hospitals, Milwaukee

Ruth Westra DO, MPH
Chair, Assistant Professor Department of Family Medicine and Community Health Duluth, University of Minnesota Medical School

SECTION I

Rural Health Care Ethics

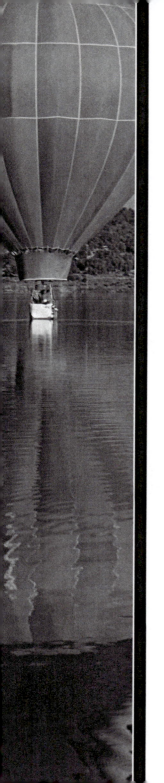

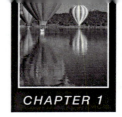
CHAPTER 1

Introduction

William A. Nelson

Introduction

William A. Nelson

from SMALL TOWN[1]

Got nothing against a big town…
But my bed is in a small town
Oh, and that's good enough for me

—John Cougar Mellencamp

Today approximately 60 million people—one-fifth of the United States' overall population—live in rural communities, which are distributed over more than three-quarters of our country's land mass.[2] Many rural residents have significant disabilities related to illness and injuries, and they may encounter tremendous obstacles when seeking needed health care. Rural Americans have limited access to clinicians, health facilities, and specialized services, and their care is hampered by geographical and climatic barriers, as well as heightened social, cultural, and economic challenges. The burden of illness for rural populations is considerable, placing great demands on a resource-poor clinical care system. Consequently, rural people are increasingly recognized as an underserved special population. Attaining an appropriate standard of care for rural people, moreover, has emerged as a major concern in the national discussion of health disparities.

With the growing understanding of rural health care has come an emerging awareness of the special ethical considerations inherent to clinical practice in closely-knit, tightly interdependent small community settings. It is difficult, for example, for a provider to protect the privacy of rural patients when the care of such patients occurs in clinics where neighbors, friends, and relatives may work. Similarly, it is difficult to establish a professional clinician-patient relationship when the patient is the doctor's former grade school teacher, or a member of the nurse's local parish. Ethical aspects of care are especially relevant and sensitive when the patient's health problem is stigmatizing, as is the case with mental illnesses, drug-abuse disorders, and infectious diseases. Because of these distinct pressures in the community context, the solutions that practitioners develop to resolve complex ethics dilemmas arising in rural areas may differ from solutions derived in urban areas. Providing health care to a family member, friend, business associate or neighbor may become necessary in a rural setting, whereas urban contexts—with the greater availability of diverse health care clinicians, facilities, and resources in the immediate area—may permit greater role separation between clinician and patient, and clearer personal and professional boundaries.

Despite the unique character of rural ethics issues, there are limited comprehensive written materials that specifically focus on assisting rural clinicians and facility administrators who are confronted with complex ethics dilemmas. Rural clinicians have expressed concerns about professional codes of ethics and ethical standards of practice that are not tailored to the dilemmas that exist in small communities. These formal documents often appear most applicable to the resource-enriched, less interdependent urban communities. Furthermore, rural clinicians have less access to local ethics committees and consultants, and fewer opportunities for ethics education. For these reasons, clinicians who are entrusted with providing competent and ethically sound clinical care in rural settings have identified a need for the development of resource documents that can offer guiding principles.

Surrounding all these ethical challenges are the basic characteristics of the rural environment. In fact, that's what rural health care ethics is about—it's about the context, the wonderful and complex rural settings that surround and foster many of the ethics conflicts. Rural health care ethics is the application of an ethics framework and ethical standards to the unique rural environment. What is unique to rural ethics is not so much the basic ethical domains, such as ethics conflicts about end-of-life decision-making or questions regarding privacy and confidentiality. Ethics challenges regarding those domains can occur in any setting, and are not unique to rural practice. What is unique is how the rural context's characteristics and features can shape and weave their way into the dimensions and dynamic surrounding the ethical uncertainty or question as well as the response to the challenge. This *Handbook* focuses on how that rural context is interwoven into the presentation of such ethics conflicts, and how the health care professional responds to the conflicts.

In 2006, a group of multidisciplinary health care professionals, including physicians, nurses, health care ethicists, and hospital administrators, gathered at a Dartmouth College retreat center in the woods of New Hampshire to share and explore a common interest in the ethics of rural health care. The participants were selected on the basis of their scholarship, teaching, and research in the field of rural ethics. Over several days, the professionals discussed many topics, such as the nature and scope of the field; ethics issues that rural clinicians and administrators experience, in contrast to their urban counterparts; the limited resources and training that are currently devoted to rural ethics; and the challenges in applying traditional ethics standards and professional guidelines to rural issues and ethics programs in small rural facilities.

The group did not agree on all aspects of rural ethics issues, but did agree that what makes rural health care unique is the context—the rural environment and culture that is woven into the fabric of the ethics issues that they all encounter. The participants acknowledged that the essence of rural health care ethics is the contextual environment that shapes and influences ethical challenges. As Dr. Tom Townsend notes in Chapter 7 of this *Handbook*, "The intimacy of rural life is a key factor to many aspects of rural health care ethics discussions. An ethical relationship with strangers is different from the ethics of close-knit relationships. The ethics issues within the patient-provider relationship change when strangers, rather than friends, neighbors, or acquaintances, are involved. This distinction is key to many of the differences between urban and rural health care ethics."

The retreat involved long discussions about what makes the rural environment unique in the United States—despite regional differences between the Northwest, Appalachia, the Southwest, New England and other rural communities, there are many common health-related characteristics that influence and create ethics challenges, including those listed in Box 1.1.

THE NATURE OF RURAL HEALTH CARE

During the retreat, in an exercise to explore the various cultural characteristics that shape rural health care ethics, participants read and discussed the book, *A Fortunate Man*—a moving description of a rural

BOX 1.1

COMMON HEALTH-RELATED RURAL CHARACTERISTICS

- Small populations and long distances from urban-based tertiary medical centers
- Overlapping personal and professional relationships between health care providers and community members
- Rural isolation which may exacerbate care providers' stress
- Limited availability of health care services, specialists and providers
- Small hospitals, many with fewer than 25 beds
- Residents with close-knit, shared connections and experiences
- Residents' strong sense of self-reliance and independent thinking
- Shared values, interdependence and culture
- Challenging economic and employment situation(s)
- Poor health status compared to non-rural populations
- Hazardous work environment(s)
- Limited rural ethics resources, i.e., a lack of rural ethics literature, rural ethicists, rural ethics training, and rural ethics committees in the area

physician. John Berger's book delivers a poignant portrait of an English country doctor caring for people in a remote community. Berger wrote that, "Landscapes can be deceptive. Sometimes a landscape seems to be less a setting for the life of its inhabitants than a curtain behind which struggles, achievements and accidents take place. For those who are behind the curtain, landmarks are no longer only geographic but also biographical and personal."[3] The doctor portrayed in this book finds a great commitment and passion for his work in the remote community, and builds strong bonds with the rural townspeople whom he supports. These positive attributes of the life of a country doctor help the protagonist transcend any professional isolation, challenges, and stressful workload as the only provider in town with no backup—he "is" the hospital.[4] Berger's writing helped to remind the retreat participants that despite the many challenges of living and working in rural communities, there is great meaning and satisfaction in being a rural health care professional.

In addition, one evening, partly for entertainment, the participants watched the film *Doc Hollywood*—the tale of an urban physician's experiences in rural America. In *Doc Hollywood*, Michael J. Fox plays the role of a young, aspiring plastic surgeon, who takes off on an adventure, driving cross-country from Washington, D.C. and heading to a high-paying new job in Beverly Hills. The doctor encounters adventure more quickly than expected when he crashes his Porsche in a tiny, remote rural community, destroying some property and ending his dreams of completing his trip uneventfully. The small town's judge sentences Fox's character to 30 days working as the town's country doctor, while the town's regular doctor goes on vacation. The rest of the comedy portrays a predictable, yet funny and believable tale of how the doctor and residents grow to know and appreciate each other.[5]

On a more serious note, the film reflects how the rural setting affects the professional's ability to deliver health care. Fox's character learns to cope with, and even comes to appreciate, the challenges and rewards of being a typical country doctor, which include professional isolation, the stress of managing a clinic single-handedly, and unexpected situations. He develops meaningful relationships with the townspeople, and becomes committed to working in this very remote, previously unknown community. Thus *Doc Hollywood* shows a glimpse of the world of the rural health care provider that is not often seen or understood by anyone, even doctors, living in urban areas.[4]

It has been suggested that the discipline of bioethics has evolved historically into a field with many wide-ranging areas of focus. The *Encyclopedia of Bioethics* noted four particular overlapping areas of inquiry: theoretical ethics, clinical ethics, regulatory and policy ethics, and cultural health care ethics.[6] Theoretical health care ethics focuses on the underlying foundations of moral reasoning that are applied to various health care topics. Clinical ethics refers to specific questions or uncertainty in individual patient care. Regulatory and policy health care ethics is the organizational and legal focus of health care-related ethics questions. Cultural health care ethics is an effort to systematically relate health care ethics to the cultural, ethnic, religious, and social context in which ethics conflicts arise. In health care ethics, one of those cultural subgroups of inquiry is the rural setting with its unique characteristics.

In both *A Fortunate Man* and *Doc Hollywood*, we are taken behind the curtain to a unique setting, the "Small Town" as John Mellencamp sings, unknown and rarely understood by many who live in metropolitan and urban settings. These works, along with the personal experiences of the gathered retreat participants, contributed to a contextual understanding of rural health care ethics. That same rural context affects the approaches that health care professionals use in their response to the ethics issues. It is this rural context that is the basis for rural health care ethics.

EVOLVING RURAL ETHICS AGENDA
There was consensus among the participants in the 2006 retreat that rural ethics has experienced a limited focus as a component of the broad discipline of health care ethics or bioethics. The participants discussed and identified a proposed rural ethics agenda to expand the needed focus on rural health care ethics. This rural ethics agenda, reprinted below, was later published in an article[7] from which the text in Box 1.2 is a direct quote.

The small group of professionals at the retreat, self-named as the Coalition for Rural Health Care Ethics, continued to communicate following the retreat. The retreat experience fostered many ongoing collaborative activities among the Coalition members—who, like most rural health care professionals, tend to work in isolation from other rural colleagues. As an example of the collaboration, Coalition members planned and implemented several presentations for the National Rural Health Association's annual meeting, the American Society of Bioethics and Humanities' annual meeting, and regional gatherings of state offices of rural health. Members also worked together on various publications and grant efforts.

BOX 1.2

RURAL HEALTH CARE ETHICS AGENDA

- "Develop a clear understanding of what constitutes the scope of rural health care ethics.
- Increase awareness and understanding of rural health care ethics issues, including the contextual nature of the ethical issues and how the issues are different from non-rural settings.
- Increase awareness and understanding of rural health care ethics decision-making, including how living and working in rural communities affects the response to ethical issues.
- In collaboration with rural health care professionals, draft guidelines for addressing common ethical conflicts.
- Explore, assess, and propose models for "doing ethics" in small rural health facilities.
- Develop training curricula and other educational resources for and with rural clinicians, administrators and policy-makers.
- Provide an ethics perspective, supported by empirical data, to administrators and policy makers who are charged with allocating health care resources.
- Foster a dialogue with the general health care ethics community regarding the unique contextual nature of rural ethical issues."[7]

HANDBOOK FOR RURAL HEALTH CARE ETHICS: A PRACTICAL GUIDE FOR PROFESSIONALS

As a direct outgrowth of the 2006 rural health care ethics retreat, a grant proposal was written, with its goal to plan, develop, and disseminate a handbook. The grant application to the National Institutes of Health (NIH) National Library of Medicine was approved, and the project was launched. Additional rural-focused ethicists, clinicians, and administrators were recruited to join in the effort to write the *Handbook*. So discussions that began in the woods of New Hampshire have continued to evolve in expanding the understanding of rural health care ethics and its agenda.

The Handbook for Rural Health Care Ethics: A Practical Guide for Professionals was conceived and written to help fill the gap in the limited ethics resources focused on rural health care. The *Handbook* is intended to help multidisciplinary rural professionals respond effectively to the complex ethics conflicts they may face each day. It addresses challenges that arise in rural settings on such issues as obtaining informed consent, establishing patient-provider relationships, adhering to treatment, boundary issues, appropriate protection of confidentiality, resolving conflicts between the interests of individual patients and the good of the overall community, distributing scarce resources equitably, and experiencing pressure to provide care in areas that are beyond the provider's usual scope of clinical competence.

The *Handbook* has been written by and for health care professionals who are living and working in rural communities. The authors are an outstanding group of physicians, nurses, administrators, and ethicists noted for their scholarship, research, and teaching in the area of rural health care ethics. The *Handbook* is divided into three main sections:

Section I: Rural Health Care Ethics Overview
This section focuses on the nature and scope of rural health care ethics. Section I includes a discussion of the ethics issues encountered in the professional life of health care clinicians and an exploration of "doing" ethics in rural settings.

Section II: Common Ethics Issues in Rural Communities
Section II contains a wide range of familiar ethics issues, including both clinical and organizational issues that occur in the context of rural communities and hospitals. Each chapter begins with brief case presentations, then delivers an overview of the relevant ethics issues, and finally provides a discussion and response to the each of the cases. Because ethics issues tend to recur, each chapter will offer suggestions for anticipating such ethics conflicts, encouraging the reader to apply the suggested strategies to decrease the likelihood that such conflicts will recur, or to make them easier to cope with if they do recur.

Section III: Rural Ethics Resources
The final section offers several chapters of practical information and approaches to expand the rural health care professional's ability to manage ethics challenges.

REFERENCES

1. Mellencamp JC. Small Town. *Scarecrow*. Mercury;1985.

2. U. S. Department of Health and Human Services, Health Resources and Services Administration. Rural Health Fact Sheet. U.S. Department of Health and Human Services. http://www.hrsa.gov/about/factsheets/orhp.htm. Accessed 1/19/09.

3 Berger J, Mohr J. *A Fortunate Man: The Story of a Country Doctor*. 1st ed. New York, NY: Holt, Rinehart and Winston; 1967.

4 Nelson WA, Schmidek JM. Rural healthcare ethics. In: Singer PA, Viens AM, eds. *The Cambridge Textbook of Bioethics*. New York, NY: Cambridge University Press; 2008:289-298.

5 Nelson WA. The challenges of rural health care. In: Klugman CM, Dalinis PM, eds. *Ethical Issues in Rural Health Care* Baltimore, MD: Johns Hopkins University Press; 2008:34-59.

6 Callahan D. Bioethics. In: Reich WT, ed. *Encyclopedia of Bioethics*. New York, NY: Simon & Schuster Macmillan; 1995.

7. Nelson W, Pomerantz A, Howard K, Bushy A. A proposed rural healthcare ethics agenda. *J Med Ethics*. Mar 2007;33(3):136-139.

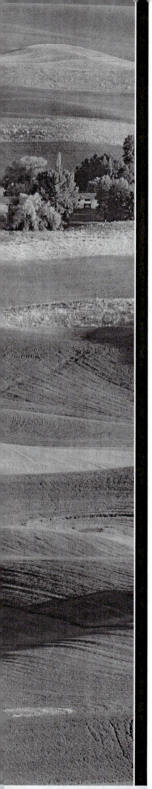

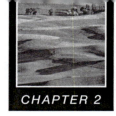

A Landscape View
of Life and Health Care
in Rural Settings

Angeline Bushy

A Landscape View of Life and Health Care in Rural Settings

Angeline Bushy

ABSTRACT

Compared with people living in more populated urban areas, residents in rural environments may experience greater isolation, have less access to health care, and identify with more traditional cultural beliefs about health and illness. Rural residents often seek care from a health professional who may also be an extended family member, neighbor, friend or professional colleague. The rural health care provider should consider these factors, along with other social, economic, and cultural contextual attributes, when he or she responds to ethical situations involving his or her patients' care. This chapter focuses on the rural contextual attributes that can impact ethical situations that arise for clinicians in this practice setting.[1, 2] The ethical situations include, among others, the often overlapping professional and personal roles of rural health care providers, and the threats to patient confidentiality and privacy that may occur in smaller communities. The rural context has factors that can cause or impact such situations, including geographic isolation, small population, and close social and/or kinship relationships among community members. These factors create unique ethical opportunities and challenges for rural health care providers. Clinicians and administrators should seek potential ethics resources, such as ethics programs and consultants, and the ethics literature, to help solve conflicts.

INTRODUCTION

Over the past two decades, there has been extensive publicity about ethics conflicts occurring, primarily, in large urban health care facilities. Ethics issues in rural health care settings have received less attention. For example, in small communities, the dynamics surrounding ethics conflicts often become extremely complicated because clinicians, patients and their families live and work in close proximity, with often overlapping professional and personal relationships. A rural clinician's patient care is provided within a context of broad familiarity and multiple relationships.[1, 2] Sometimes an ethics case has intense emotional aspects, especially if there is a stigma associated with a particular condition, such as substance abuse, domestic violence, mental illness, or sexually transmitted diseases.[3] It is this rural context that makes rural health care ethics unique. Some rural contextual features that contribute to ethical conflicts are listed in Box 2.1.[4, 5]

BOX 2.1

FEATURES ENCOUNTERED BY THE RURAL PROVIDER

- Limited health care services and resources
- Geographic barriers to health care services
- Conflicts between community values and professional guidelines
- Challenges to privacy and confidentiality
- A clinician providing care to a neighbor, a friend, or a family member
- A provider trying to deliver quality care, despite being professionally isolated, with limited access to peers and specialists
- Overlapping professional and personal boundaries
- Community expectations and professional stress

Despite the uniqueness of every rural community, there are several general characteristics that influence ethics conflicts in all rural communities. There are limited resources in the rural setting, including various health care specialties as well as experts in the field of ethics. Clinicians often work in isolated situations, away from peer colleagues. There are geographic barriers such as challenging roads, limited public transportation, and weather conditions that may impede patients' access to health care services. Rural clinicians commonly experience the phenomenon of overlapping or dual relationships with patients. Because everyone knows each other, disease stigma is frequently encountered, especially associated with conditions like substance abuse, mental illness or sexually transmitted diseases.

Professional isolation and high demands for the clinician's services can create provider stress. In some cases a doctor or nurse is on call 24x7 with no real backup. These general contextual features regularly surround and shape the ethical issues that are encountered by rural clinicians.[3]

When ethical issues occur in small towns, they are often not easily remedied using professional guidelines that were, in many cases, developed and applied in urban-based and resource-rich health care facilities. The rural clinician's response to ethics conflict is based not only on his or her training, experience, and professional guidelines, but also on the community's values. The social, economic, and cultural characteristics of small communities reflect the values of their residents. Understanding the health care ethics conflicts that have occurred in the past in the rural community can provide insights to clinicians, enabling them to more effectively respond to ethics conflicts and anticipate potential conflicts.[1]

Defining Rural Communities
The term "rural" can be defined in many ways, depending both on who is defining it, and why he or she is defining it, which can result in sometimes confusing and conflicting statistics. In fact, the National Rural Health Association does not provide a definition of rural, but instead encourages individuals to tailor the term to meet the needs of a particular program.[6]

Population is a common way to define rurality. According to the U.S. Bureau of Census, about 60 million people live in areas defined as "rural."[7] Rural residents make up about one-fifth (20%) of the total U.S. population and are spread across four-fifths (80%) of the U.S. land area.[8]

Another common definition of rural is based on the geographic size of a community relative to population density; for example, the number of people living in a square mile. More remote regions having fewer than six people per square mile are defined as frontier areas, although this statistic varies as well, depending on the program.[9] Of the total U.S. rural population, about 5% live in towns of 2,500 residents or less. Some definitions of rural also consider the distance to services and/or "time to access services" (e.g., greater than 30 minutes or more than 20 miles to a certain destination).[10] It is important to note that the time to access health care may also impact residents who live in inner city or suburban areas due to transportation challenges.[6]

Perceptions of "rural" and the available resources within a particular region are relative in nature. For example, some communities with a population of approximately 25,000 may statistically be defined as rural, yet have features that one expects to find in a large city. Or, in a relative sense, residents in a town of fewer than 2,500 may perceive a community with a population of 10,000 as a city. Likewise, a family living in a frontier region may not feel isolated, because urban-based services are relatively easy for them to access via telecommunication and reliable transportation.[1, 11]

Rural Demographics
American rural communities have a diversity of geographical regions, population dynamics, age stratification, and other features. For instance, a higher proportion of African-Americans reside in the southeast, more elderly live in the rural Midwest, while Native Americans tend to reside on or near reservations (usually located in more remote parts of the United States). Rural communities also have diverse population trends; some have experienced a declining population in recent years, and others have had an economic revival and population growth.

Demographically, the population in rural communities sometimes is described as bipolar; rural residents tend to be under the age of 17, or over 65 years of age. This may be because many rural communities have strong schools and are safe places to retire, but lack the employment options needed to sustain groups of young and middle-aged adults. Consistent with national trends, there has been an increase in racial and ethnic minorities in rural areas, who now comprise about 17% of the overall rural population. Overall, compared to urban residents, a greater proportion of rural residents are married, have fewer years of formal education, have lower incomes, and fewer have completed high school.[12-16]

HEALTH STATUS OF RURAL RESIDENTS
Health and illness are defined in various ways, as influenced by individuals' cultural background. Among some rural residents, health is defined as "the ability to work; to do what needs to be done," reinforcing a work ethic. Thus, a patient with such views may not seek "formal" health care until he or she becomes too ill to work. Further, the practical limitations of time and work in a rural community mean that residents may wait to seek medical care until they can combine it with other business requiring a trip to town.[11] Box 2.2 provides a brief overview of some urban-rural comparisons regarding health status.

BOX 2.2

HEALTH DISPARITIES OF RURAL AREAS AS COMPARED WITH URBAN AREAS[12-16]

- Higher infant and maternal morbidity rates
- Higher rates of chronic illnesses, such as hypertension and cardiovascular disease
- Higher rates of mental illness and stress-related diseases (especially among the rural poor)
- Lower rates of health insurance and pharmacy coverage plans
- Greater expenditures on prescription medications, associated with lack of pharmacy insurance benefits and/or more out-of-pocket costs for drugs because of lower insurance coverage
- Problems unique to rural occupations, such as machinery accidents, and skin cancer from sun exposure in farming or outdoor labor

A recent U.S. Department of Health and Human Services (HHS) report indicated that "rural residents are more likely to report fair to poor health status than urban residents, and are more likely to have experienced a limitation of activity caused by chronic conditions than urban residents."[17] Rural residents have a higher prevalence of long-term health problems as compared to urban residents; this is primarily attributable to rural areas having a higher proportion of poor and elderly residents, as well as more accidents and trauma.

Mental health needs appear to be particularly significant in rural settings where residents struggle with significant substance dependence, mental illnesses, and psychiatric-medical co-morbidity. It has been noted that suicide rates in rural areas have surpassed urban suicide rates for over 20 years.[18]

Yet, rural residents have relatively low mortality in light of their high rate of chronic illnesses. A serious gap exists in the health-status data of vulnerable and at-risk populations like those in rural areas. Knowledge of a community's demographics is particularly important, because health status can affect health care ethics conflicts. The HHS report concludes, "a scant provider network, lack of adequate and affordable health coverage, and difficulty accessing high-quality care can lead to worse health among rural populations."[17]

RURAL CHARACTERISTICS AND LIFESTYLE

Even though each rural community is unique, the overall experience of living in a small rural town tends to be similar, characterized by certain features, a list of which is shown in Box 2.3.[1-5, 11]

BOX 2.3

CHARACTERISTICS OF THE RURAL LIFESTYLE AND CULTURE

- Extensive distances between people and services
- Work and recreational activities are often cyclic and seasonal in nature
- Prominence of high-risk land-oriented occupations and activities
- Social interactions that facilitate frequent, informal, face-to-face contacts
- Close social or kinship relationships among community members
- Preference for informal support systems in times of need
- Individual and community self-reliance
- Small towns as centers of trade
- Churches and schools are centers of socialization for residents
- Importance of local health systems, especially hospital and long-term care facilities, to the local economy
- Overlapping roles and relationships for clinicians as community members

It's always risky to generalize about a particular group, as this can perpetuate stereotypes. Furthermore, the belief systems of rural residents are complex, and there is wide diversity among and within communities. However, some authors describe a "rural culture" associated with local belief systems and values, including some rural residents' sense of fatalism and subjugation to nature associated with nature-oriented businesses (e.g., agriculture, mining, timber production). Weather also tends to play a prominent role in these residents' lives, because of its effect on economic activities and the ability to travel.[2, 11-14]

Conservative Values and Perspectives

Members of small and homogenous communities tend to be conservative politically and socially, with some exceptions. They tend to be "church-going," i.e., actively involved in a faith community's activities. Residents in rural communities are likely to adhere to traditional gender-role expectations, holding precise ideas about what constitutes "men's work" versus "women's work." Men are expected to work outside the home for money and to support their families without public assistance. Women are expected to manage the household and to nurture and support their husbands and children without monetary compensation.[11-14]

Such old-fashioned, or (what some might call) sexist expectations shape some rural people's views about medical providers. Regardless of their actual education, women tend to be viewed as the "nurses" while men are considered "doctors." Female clinicians living in a rural community may be expected to serve as a community resource, and volunteer their professional expertise. Community members may look to nurses and other clinicians to provide no-cost consultations, to respond to local emergencies, or even to provide home-care services that are otherwise unavailable.[1, 11]

Self-Reliant Behaviors
Self-reliance is another characteristic often attributed to rural residents. Historically, and today, the trait of self-reliance has helped families to survive in austere, isolated, and rugged environments. Self-reliance can help a patient through illness, with informal support from family, neighbors, or community groups; however, it can undermine healing if the patient and family avoid formal health care treatment and "tough it out." For example, a man abusing alcohol or chemical substances may avoid acknowledging his problem and from seeking much-needed professional services, due the enabling behaviors of his family. Or the community may view a woman with a mental illness as exhibiting a character flaw or weakness typical of her family, about which nothing can be done. Hence the admonition, "What happens in the family, stays in the family." To preserve family integrity, it becomes important to maintain secrecy, and not let others know about the problem (e.g., substance abuse, domestic violence, incest, rape, emotional disorders, stigma laden-illnesses, or unplanned pregnancy). Additionally, professional values and guidelines may conflict with family expectations, and coupled with community-defined standards of behavior or values, can impose stress for residents and the clinicians who care for them. Such scenarios can lead to patient-provider-family conflicts and, subsequently, ethics conflicts.[2, 11-14]

Rural Social Support Systems
The literature describes three levels of social support for patients in rural settings. The first level includes assistance volunteered by a patient's immediate and extended family, friends and neighbors. Although this type of support is not monetarily reimbursed, there is an expectation of reciprocity

by those rendering the services. The second level includes support provided by a group or organization (e.g., civic organizations, homemakers' clubs, faith community, youth groups) in which members assist each other in the network during times of need (e.g., volunteering expertise, providing food, contributing financially, assisting with field work and farm chores).[2, 11-14] Essentially these levels offer an "insurance policy" should a catastrophic event occur to anyone belonging to one of these community or faith groups. These care systems are a resource for rural residents who are coping with hardships and geographical isolation; yet they also reinforce perceptions of self-reliance. The third level of care consists of formal support, such as services provided by health departments, home health and hospice agencies, community nursing services, mental health centers, physicians, and hospitals. Financial remuneration is expected for these services, albeit in some cases on a sliding scale.[4, 5]

Urban residents often prefer the third level of support, since they may not have access to the informal care systems that characterize small towns. Rural communities, however, historically rely on the first two levels of support. In day-to-day activities, rural residents prefer to deal with someone they know ("kith and kin") rather than a stranger ("bureaucrat"), such as providing child care to a family during an illness, or preferring to receive care in the local hospital from the doctor and nurses who are neighbors, friends or relatives.[11]

Rural Economics
Rural economics can impact a sick person's care-seeking behaviors. Generally, in small towns, salaries are low; there are limited benefits, including employee health insurance benefits, which results in a high rate of uninsured and under-insured.

The 2008 *Health Disparities: A Rural-Urban Chartbook* pointed out that, "Rural residents were more likely to be uninsured than were urban residents. The proportion of uninsured persons increased as the level of rurality increased, with residents of remote rural counties having the highest rate of uninsurance."[19] The *Chartbook* further noted that, "Rural residents were more likely to report that cost had kept them from seeing a doctor than were urban residents. The proportion of adults who reported deferring care because of cost increased with the level of rurality."[20]

According to the Rural Assistance Center (RAC), "The uninsured in remote rural counties are not a peculiar sub-population of their communities:

68 percent come from families where there is at least one full-time worker; 30 percent are children; and almost two-thirds come from low-income families (less than 200 percent of the federal poverty level—less than $37,700 for a family of four). Families with two full-time workers, married couples, and the employed are also at greater risk of being uninsured if they live in a remote rural county."[21]

The RAC also reports: "Remote rural residents are less likely to be offered health benefits through their employment: approximately 59% of workers in rural non-adjacent counties are offered employer-sponsored health insurance, compared to 69% of urban workers, and less than half of workers in rural nonadjacent counties are covered by their employers (compared to nearly 60% of urban workers)."[21]

In addition to the economic issues that impact individual residents' use of health care services, rural health care facilities are a main economic driver in small communities. In most rural communities, the largest employers are the school system and the health care facilities. Because rural health businesses may experience frequent financial challenges, these financial issues are passed on and can significantly impact the broader community. For example, the closure of one rural hospital can create a dramatic ripple effect on the economic status of the community, many of whom may have had jobs there.

RURAL HEALTH CARE

Even in the most remote rural areas, communities have some health care system that includes formal organizations and providers, as well as informal support systems. Rural health care professionals work in a variety of settings, including those listed below.

- *Federally-Qualified Rural Health Centers (FQHC, also known as Community Health Centers):* FQHCs qualify for enhanced reimbursement from Medicare and Medicaid, as well as other benefits. FQHCs must serve an underserved area or population.
- *Critical Access Hospitals (CAH):* These are small (25 beds or less) federally designated facilities. CAHs provide essential services to a community and are reimbursed by Medicare on a "reasonable cost basis" for services provided to Medicare patients.
- *Rural Health Clinics:* These must be rural and in a designated shortage area, eligible for cost-based reimbursement. The Rural Health Clinics (RHCs) program is intended to increase primary-care services for Medicaid and Medicare patients in rural communities.

RHCs can be public, private, or non-profit. The main advantage of RHC status is enhanced reimbursement rates for providing Medicaid and Medicare services in rural areas. RHCs must be located in rural, underserved areas and must use midlevel practitioners, such as a nurse practitioner (NP) and physician's assistant (PA).

- **Community Mental Health Centers:** Federally enabled centers providing a safety net for mental health care in underserved areas.
- **Private Practice Settings Clinics:** Private clinics, providing primary care. Some private clinics are affiliated with CAHs.

Despite federal assistance, many of these various health care mechanisms continue to struggle economically. Low population density often means there is not a critical mass of consumers for a particular health care service; thus, rural facilities and services often are challenged financially due to the lack of a specialized-care revenue stream.[12-15, 22]

Although there have been hospital closures nationwide in recent years, the rate of closure has been higher among rural hospitals.[12-15] Rural closures have been related to the lack of physicians in a small community, coupled with tenuous finances. For instance, if the small town's only physician leaves the community, it could mean the local hospital must close - even if there are other health professionals, particularly nurses, in the area. Of note is the federal designation Health Professional Shortage Areas (HPSAs) characterized by insufficient numbers of providers in a geographical area.[15, 22] With this federal designation, a community is given priority in seeking a health care provider replacement.

The contextual realities at these various health care settings have implications for health care professionals in rural areas. Clinicians in the rural context often are expected to function as generalists, because they care for individuals of all ages with a wide variety of health problems. For example, in one day at a rural hospital, a primary-care clinician may care for an obstetrical family (mother and newborn infant); a patient with postoperative complications from recent surgery; and an elderly person, who has a life-threatening chronic health problem.[1, 3, 11] Such diversity in a practice can be perceived as a positive benefit by many rural health care professionals, just as it can produce caregiver stress. To manage the inherent stress and ethics situations in rural settings, clinicians must be aware of both the formal and informal resources that make up the local health care system, as well as how the two interface, and what it takes to connect with these services.

Availability of Health Care Services

Availability refers to the existence of services and the presence of sufficient personnel to provide those services. Rural areas have fewer physicians and clinicians, nurse practitioners, and specialists; especially obstetricians, pediatricians, psychiatrists, and social-service professionals.[12-15, 22] Economically, a sparse population limits the number and array of services in a given region, as the cost of providing services to a few people may be prohibitive.

Access to Health Care Services

Accessibility refers to whether a person has the means to obtain and afford needed services, or is impaired by certain barriers to accessing health care. It has been noted that, "rural residents were more likely to report that cost had kept them from seeing a doctor than were urban residents. The proportion of adults who reported deferring care because of cost increased with the level of rurality."[20] A person in need of health care can encounter various barriers ranging from economic to transportation barriers; some of these are shown in Box 2.4.[12-15, 22]

BOX 2.4

BARRIERS TO ACCESSING HEALTH CARE

- Long travel distances
- Lack of public transportation
- Limited telephone and Internet services
- Shortage of health care providers
- Limited economic resources—income and insurance
- Challenging roles and unpredictable weather conditions
- Inability to seek or obtain entitlements

Two other barriers which, like economic barriers, can limit access to health care include geographical and physical barriers. Consider the case of a rancher with a high income, who lives in a medically underserved frontier area, and who suddenly suffers a heart attack. He may not have access to the most basic emergency care because of his geographic distance from the hospital, even though he has comprehensive medical insurance.

In addition to economic and physical barriers to health care, there are cultural and educational barriers that result when rural individuals lack a particular skill or element of education. Perhaps a small clinic is seeking a grant to access funding to implement a health program. However, the staff is hampered because they lack grant-writing skills. Or there may be a community perspective that opposes the use of federal or state welfare programs. Rural-based clinicians must recognize the stigma attached to the use of some types of services, and then adapt delivery approaches to try and assure anonymity and confidentiality within a rural context where people tend to be acquainted or related.[12-15, 22]

Acceptability of Health Care Services

Acceptability refers to whether a particular service is offered in a manner that agrees with the values of a target population. With the wide diversity among rural residents, acceptability of available services, like community nursing services, can be hampered by any of several factors, as described in Box 2.5.[5, 12-14]

BOX 2.5

BARRIERS TO ACCEPTING HEALTH CARE SERVICES

- Self-reliance leads to self-care for health issues (e.g., patients preferring to self-treat with over-the-counter medications, exercise, rest, or prayer)
- Beliefs about the cause of an illness and the appropriate healer for it (e.g., patients prefer to see a "medicine man/woman," curandero, shaman, or clergyperson)
- Community values about illness (e.g., patients being stoic and suffering in silence rather than seeking care)
- Lack of knowledge about a physical or emotional disorder, or of the importance of formal services for prevention and treatment
- Difficulty in maintaining confidentiality and anonymity in a setting where most residents are acquainted

Geographic, demographic, social, and economic factors will impact a clinician's practice as well as the health status in a particular rural community. In turn, ethics conflicts in rural settings generally are associated with these characteristics.

ETHICS ISSUES AND THE RURAL CONTEXT

The features of rural lifestyle (geography, population density, cultural values, and health care systems and services) influence the ethics situations that rural clinicians encounter.[1-5, 11] Many of the previously described rural characteristics that influence ethics conflicts are listed in Box 2.6.

BOX 2.6

RURAL CONTEXTUAL FEATURES THAT INFLUENCE HEALTH CARE ETHICAL SITUATIONS

- Community values and beliefs that differ from professional standards
- Overlapping personal and professional roles within the community
- Threats to confidentiality and privacy
- Real and perceived geographic and professional isolation
- Limited access to, and availability of, health care services and providers
- Economic limitations, such as low income and lack of adequate insurance
- Clinician stress associated with community expectations, professional workload, and isolation
- Reliance on informal, non-professional community health care support networks
- Limited ethics resources

Overlapping Professional and Personal Roles

Probably the most common part of the rural context that can foster ethics conflict is the role of overlapping relationships between clinicians and patients. Due to the geographical and social structure of rural communities, rural health care providers commonly interact with members of the community in more than one relationship—i.e., a nurse may serve on a school committee which also has one of her patients on the board; a doctor's children may play with the children of his patient; a psychiatrist may attend a house of worship where some of her patients also go. Generally, rural providers live and work in the same place, and everyone knows one another. Everyone knows the community's physician and/or nurse, and it is difficult to escape that role. Rural health care professionals frequently interact outside the office with community members. These multiple relationships can enhance and complicate the patient-clinician relationship.

This regular contact allows rural clinicians to have a knowledge of their patients that is unlikely in more urban settings. Rural clinicians have the unique opportunity to understand their patients in depth, including the patient's personal values and perspectives. The patient-provider relationship is formed and cultivated in both the examining room and in the general store. This can be very beneficial for treatment; however, ethics issues can also arise in maintaining professional boundaries with patients. Almost every rural ethics issue encountered is influenced and shaped by provider familiarity and overlapping roles. Patient-provider relationships and overlapping roles are discussed in more detail in Chapters 5 and 6, respectively.

Community Values Can Differ From Professional Practices

Authors have noted that rural residents from various cultures hold different views of pain, the etiologic explanations for sickness, tolerance of illness, and the use of folk healers. When the pervasive community values about illness differ from the traditional practice and ethos of clinicians, it is more likely that ethics conflicts will arise. Ethics conflicts may occur if providers show insufficient respect for cultural and community values. Recognizing community values and openly communicating with patients about how those values and beliefs differ from traditional health care clinical and ethics practices are key to the provider in addressing potential conflicts. Clinicians should also consider approaches to patient care that apply community values to their professional standards of practice. For example, a community value may be that an individual nearing death is allowed to remain in his or her home, with family, friends and neighbors supporting the family during this life transition.

Cultural insensitivity can also exacerbate a mistrust of clinicians. More specifically, a clinician's attitude can impact the long-term health status of a patient who may be embarrassed about his or her health problem(s). Embarrassment may be evidenced in certain ethnic or cultural groups, who may minimize symptoms of illness, not acknowledge self-care practices, or not seek care when it is needed. In such groups, health care is sought only for an acute illness or an emergency.

To diminish ethics issues related to cultural and community values, it would be beneficial for all health professional programs (medical training, nursing schools, technologist training, etc) to expose students to the rural environment and the cultural perspectives that they will encounter. For example, a rural-focused elective course could promote cultural competency in relationship to health care issues. Rural-based experiences and cultural understanding could go a long way to create a climate of mutual sensitivity and trust between clinicians and rural patients that could prevent health care ethics situations from occurring.[5, 12-14]

Threats to Confidentiality and Privacy

Closely related to overlapping relationships are threats to confidentiality and privacy. Breaches in confidentiality and privacy can be both intentional and unintentional, due to the close-knit nature of rural settings. It is not unusual for rural residents to report that even though they are well acquainted with most residents in the community, they feel there is no one they can trust, or with whom they can discuss personal problems. This experience is in part attributable to small town residents' genuine interest in the lives of neighbors, friends and relatives.[1-5]

Regardless of the setting, it can be devastating for those involved if their personal problems become public knowledge. Informal social structures, such as a church or extended family, in turn, can impose restrictions for those who desire to seek professional help for issues with moral overtones, such as drug and alcohol dependency, an unplanned pregnancy, sexuality issues, conflicts in personal relationships, or behaviors associated with mental illness. Further complicating the issues is the reluctance of some rural patients to access urban-based outreach services provided by professionals who are strangers, while services provided by the parish nurse may be openly welcomed.

A threat to confidentiality and privacy is a concern for rural residents, even for those who enjoy being personally acquainted with others in the community. As with all facets of professional life, familiarity has advantages and disadvantages. One provider's positive experience is described in this statement:

> *"Personally knowing a client and his or her family's lifestyle helps me to provide total care. After I provide care, I'm also able to keep track of the person's progress from direct reports by the person when I meet him or her in the store or on the street. Or, if the client is home-bound, I get word of mouth reports from his or her family, friends, neighbors, or other members of his or her church."[1]*

Personally knowing a patient creates some concerns and frustrations for clinicians, as well, as illustrated by the following comment:

> *"Sometimes knowing your patients well allows you to make assumptions without a really valid evaluation...You can miss something that should actually have been caught...I just*

*think other emotions can get in the way when you know
someone well.*[23]

Maintaining confidentiality is often difficult, particularly when the clinic
or agency is located in a public facility, such as the county courthouse.
Often the waiting room may be in a common hallway or an area where
patients are likely to be recognized. Moreover, announcements of
"specialty services" such as prenatal or family planning clinics, HIV
testing, Women, Infants and Children programs and immunization clinics
often are publicized in the local media (newspaper, church bulletins,
radio, television) and sometimes posted in public places such as grocery
stores, service stations, and grain elevators. People in small towns
often are recognized by the car they drive and thus, even parking lots
can jeopardize confidentiality. If a family planning clinic is held on Friday
mornings, for example, assumptions may be made about anyone seen
parking in front of the building—even if it is not to attend the clinic. Leaks
in confidentiality can result from such chance encounters and quickly
become public knowledge through the local rumor mill. Maintaining
confidentiality must always be a consideration in the rural context.
For example, prenatal or family planning clinics could be scheduled to
coincide with an immunization clinic, and STD clinics and HIV testing
could be offered on a walk-in basis. Innovative approaches are required
on the part of clinicians in rural practice to address the community's
concerns surrounding anonymity and confidentiality.[1-5]

Limited Access to Health Services
The limited availability, accessibility, and acceptability of health care
services can foster ethics challenges that are regularly encountered in
rural settings. The lack of services and specialists, such as mental health
professionals, creates situations where the general practitioner may need
to provide specialized mental health care. Other health care professionals,
including nurses and social workers, may become the *de facto* primary-
care provider in settings with limited resources. Many rural communities
have no hospitals; yet travel to the large, distant medical centers can
create burdens on both the patients and the rural providers. For example,
a patient may need to travel long distances over challenging roads to
find needed emergency care. Or a patient may need specialized cancer
treatment at the distant medical center, but opts out of the care because
of the distance and lack of support. Such situations place a great burden
on rural primary-care clinicians who may be forced to provide care outside
their areas of expertise.

Taken together, these factors (limited availability, accessibility, and acceptability) conspire so that small communities may have few health care services, lesser expertise, tremendous professional shortages, heightened ethical binds, and greater risk for errors and quality issues.

Community Economic Limitations

The economic status of rural residents can influence their use of health care services. A community member's willingness to accept needed care may be restricted by his or her economic situation. For example, patients requiring care may be underinsured or uninsured. Ethical questions can arise as a result of these situations. Rural health care professionals regularly encounter situations where they must decide whether to provide needed care with little or no reimbursement, which may potentially jeopardize both their patients' health and their own overall practice and standing within the community. Not providing needed services is a difficult decision, because it may be contrary to community values and the perceived role of the clinician. Because everyone in the community knows the physician, such decisions can never be made in a confidential manner. Resource allocation and access to health care are areas of great ethical challenge for rural physicians.

Clinician Stress

Clinicians tend to be held in high esteem by residents in small towns, but this can make it difficult to have a life outside of work. A nurse offers these insights about her practice:

> *"In an urban setting, when you leave work and drive your car out of the parking lot, you are just one more person in a city of a million people. In a rural area when you move your car out of the parking lot... you are the same person as when you were in the parking lot. Everywhere you go you are seen as [a nurse]...This affects how you conduct yourself when you are downtown, too."[23]*

Another component of health care provider stress is professional isolation. Geographic isolation poses challenges to rural clinicians because patients probably do not live nearby, as described in the following:

> *"We had a situation...where we had a man coming home from the hospital after having a CVA-stroke. He was completely paralyzed on his left side. He came home one evening, and a*

*nurse went out to the ranch the next morning to start servic-
es. We thought physical therapy and nursing and some aide
services would be appropriate.*

*When she got there (at) about 10 o'clock in the morning,
and was taking the history and assessment, she found out
that the man had driven into [the nearest town] the afternoon
before. She asked him how he had driven with [his] left side
completely paralyzed. He said when he got home he realized
that unless they drove that pickup, they were stranded. There
wasn't anybody around for miles and miles.*

*So he thought it over, and he got a couple of his leather belts
and put them together, climbed into his pickup, which was
a feat in itself, and got it into first gear, got out on the road,
slipped the belt around his left foot and when he was ready to
change gears he just reached over with his right hand, pulled
his foot up with the belt, dropped it on the clutch, put it in
second, and went down the road.*

*Right away that precludes him from meeting the home bound
criteria for Medicare. All (of) those services were not available
to him. We provided services (in) some other ways, but we
were not able to get any Medicare benefits for him."[23]*

Although this account does not reveal the reason why the patient went into
town, the account does suggest a degree of self-sufficiency and autonomy as
a way of coping with the isolation. Self-sufficiency in this case, however, cost
the patient his Medicare benefits. Knowing the patient could have used those
benefits likely caused stress to the clinician, who could not provide all the care
that might have been necessary. Rural providers might also feel stress in these
situations because they are isolated, and urban-based health care workers do
not understand the unique rural patient or provider experience.

Isolation for a rural health care professional also assumes not having an
immediately accessible network of peers who can provide support and
consultation on a particular concern. Professional, and sometimes social,
isolation may be associated with geographic isolation. Isolation can be
perceived by the clinician as positive, negative, or a combination of the
two. Some rural clinicians appreciate the opportunity for developing
professional autonomy and creativity, while others find the expectations and

responsibilities in rural practice to be stressful and overwhelming. Likewise, the lack of immediately available opportunities for establishing relationships with other professionals, or not having the central office nearby, can reinforce feelings of isolation.

Perceived professional isolation requires the clinician to evaluate and prioritize needs and types of services that can be provided to the local population. The clinician can experience considerable professional strain and stress from the lack of geographic access to other specialist providers, as well as the lack of continuing education, current telecommunications, and medical technology. Individuals who are uncomfortable when working alone, or who lack the confidence to make independent clinical decisions, probably would not fare well in a remote rural area. These individuals would likely be more comfortable in a less isolated setting with more support.[1-5, 11]

Limited Ethics Resources

Unlike their urban counterparts, many rural facilities and health care profes-sionals have limited access to ethics resources (see Box 2.7) to help them address ethics conflicts, including rurally focused ethics literature, ethics committees, and health care ethicists. As Nelson has noted, this further supports the viewpoint that rural America is underserved.[24, 25]

BOX 2.7

LIMITATIONS IN RURAL ETHICS RESOURCES

- Rural-focused ethics literature
- Rural ethics committees
- Rural-based health care ethicists
- Rural-focused ethics training

Using an established methodology for conducting literature searches, Nelson *et al.* identified only 55 publications between 1966 and 2004 that specifically and substantively addressed rural health care ethics. The majority of publications, 30 (55%), were clinically focused; 15 (27%) addressed organizational ethics; and 10 (18%) addressed ethical ramifications of policy at a national or community level. Only seven (13%) of the publications were original research publications.[26]

A survey of hospitals in six western states by Cook *et al.* found that out of 117 respondents, 59% did not have ethics committees or other formal

models for ethics services.[27] For hospitals with 25 or fewer beds, 85% lacked
an ethics committee. The data also suggested a predictive association
among the size of the hospital, the presence of an ethics committee, and
Joint Commission accreditation. The study also revealed that only 59% of
those with committees met regularly; most of these committees engaged
primarily in educational efforts, with the skill and knowledge development of
their own committee members as their central focus. Having et al.[28] reported
that only 37% of the rural health facilities among their sample of 79 health
care facilities listed on the Illinois Department of Public Health Web site had
formal ethics committees. Where rural committees existed, the literature
emphasized the lack of basic ethics training and expertise for committee
members. When rural providers did seek training or consulted the ethics
literature about clinical conflicts, the training and material had such an urban
focus that it proved to be unhelpful.[29, 30]

A study by Nelson and Weeks[31] suggests that there are a limited number
of bioethicists working or living in rural communities. This study used the
American Society for Bioethics and Humanities (ASBH) membership as
a representative cross-section of professional health care ethicists, to
determine how members are distributed along the rural-urban continuum.
The results note that, "while 91% of ASBH members live or work in urban
settings, only 66% of the U.S. population did so. In contrast, 2% of ASBH
members live or work in rural settings compared to 13% of the population.
ASBH members were 10.7 times (95%) more likely to be represented
in urban as compared to rural settings when compared to the general
population, 25.6 times (95%) more so when compared to hospital facilities,
and 6.9 times (95%) more so when compared to hospital beds. Using
various comparisons, the authors consistently found that ASBH members
are under-represented in rural, as compared to urban settings."[31] Even
though not all health care ethicists are ASBH members, the authors'
findings suggest that the availability of professional ethics resources is
limited in rural America.

As a result of limited ethics committees at rural facilities, and limited rurally focused ethics publications, rurally based bioethicists, and rural resources and
training, there is a need for increased rural health care resources and training that
integrates rural culture and values into ethical reflection and decision-making.

To address these limitations, several strategies may help the rural clinician
to identify rural ethics resources (see Box 2.8). Often the local health
care facility is part of a larger network that has an ethics committee, an

ethics consultant, and continuing education opportunities for participating members. Rural clinicians should ask and become informed about what is available to system members. Other small communities within a given geographical setting have combined resources and developed their own health care ethics committees and educational resources. In some cases, health care providers in small communities have partnered with institutions of higher learning to educate local health professionals about ethical principles and decision-making. It is important that rural health care providers consider, though, that educational programs for health professionals generally are located in urban areas, and most clinical experiences occur there. In turn, students are not necessarily exposed to rural patients and rural health care systems. In these cases, rural clinicians must become proactive and educate urban-based educators about rural contextual features that can impact ethical situations occurring in more austere and remote environments.[2]

BOX 2.8

POTENTIAL ETHICS RESOURCES

- Local health care facility's ethics committee
- State network of ethics committees
- Multi-facility ethics committee
- Academic medical center ethics program
- University or college ethics department
- On-line resources offered by health professional organizations

CONCLUSION

Health care ethics or bioethics has evolved historically from many wide-ranging areas of focus. The *Encyclopedia of Bioethics* has indicated that there are several areas of inquiry which make up the discipline of bioethics—theoretical, clinical, regulatory and policy, and cultural.[32] *Theoretical health care ethics* deals with the foundations of moral reasoning that are applied to a variety of health care issues. *Clinical ethics* refers to challenges in individual patient care. *Regulatory and policy health care ethics* is the organizational and legal reflection of health-care-related ethics questions. *Cultural health care ethics* refers to an effort to systematically relate health care ethics issues to the cultural and social context in which ethics conflicts arise. One of the important cultural subgroups of inquiry is the rural setting; specifically, how the rural environment influences the ethics conflicts encountered in rural America.

In sum, living and working as a health professional in a rural environment is unique, and most would describe it as a highly rewarding personal and professional experience. Compared to people in more populated settings, rural American residents often experience greater isolation; have less access to health care; espouse traditional cultural beliefs related to health and illness; and may need to obtain care that is provided by a clinician who could be a neighbor, family member, friend or professional colleague. These and other contextual features significantly influence the health care ethics challenges, and the manner in which health care professionals respond to those challenges.[1, 2, 11]

REFERENCES

1. Bushy A. Rural nursing: practice and issues. American Nurses Association Continuing Education Program Module. http://nursingworld.org/mods/mod700/rurlfull.htm. Accessed July 2, 2009.

2. Bushy A, ed. *Rural Nursing.* Newbury Park, CA: Sage Publications; 1991.

3. Bushy A. Nursing in rural and frontier areas: issues, challenges and opportunities. *Harvard Health Policy Review.* Dec. 14, 2008 2006;7(1):17-27.

4. Bushy A, Baird-Crooks K. *Orientation to Nursing in the Rural Community.* Thousand Oaks, CA: Sage; 2000.

5. Bushy A. *Rural Minority Health Resource Book.* Kansas City, MO: National Rural Health Association; 2002.

6. How is "rural" defined? National Rural Health Association. http://www.ruralhealthweb.org/go/left/about-rural-health/how-is-rural-defined. Accessed April 5, 2009.

7. US Census Bureau. United States — Urban/Rural and Inside/Outside Metropolitan Area. GCT-P1. Urban/Rural and Metropolitan/Nonmetropolitan Population: 2000 http://factfinder.census.gov/servlet/GCTTable?_bm=y&-geo_id=01000US&-_box_head_nbr=GCT-P1&-ds_name=DEC_2000_SF1_U&-redoLog=false&-mt_name=DEC_2000_SF1_U_GCTP1_US1&-format=US-1&-CONTEXT=gct. Accessed Dec. 6, 2008.

8. Rural health fact sheet. Health Resources and Services Administration, US Dept of Health and Human Services. Available from: http://www.hrsa.gov/about/factsheets/orhp.htm. Accessed Jan. 19, 2009.

9. Rural Assistance Center. Frontier Frequently Asked Questions: What is the definition of frontier? http://www.raconline.org/info_guides/frontier/frontierfaq.php. Accessed April 5, 2009.

10. WWAMI Rural Health Research Center. RUCA Data: Travel Distance and Time, Remote, Isolated, and Frontier. http://depts.washington.edu/uwruca/travel_dist.html. Accessed May 23, 2009.

11. Long KA, Weinert C. Rural nursing: developing the theory base. *Sch Inq Nurs Pract.* Summer 1989;3(2):113-127.

12. Gamm LD, Hutchison LL, Dabney BJ, Dorsey AM, eds. *Rural Healthy People 2010: A Companion Document to Healthy People 2010. Volume 1.* College Station, TX: The Texas A&M University System Health Science Center, School of Rural Public Health, Southwest Rural Health Research Center; 2003.

13. Gamm LD, Hutchison LL, Dabney BJ, Dorsey AM, eds. *Rural Healthy People 2010: A Companion Document to Health People 2010. Volume 2.* College Station, TX: Texas A&M University System Health Science Center, School of Rural Public Health, Southwest Rural Health Research Center; 2003.

14. Gamm LD, Hutchison LL, eds. *Rural Healthy People 2010: A Companion Document to Healthy People 2010. Volume 3.* College Station, TX: Texas A&M Univerity System Health Science Center, School of Rural Public Health, Southwest Rural Health Research Center; 2004.

15. *One department serving rural America: HHS Rural Task Force report to the Secretary.* Washington, DC: Health Resources and Services Administration, US Dept of Health and Human Services;2002.

16. US Department of Health and Human Services. *Tracking Health People 2010.* Washington, DC: US Dept of Health and Human Services; 2000.

17. Seshamani M, Van Nostrand J, Kennedy J, Cochran C. *Hard times in the heartland: health care in rural America.* Washington, DC: US Dept of Health and Human Services;2009: 3.

18. Roberts LW, Battaglia J, Epstein RS. Frontier ethics: mental health care needs and ethical dilemmas in rural communities. *Psychiatr Serv.* Apr 1999;50(4):497-503.

19. Bennett KJ, Olatosi B, Probst JC. *Health Disparities: A Rural-Urban Chartbook.* Columbia, SC: South Carolina Rural Health Research Center;2008: 17.

20. Bennett KJ, Olatosi B, Probst JC. *Health Disparities: A Rural-Urban Chartbook.* Columbia, SC: South Carolina Rural Health Research Center;2008: 20.

21. Uninsured and underinsured frequently asked questions. Rural Assistance Center. http://www.raconline.org/info_guides/insurance/uninsuredfaq.php. Accessed July 2, 2009.

22. Shortage designation: HPSAs, MUAs & MUPs. Health Resources and Services Administration, US Dept of Health and Human Services. http://bhpr.hrsa.gov/shortage/index.htm. Accessed June 2, 2009.

23. Davis DJ, Droes NS. Community health nursing in rural and frontier counties. *Nurs Clin North Am.* Mar 1993;28(1):159-169.

24. Nelson WA. The challenges of rural health care. In: Klugman CM, Dalinis PM, eds. *Ethical Issues in Rural Health Care* Baltimore, MD: Johns Hopkins University Press; 2008:34-59.

25. Nelson WA, Schmidek JM. Rural healthcare ethics. In: Singer PA, Viens AM, eds. *The Cambridge Textbook of Bioethics.* New York, NY: Cambridge University Press; 2008:289-298.

26. Nelson W, Lushkov G, Pomerantz A, Weeks WB. Rural health care ethics: is there a literature? *Am J Bioeth.* Mar-Apr 2006;6(2):44-50.

27. Cook AF, Hoas H, Guttmannova K. Bioethics activities in rural hospitals. *Camb Q Healthc Ethics.* Spring 2000;9(2):230-238.

28. Having KM, Hale D, Lautar CJ. Ethics committees in the rural Midwest: exploring the impact of HIPAA. *J Rural Health.* Summer 2008;24(3):316-320.

29. Cook AF, Hoas H. Where the rubber hits the road: implications for organizational and clinical ethics in rural healthcare settings. *HEC Forum.* Dec 2000;12(4):331-340.

30. Cook AF, Joyner JC. No secrets on Main Street. *Am J Nurs.* Aug 2001;101(8):67, 69-71.

31. Nelson W, Weeks WB. Rural and non-rural differences in membership of the American Society of Bioethics and Humanities. *J Med Ethics.* Jul 2006;32(7):411-413.

32. Reich WT, ed. *Encyclopedia of Bioethics.* New York: Macmillan; 1995.

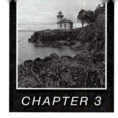

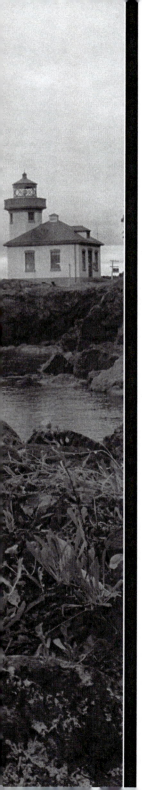

The Ethical Life
of Rural Health Care
Professionals

Ruth B. Purtilo

CHAPTER 3

The Ethical Life of Rural Health Care Professionals

Ruth B. Purtilo

ABSTRACT

The study of ethics helps professionals to recognize ethics situations, to reason about them, and to seek resolution of challenging situations. Each function can be put to use within one's professional life. This chapter introduces rural health care professionals to the difference between, and the significance of, morality and ethics in the rural professional's life. Each professional confronts three realms of morality: personal, professional and societal. Ethics tools can ease the navigation through each of these realms by ensuring integrity. In addition to defining ethical mechanisms, this chapter presents the relationship between ethics issues and ethics problems. Three basic types of ethics problems help the clinician recognize which components of morality are embedded in a situation: ethical distress, ethics conflicts, and appropriate locus of moral authority. Health care ethicists and others have concluded that ethics problems arise when moral values and goals compete. Ethical principles can act as intermediaries between general moral considerations and the specific situation, lending an enhanced opportunity to reason through the situation. Common principles include autonomy, beneficence, nonmaleficence, fidelity, veracity, and justice. Ethics theories centered on duty-based (deontological) reasoning tend to treat the principles as explanations of duties, while those based on utilitarian reasoning tend to consider the overall usefulness or "utility" of conduct governed by one principle in contrast to another. In addition to principles, character traits and attitudes of professionals must be taken into account. This chapter concludes with practical suggestions for sustaining ethical practice by fostering self-care and the use of available resources.

INTRODUCTION
Like many of my colleagues in health care ethics, my familiarity with the
rural environment is spotty. Mine is also largely second-hand, though
my "roots are rural. My father grew up in rural Minnesota, the only son
among six children, and became the breadwinner at an early age when my
grandfather succumbed to a stroke. At 30, he left the small farm, with his
mother now in the care of an unmarried sister, and went to the city. There
he found a wife who had been "born and bred" in an urban environment.
I anticipated my rural experiences with great enthusiasm as a child when,
four or five times a year, we visited my father's sisters—all of whom had
stayed on or near their rural birthplace. To me these times represented
sunshine and fresh air, the smell of the barn, running free in the fields and
woods with cousins, amazing encounters with nature, and sumptuous
amounts of food, all served against a backdrop of women's chatter. I also
recall them as the times when my father laughed more openly during the
visit, and grew more silent on the trip home. Now I understand that one
great gift he gave to his children was his attempt to share that country life
and what it meant to him, as a rural man to the core.

Many years later, when I became the director of a health care ethics
center in a largely rural state, I received a grant to travel across that
state and the neighboring states, visiting with rural practitioners, health
care administrators, and patients. I wanted to get my bearings about the
environment from which most of my students had come and to which
they might return after completing school. I wanted to understand the
special needs and strengths that rural patients and their families brought
to the university hospital, as well as to better understand the small
towns and clinics to which they would return. These travels taught me
that rural life had many blessings, but such life was not just sunshine
and fresh air.[1, 2] Today when I visit the remaining aunts and cousins,
or read the newspapers and other literature on rural life, I see rural
communities being as diverse as the unique neighborhoods in the city in
which I live.

Living and working with health care professionals in both rural and urban
settings, I have come to conclude that all professionals struggle with ethics issues in their practices. I have also learned that geographic context,
such as a small rural setting, can significantly impact the ethics issues we
all face as tenants-in-common sharing the larger landscape of the human
condition. Some of the questions that a professional will encounter on the
journey of a rural health care provider are found in Box 3.1.

BOX 3.1

QUESTIONS ENCOUNTERED BY THE RURAL PROVIDER

- What is the significance of morality and ethics to the rural professional?
- How can ethics be useful to rural professionals?
- How can one balance competing values?

In this chapter I examine these questions, and make a few practical suggestions for nurturing the deep values that guide each provider's professional life.

WHAT IS THE SIGNIFICANCE OF MORALITY AND ETHICS TO THE RURAL PROFESSIONAL?

Fortunately, health professionals in any environment can usually rely on common sense, counsel with professional colleagues, and lessons from past experience to provide sufficient moral traction for the clinician to address the day's many decisions with confidence. When decisions serve the patient's best interests, and are consistent with personal values and society's moral guidelines, a clinician usually can conclude that the attitude or conduct was morally correct. Even so, under scrutiny, this may not always be the case. Thoroughly taking stock throughout the day requires the clinician to use ethics as a tool. Occasionally, providers become aware that the gears of personal or professional values and goals are beginning to grind, and something is wrong. Any time the feeling that "something is wrong" threatens to mire your confidence in doubt, ethics is an essential tool.

You've heard it said, "This is the moral and ethical thing to do." Sometimes moral and ethical are used interchangeably. They are deeply related but not synonymous. A distinction between morality and ethics is useful for understanding why both are necessary. *Morality* is the sum of attitudes, conduct and character traits that describe how humans in a particular setting have agreed to live so that everyone can exist in harmony.[3] Morality helps to delineate basic shared values and goals. Beauchamp and Walters describe morality as "certain things [that] ought or ought not to be done because of their deep social importance in the ways they affect the interests of other people."[4] An individual's morality becomes integrated into his or her identity as the individual grows, absorbing the influence of parents, mentors, the media, social norms, and other diverse sources.

Ethics is a systematic study of and reflection on morality. It is systematic because it is a discipline that uses special methods and approaches to examine moral situations; it is also reflection because it consciously calls into question assumptions about existing components of our morality.[5]

But no person lives in a social vacuum, least of all the professional. Health professionals know that they are expected to conform to certain moral expectations of themselves, their patients, and society. Whether or not a clinician agrees with everything society expects of him or her, at least he or she acknowledges the need to reconcile personal morality with societal morality. Doctors learn that professions themselves have a morality, one expression of which is in the public "professing" that is offered to society in code or shorthand form, each profession's code of ethics. So even as one hits the road as a health professional, one deals with at least three realms of morality: personal, professional, and societal. In fact, every time a doctor makes a patient-care decision in his or her professional role, he or she deals with all three realms.

Consider the following story, focusing on the personal, professional, and societal moralities that Dr. Siegel encounters within one relationship:

Dr. Kim Siegel is very excited about being invited into the rural group practice. During her hiring interview with the group, she finds that the team of physicians, nurses, technologists, therapists, and others are compatible with her own commitment to high-quality health care. She tells them that she has grown up in a small town in another state, and, although she enjoyed the opportunity to attend medical school in a large metropolitan center, she realized as she neared the end of her residency that she wanted to return to a rural area. The group is impressed with her enthusiasm and with the several academic and humanitarian awards she has received during her training, and offers her the job, which she accepts.

After a short time on the job, Dr. Siegel accidentally misdiagnoses the asthma symptoms of one patient, Mr. Ortega, as a temporary allergic response attributable to a high pollen count. She remembers having been exhausted on the evening when Mr. Ortega came in, and then feeling relieved that he was just another person reacting to pollen. She had wanted to be available that evening to serve at a community church supper. When asked if he had ever had such a reaction before, Mr. Ortega had said no. But when Mr. Ortega returns two months later, again complaining of difficulty breathing, it dawns on Dr. Siegel that she should probe further. She is aware that the allergy medication she previously prescribed probably has not done Mr. Ortega any harm, but also knows that untreated asthma can have severe and sometimes fatal consequences. The doctor conducts additional tests that confirm Mr. Ortega's asthma. She finds herself uncertain about whether to tell him that she had misdiagnosed him two months earlier, because she knows from experience that acceptance of new young doctors in a rural community is slow and that word travels quickly. "Why am I hesitating?" she asks herself; "I am an honest person!" She concludes that part of her hesitance stems from not wanting to disturb the trust she feels she has been building with Mr. Ortega and his ethnic community, many of whom have been suspicious of the "white doctors" and therefore have failed to come for care. To further complicate things, Dr. Siegel feels an increasing need to hold on to patients who might otherwise go to a larger facility 30 miles away.

One can readily see some of the moral considerations that face Dr. Siegel. Her personal morality counsels her to do her duty well, honestly, and fairly. Her professional morality requires competent patient care as well as concern about how her disclosure of the mistake may affect this patient and others. And the morality of the community expects that access to high-quality care would be available for all groups of patients.

The function of ethics as a tool is also highlighted in this incident. Thus, when people say it was "the moral and ethical thing to do," it means that the realms of morality are identified as well as reflected upon, using appropriate methods of ethics designed for that purpose.

As the reader moves through this chapter and others, it might be helpful to break the idea of "reflection" into three components, so that ethics becomes a tool for the health care provider. The three forms of ethics reflection are defined in Box 3.2.

BOX 3.2

FORMS OF ETHICS REFLECTION

Recognition: Being aware of morality in its three realms within the context of everyday practice

Reasoning: Analyzing the conflicts that might move an ethical issue into the category of an ethical problem or conflict

Resolution: Seeking to evaluate and propose potential solutions

I find the forms of reflection so fundamental that I think of them as the three "Rs" of ethics deliberation—ultimately making ethics useful in practical situations. We turn now to some of those methods. In this chapter, the major focus is on the first two "Rs," and in Chapter 4 they are further elaborated into a full deliberative process that helps move the rural health care professional towards the third R.

HOW ETHICS CAN BE USEFUL TO RURAL PROFESSIONALS

In learning to recognize the moral dimensions of a situation, I have found it helpful to distinguish ethics issues from ethics problems:

Ethics Issues

Ethics issues are situations or themes that are embedded with questions of morality that deserve reflection so the decision-maker is assured of continuing on a path consistent with the correct moral direction or disposition. The process that Dr. Siegel engages in during her first meeting with Mr. Ortega illustrates this. On the first encounter, she is a reflective practitioner, acting consistently with her personal morality; consciously aware that in spite of her fatigue, she has a professional moral duty to treat her patient competently and humanely. She is pleased to be able to keep her societal commitment at the church supper as well.

Ethics Problems

Ethics problems are on the horizon when there is no way to act according to the three realms of morality in a situation without something of moral worth being compromised in one or more of the realms. There are three general types of ethics problems. They include:

- *Ethics Distress:* The health care provider recognizes what is right, but can't act on it
- *Ethics Conflicts:* More than one right or wrong option is presented to the professional, but to act on one will compromise the other
- *Locus of Authority:* The clinician must ascertain who has the ultimate moral authority in this situation

In Dr. Siegel's situation, her confidence is shaken when Mr. Ortega returns after two months and she realizes she has diagnosed his condition incorrectly. This moment also raises serious questions about the relative weight each of the three realms of morality should have on her at different times in her relationship with Mr. Ortega. In short, she is coming to grips with the fact that she has an ethical problem.

Ethics Distress: Ethics distress occurs when the decision-maker (usually a team) knows what should be done to uphold the professional's personal moral values, as well as to support the patient's and society's values and goals, but external constraints keep the right thing from being accomplished. The constraints may come from scarce resources, policies, laws, or other sources. Scarce health care resources (e.g., limited personnel, equipment, time, space, money) are common reasons for such distress in rural health care environments. Ethics distress may occur when the wishes of patients or their families stray from what the medical team considers sound clinical practice, or when the health care team doubts that the family is reflecting the patient's true wishes. In Dr. Siegel's case, we have no clear indication that she has this type of ethics problem.

One thing that does deserve mention here in regard to Dr. Siegel's situation is the term "ethics distress" itself or, as some term it, "moral distress." Since the health professional actually knows what to do, his or her experience of distress is a helpful feeling, as a marker that more attention is needed. In this respect, Dr. Siegel is tuning in emotionally to the fact there is a problem when Mr. Ortega returns after two months and it dawns on her that she has made a mistaken—and perhaps hasty—diagnosis.

Ethics Conflicts: In ethics conflicts, the decision-maker is confronted with more than one right (or wrong) course of action that honors personal, professional, and societal morality, but acting in accordance with one will compromise the other. For example, rural practitioners often face confidentiality conflicts. They must adhere to a professional moral dictum to honor confidential patient information. At the same time, the close web of families, neighbors, and the community as a whole may make sensitive information recorded on a patient's medical record public knowledge. But not to document such information may compromise the patient's best interests if he or she requires care outside of the immediate environment.

Another type of ethics conflict involves implementing life-sustaining technologies that would require a patient to be moved from the local community to a distant site. This can compromise local support systems, often adding burdensome expense to the family and generally disrupting the lives of patients and their families. Similarly, limited resources create ethics conflicts, because energy and financial resources can be spent only once, even though an equally compelling need exists.

Dr. Siegel has identified an ethical conflict during her deliberation following the return of Mr. Ortega. Both her personal and professional moral compasses direct her to be honest about her mistake. Still, she fears that this disclosure may have a negative effect on the complex relationships that she and the group's facility have with Mr. Ortega and his community of patients. She also knows that if enough patients were siphoned off to the competing facility down the road, her office might be forced to close, leaving many of the already underserved patients without health care access.

Locus-of-Authority Conflicts: Locus-of-authority conflicts, like those experienced by Dr. Siegel, are not unique to the rural situation, although when they arise, the long-standing practices of the rural community are likely to prevail over hard-and-fast policies. This type of problem shifts attention from quandaries regarding what should be done, to a consideration of who has the morally authoritative voice. For example, in situations where it is uncertain how to proceed with treatment, the opinion of a therapist who has served the area for years likely will trump the judgment of a new clinician. This might occur even though the health care team and/or an objective outside reviewer may believe the new clinician is more equipped to make the call. Customary and long-standing practices also spill over into the relationship within families. If a professional were to encourage the wife of an incapacitated man to speak on her husband's behalf, she might balk if she feared that the whole community would judge her negatively if she attempted to express her own preferences. Or a local religious leader might hold almost complete sway over reproductive care, end-of-life care, or other types of health care decisions, and it might be futile for a clinician to present alternatives to a patient or family without the leader's input.[6]

Locus-of-authority questions also take another turn. With the increasing ethnic and religious diversity in many rural communities, the professional health care provider may be confronted with customs that seem foreign, and contrary to the customary rural practices. Dr. Siegel's story does not suggest whether she has considered consulting anyone for insight regarding her concern about disclosure on the basis of Mr. Ortega's ethnic community. She has assumed that it is up to her to decide whether and how much to say. In this case she has seen herself as the sole team member involved in this situation. She has not lost moral direction, but may be cheating herself of valuable ethnically knowledgeable professional resources who might advise her after learning the news that a mistake has been made.

Not all challenges involving the recognition of ethics issues and ethics problems are embedded with one of the three types of problems outlined above (ethics distress, ethics conflicts or locus-of-authority problems). For instance, a dilemma about the withdrawal of a life-sustaining technology, such as a feeding tube, may be resolved by including active debate about who holds the appropriate moral and legal authority to have the final say.

In summary, learning to recognize these three major types of ethics problems provides one ethics tool that a clinician can utilize when reflecting upon the morality of his or her professional role, the need to integrate it into personal morality, and the expectations of society. Moreover, this tool will begin to allow the rural professional to steer through the first "R," recognition, towards reasoning. To complement ethics work, the next section outlines another type of ethics tool by describing some basic ethical principles.

HOW PROFESSIONALS BALANCE COMPETING MORAL VALUES AND GOALS

Several ethical principles are used widely in medical and professional ethics circles to help professionals reason about the moral components present in a given situation. These principles are often viewed as conceptual tools, which are helpful for reasoning among the duties, rights, character traits, and other components of morality and the particularities of a specific situation. A short definition of each ethical principle is found in Box 3.3.

These principles are especially useful when a physician recognizes a potential ethics problem and needs some conceptual tools to help sort out what's going on. For example, when the principle of justice cannot be accomplished because of policy constraints, a clinician has a situation of ethics distress. An ethics conflict exists when patient autonomy conflicts with a physician's best judgment about what will prevent harm. Thus, conduct according to one would preclude also honoring the other. Taken alone, each principle is worth honoring, but the particular situation puts a professional between a rock and a hard place.

A detailed deliberative process is required to move from reasoning at this level to possible resolution of an ethics problem. Such a complete process is presented in Chapter 4 of this *Handbook*. However, this chapter gives professionals an opportunity to familiarize themselves with the most frequently used ethical principles in health care ethics.

BOX 3.3

BASIC ETHICS PRINCIPLES

Autonomy

Autonomy is when an individual has the final say in decisions affecting his or her well-being, even at times of life-and-death decisions

Beneficence

Beneficence, meaning "bene" or "good," implies that health professionals must act with the patient's interests as the top priority

Nonmalefience

Nonmaleficence is the stringent moral claim on health professionals not to put a patient in harm's way

Fidelity and Veracity

Fidelity is from the root fides, faithfulness. Veracity is the devotion to truth. In the patient-clinician relationship, faith and truth combine in the form of trust

Justice

Justice helps clinicians make moral choices when one claim for resources trumps others, using criteria including relative degrees of merit, contribution, or need among people or groups

Autonomy

Autonomy is when an individual has the final say in decisions affecting his or her well-being, even at times of life-and-death decisions. In western societies, where independence of thought and action is considered the norm, the term "self-determination" is commonly used. Professional autonomy, as a guide for health professionals, is necessary in order for a clinician to make informed and accountable decisions. A patient's autonomy may be expressed through his or her own words, or through surrogates, in instances when the patient can't personally express his or her informed preferences. No one would argue with trying to determine the patient's informed preferences as a tool for directing the health professional's decision-making. One caveat regarding traditional interpretations of patient autonomy as a reliable ethical principle is the emergence of groups whose understanding of their individual well-being are not viewed as dependent on individual preferences. This is particularly important in rural communities where new ethnic and religious groups are becoming more prevalent against the backdrop of individualism.

Beneficence
Beneficence is from the Latin root "bene" or "good." In common health care ethics and health care usage, this term implies that action by health professionals and others must be conducted with the patient's interests as the top priority. Some writers break beneficence down into at least three components: doing good, preventing harm, and removing harm.[7] Health care teams today are faced with a lot of ethical distress, due to limited resources and other constraints on what they believe would support care consistent with the patient's best interests. Also, a patient's informed preferences may sometimes depart from the ideas of health professionals or ethics committees about how to best help patients and prevent or remove harm. When Dr. Siegel weighs the benefits of disclosing her mistake against the benefits of withholding it, she is making beneficence-based deliberations.

Nonmaleficence
Nonmaleficence is the stringent moral claim on health professionals not to put a patient in harm's way. This, too, can bump into other principles. Take the simple example, not uncommon in rural settings, where good clinical judgment suggests moving a patient to a distant tertiary-care facility for life-saving interventions that are not available locally. Not to do so, the professional argues, makes him or her agent of potential harm to the patient. However, viewed from the larger social fabric of the patient's life in this dire circumstance, to remove the patient from his or her local support network also may cause harm. Though Dr. Siegel does not face this situation, it is so prevalent in the rural setting that it is likely a part of her everyday reflection on her moral life as a health professional.

Fidelity and Veracity
Fidelity is from the same Latin root, fides, as faithfulness. *Veracity* is the devotion to truth. On the journey of the patient-clinician relationship, faith and truth combine to form a main road marker in the form of trust. Both terms reflect the insight that honoring reasonable expectations of a relationship is a good thing. Understandably, Dr. Siegel is concerned about any course of action that may involve withholding the truth about her mistake from Mr. Ortega. Our moral intuition and historical reflection support the idea that faith and truth support human life. Still, every reader is familiar with the ethics conflict that arises when conveying the truth also carries the possibility of harm, and Dr. Siegel is face-to-face with that concern.

Justice
Justice is a reminder to take into account the fact that moral claims for
resources may not be equal in moral weight. The concept of justice
provides criteria regarding how to make moral choices when one claim for
resources trumps others. Some common criteria include relative degrees
of merit, contribution, or need among people or groups. Justice is different
from the other principles insofar as the unit of consideration is a group or
population with similar characteristics. However, the clinical decision-maker
experiences justice in a manner similar to how he or she experiences other
ethics problems. For instance, ethics distress would result if a doctor were
unable to offer effective treatment to a child with a rare metabolic disorder,
because policies did not support the cost of treatment. The same clinician
or ethics committee might face an ethics conflict when considering whether
to support expensive life-saving treatment, knowing that the drain on a
limited pool of financial resources would harm future patients.

These basic ethics principles are included in the classic ethics theories and
are imbedded in health professionals' codes of ethics. For a fuller discussion
of these ethical principles see Beauchamp and Childress' book *Principles
of Biomedical Ethics*.[8] This list is by no means exhaustive. For example, the
moral concept, "do your duty," as noted by Bernard Gert in his book *Common Morality*, relates to one's duty as a member of a particular profession.[3]
This has also been referred to as professional ethics or group-specific ethics.
If one elects to be a member of a particular health profession, such as nursing, occupational therapy or health care administration, the person should
accept the ethical standards and guidelines that reflect the expectations of
the profession. Applying these various ethics principles to one's work can
help to highlight the basic ideas about harm and good, right and wrong.

Weighing Ethics Principles
There are two common, conduct-oriented ethics theories that propose how
to weigh the aforementioned principles against each other when ethics
questions arise. They are the deontological and utilitarian approaches.

Deontology, from the Latin root "deonto" or duty, focuses on principles as a
means of delineating duties. This approach does not provide hard-and-fast
rules about which duty is the most binding, though the history of medical
ethics places a high priority on nonmaleficence.[6]

The *utilitarian* approach, is from the Latin root meaning "utility" or
"usefulness," considers options by which a course of action will bring about

the best overall consequence. This good is not just moral, but positive, in terms of its widely considered consequences.

While this is a great oversimplification of these two rich theories, my intent is simply to give professionals a basic idea of where they may see the principles popping up in writing in the fields of health care ethics, professional ethics, and other health care publications and policies.

The essential idea in ethics is that the moral character of any decision-maker has relevance along with the course of action that he or she chooses (or that a group of decision-makers jointly choose). In addition to ethics principles and theories, it is important to consider the character traits of clinicians, administrators, and others who are involved in reflection and decision-making. The list of potential character traits is long, and traits that are often named as particularly relevant include respect for human life, commitment to competence, compassionate disposition, patience, sympathy, honesty, trustworthiness, kindness, humility, and fairness. A professional may make his or her own appraisal of which character traits Dr. Siegel seems to exhibit as she moves through the visits with Mr. Ortega. Are there other traits that might be helpful? Are there other traits that she may have to work to cultivate for future situations of this type? These types of questions are useful in the process of ethics reasoning. Ethics tools for reasoning are described in Box 3.4.

BOX 3.4

ETHICS TOOLS FOR REASONING

- Ethics principles help make a link between personal moralities or values and specific situations
- Ethics principles can enhance reasoning about ethics issues/problems
- Conduct-oriented ethics theories, such as deontology and utilitarian theories, highlight the importance of duty and the outcomes of one's acts
- Character traits of decision-makers help position them for morally right action

Using these tools, rural health care professionals can better navigate ethics situations and reflect on their own ability to provide ethically grounded care.

CARING FOR YOURSELF AS A RURAL HEALTH PROFESSIONAL
I have rarely met a health professional who puts self-care on even par
with the demands of caring for others. This is not surprising, since health
professions' codes are built on the idea of putting others first. Health
professionals' education has been less than successful in preparing
professionals for the relationship between self-care and the ability to
care for others effectively. As a result, there is a deeply disturbing profile
of the health professions as a career line, with a disproportionately high
percent of burnout, stress-related illnesses, addictions, divorce, and
even suicide. These are often the sad end-points that result from a health
care professional overextending for others at the price of his or her own
health over a period of months or years. Fortunately, some professional
preparation programs are now recognizing the high human, social, and
economic price that such a lifestyle exacts, and are placing more attention
on helping future professionals create the time, space, and skills to engage
in health-sustaining and stress-relieving activities.

Rural health care practice can be a special challenge, because the rural
environment promises to provide some of the most healthy and relaxing
lifestyles on the planet. Examples include physical beauty, relatively clean
air, and an abundance of nature. I have talked to many former students
who would not trade those energizers for the "lights and excitement
of the big city." But against this stereotypical backdrop, the rural
health professional is vulnerable to the pressures of close, overlapping
relationships, concerns about unfinished tasks and unmet duties, and other
vicissitudes of life. The rural health professional inevitably is in the eye of
the storm whenever natural disasters, major accidents, or violence occur.
When these events are compounded by clinician exhaustion or illness,
it can be difficult for both the patient and for the clinician. And when the
clinician needs self-care, it is often even more difficult to allow the roles to
be reversed.

There is a story of the famous psychoanalyst Carl Jung, who refused to
see a distraught client when she called to beg for an appointment the next
day. He told her that he already had an important appointment that he did
not want to change. And so her anger was fueled when the next day, she
saw him sitting quietly beside a stream in the local park. She gathered up
her courage and confronted him with his apparent disregard for her need.
He turned to her quietly and said, "Today I had an important appointment
with myself." I would wager that this is one of the most difficult decisions
any reflective professional makes, no matter how justified the need is for

keeping an important appointment with oneself. It is impossible to fully assess from the story of Dr. Siegel whether or not she felt that her evening appointment at the local community supper was a way to help restore her flagging energies from the long days at the clinic, or if this, too, would be an energy drain, a commitment undertaken only because of her belief that she should be a good community participant. We do know that she acknowledged feeling exhausted when Mr. Ortega first came to the clinic, and remembered that fatigue when she reflected on her diagnosis.

Taking good care of one's self is an intentional decision and discipline, more than the task of carrying out any prescribed activity. Depending on personal circumstances and personality, one professional may find a fast hike restorative, while someone else needs to "veg out" in front of the TV, enroll in a class to learn a new skill, or cook up a good meal. It is almost always a good idea to plan time out from the immediate physical environment in which one works, especially in the fishbowl setting of most rural health care clinics.

I don't offer these suggestions because I believe that the rural health care professional's status in the community, or his or her work habits, make him or her deserve privileges not available to others. To the contrary, self-care is essential for all. Self-respect for one's true needs is manifested through simple acts of self-care, and from that strength, true respect and regard for others' needs are optimized.[9] In other words, self-care is essential to ethical practice.

Allowing Others to Care For You
Using and celebrating the availability of support and counsel from various resources is another vital part of a sustainable ethical practice. Accepting care from others seems almost an impossible task for many professionals. Dr. Siegel is like many other health professionals when she goes through the decision process alone in determining the best course of action regarding disclosure of her mistake without seeking help. There is little mention of the nurses and others in the clinic who may have met several situations similar to hers, might be more familiar with the local ethnic community of which Mr. Ortega is a part, might know the foreman who brought him back to the clinic the second time, might be cognizant of the likely reactions, and who also might be able and willing to support her decision about how to proceed.

Not every clinic, particularly those in rural areas, may have an ethics consultant or ethics committee. However, advice and assistance with reasoning through thorny ethics problems are almost always available in the vicinity. Much more is said about these resources throughout this *Handbook*. It is enough of a reminder for the health care professional that allowing others to help is not negotiable, if one is to sustain an ethical professional life. It is essential.

CONCLUSION

I occasionally travel to the rural northern Minnesota community where some of my relatives live. If you are from the Midwestern United States, you will know that I am heading "up north." But this "up north" rural community is one of several thousand in the U.S., and of tens of thousands in the world, each possessing its own special characteristics and contours. What I will find there, that is shared in common with all rural communities, are good people working together to address the moral challenges presented by personal, professional, and societal moralities, including ethics problems. In that we can rejoice, share whatever each of us can bring to human survival, and flourish as we welcome these challenges and address them with all of our potential.

REFERENCES

1. Purtilo RB. Rural health care: the forgotten quarter of medical ethics. *Second Opin.* Nov 1987(6):10-33.

2. Purtilo R, Sorrell J. The ethical dilemmas of a rural physician. *Hastings Cent Rep.* Aug 1986;16(4):24-28.

3. Gert B. *Common Morality: Deciding What to Do.* New York, NY: Oxford University Press; 2004.

4. Beauchamp TL, Walters L. *Contemporary Issues in Bioethics.* 7th ed. Belmont, CA: Wadsworth Pub; 1999.

5. Purtilo R. *Ethical Dimensions in the Health Professions.* 4th ed. Philadelphia, PA: Saunders; 2005:15-16.

6. Purtilo R. *Ethical Dimensions in the Health Professions.* 4th ed. Philadelphia, PA: Saunders; 2005:46-76.

7. Beauchamp TL, Childress JF. *Principles of Biomedical Ethics.* 5th ed. New York, NY: Oxford University Press; 2001:293-312.

8. Beauchamp TL, Childress JF. *Principles of Biomedical Ethics.* 5th ed. New York, NY: Oxford University Press; 2001.

9. Purtilo R. New respect for respect in ethics education. In: Purtilo R, Jensen GM, Royeen CB, eds. *Educating for Moral Action: A Sourcebook in Health and Rehabilitation Ethics.* Philadelphia, PA: F.A. Davis; 2005:1-10.

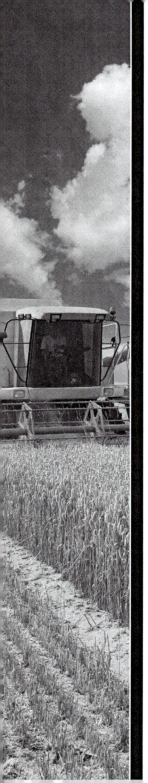

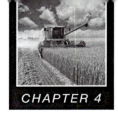

"Doing" Ethics
in Rural Health Care Institutions

Jacqueline J. Glover

"Doing" Ethics in Rural Health Care Institutions

Jacqueline J. Glover

ABSTRACT

Ethics is often a scary term for health care professionals, because it is a word that may evoke accusations of wrongdoing. But ethical values are an important part of everyday clinical decisions. The provider's ability to identify ethics issues, and to work to resolve them, is an important part of delivering quality care. Ethics issues arise for administrators and health care clinicians in both rural and urban settings. However, access to ethics resources is often limited in a rural setting. This chapter provides basic information about ethics and ethics deliberation. "Ethics" is defined and distinguished from the law. The challenges to ethics deliberation in a rural context are discussed, and three mechanisms for supporting ethics deliberation in rural settings are provided. A practical model template for ethical decision-making is provided and applied to a sample case. The template mirrors clinical-care decision-making and includes eight steps:

1. What is/are the ethics question(s) or issue(s)?
2. What is your gut reaction?
3. What are the facts?
4. What are the values at stake for all involved?
5. What could you do?
6. What should you do?
7. What is the justification for your choice?
8. Could this question or issue have been prevented?

ETHICS IS A PART OF EVERYDAY DECISION-MAKING

Every day, health care professionals make ethical decisions as an integral part of clinical decision-making. Clinical decision-making incorporates profession-grounded values. This is evident when physicians, dentists, nurse practitioners or physician assistants solicit a patient's views out of respect for his or her preferences, or recommend therapies aimed toward the patient's well-being; or when nurses or social workers raise questions about the safety of a discharge plan. Additionally, ethics discussions go on every day without necessarily being called ethics discussions. For example: the staff of a clinic is discussing whether to recruit an interventionist cardiologist, and the conversation revolves around whether they would have enough patients to keep doing procedures well, and whether the money spent on this procedure is more appropriately spent on other things. This is an ethics discussion that involves the values of beneficence (promoting well-being) and justice (fair distribution of resources.)

Unfortunately, a discussion of ethics and ethics committees makes some people nervous. When "ethics committees" are mentioned in the news these days, it is often in the context of government officials, accusations of wrongdoing, conflicts of interest, and taking the claim to an ethics board. Some people assume that to raise ethics issues at all, in the health care arena, is to accuse clinical professionals of being unethical, or in special need of ethics remediation. This *Handbook* is not intended for either of these situations; rather, it is meant to aid in ethics discussion and ethics conflict-resolution for rural health care providers.

DEFINING ETHICS AND THE NEED FOR ETHICS DELIBERATION

If ethical values are already included in day-to-day clinical decision-making, why do we need a more formal mechanism for ethics deliberation? Can't we just assume that good people will make good decisions? Yes and no. Personal values are an important factor in making reliable moral judgments and following through with them. However, many professionals may want to answer health care ethics questions or conflicts according to their personal values—which may differ from their professional values. Historically, many ethics scholars have distinguished between personal morality and ethics reasoning. Morality refers to one's personal moral choices that come from family upbringing and traditions, culture, and/or religious beliefs—whereas ethics reasoning is a more formal conflict-analysis process. A clinician's personal values may be in conflict with his or her patient's values, professional ethics, the organization's ethical standards, or even society's common morality (do not kill, harm, deceive, do your duty, etc).[1] How does a health care provider resolve the conflict? Resolving ethics conflicts in health care requires the more formal mechanism of ethics reasoning, defined below.

ETHICS REASONING

Ethics reasoning refers to a formal process of analyzing the basis for moral judgments of ethics conflicts or uncertainty. Ethics conflicts or uncertainty occur when personal values, professional and organizational values, and society's common morality compete. Ethics reasoning provides a formal way to step back from the conflict or uncertainty and to apply this reasoning in future situations. Sometimes in health care situations, the values are in such conflict that a plan of care cannot be developed until the conflict is resolved. That's when it's important to have a more intentional way to identify and resolve the ethics issue (moral value conflict) involved.

LAW AND ETHICS DIFFERENCES

Many people turn to the law to resolve ethics issues. The law is one expression of the shared values in communities and society, and it is important to obey the law. But even though the law does have ethics content, it is a kind of minimalist expectation of obligations to others. Ethics strives to inspire the best professional behavior and the law demands only a basic minimum. For example, the law would require professionals not to abandon patients that they no longer wish to have in their practice. Ethical values would require a professional to try to work with patients until a point where it is judged that the patient would be better served in someone else's practice.

Additionally, the law can be ambiguous, and it is not always clear what the law actually says about a certain question. Laws also can vary in different jurisdictions. The law is often not capable of subtle distinctions in specific situations. For example, all states have laws about who can be held on an emergency mental health hold and what that process entails. Some states have clearer language than others about what is the specific mental health criteria for detaining or committing someone against their will, and how other conditions, like substance use disorders or dementia, are to be viewed.

The law does not address many of the issues that are important in ethics. The study of ethics is concerned not only with what a decision or action a person makes, but also with the kind of person he or she is or what kind of character he or she has. In the above example about mental health law, the law is more concerned that a professional acts in a way that does not violate another person's legal rights. Ethics is concerned that providers are also compassionate and caring, and that they communicate in an honest, clear and respectful manner. And finally, ethics is more fundamental than the law. We can always ask from an ethical standpoint, "Is this a good law? Should I conscientiously disobey the law or should I work to change it?" For example, some clinicians believe that the mental health laws in their states impede patients from receiving needed, appropriate treatment because the laws respect patient rights to refuse forced treatment. A number of clinicians are working to change state laws, to use the same process as psychiatric emergency holds to allow emergency psychiatric treatment.

When making ethics decisions, it is important to have clear and accurate information about the relevant laws. But it is also important not to stop there. If a provider involves attorneys in any ethics deliberations, everyone must be clear on his or her role. Attorneys, like other individuals and professionals, certainly bring a different and valuable viewpoint to the discussion. They can be an important resource to provide helpful information about the relevant laws. But they are only one voice among many, and subject to the same rational deliberation regarding the ethics issues. Attorneys should not be allowed to trump important ethics deliberation.

CHALLENGES TO ETHICS DELIBERATION IN A RURAL CONTEXT
Ethics deliberation is influenced by the rural context. Even though there are some contextual differences among various rural communities, rural life in general, as noted in Chapter 2 of this *Handbook*, is characterized by the following factors: limited economic resources; reduced health status of patients and clinicians; limited availability of, and accessibility to, health care services; dual and overlapping professional-patient relationships; distinct cultural and personal values; and clinician stress.

The rural context described in Chapter 2 affects the kinds of ethics issues that are identified and discussed during the deliberative ethics analysis process. Section II of the *Handbook* (chapters 5-14) elaborates on specific issues in a rural context, including confidentiality, truth-telling, shared decision-making, boundary issues, justice, and access to quality health care services.

The rural context also affects the mechanisms by which ethics deliberation takes place. Ethics committees are an important mechanism, but they are mostly found in large, urban, tertiary care centers. A traditional ethics committee consists of different health care professionals who meet on a regular basis to address hospital policies, such as a resuscitation policy; to develop educational programs and materials; and to provide ethics case consultation. An emerging trend is to have a separate organizational ethics committee to deal with ethics issues that arise from the business decisions of a hospital.[2-4] Small rural health care facilities are less likely to have ethics committees. Survey data from 117 hospital administrators from six western states indicated that only 42% of the small hospitals had created ethics committees, or other formal mechanisms for providing ethics services. Surveys of physicians and nurses indicated that only 29% and 22% of these groups, respectively, have access to ethics resources. In another survey of 600 randomly selected rural physicians from Montana, Wyoming, and North Dakota, only 29% reported having access to any ethics-related resources, and 75% of the physicians had never referred a case to an ethics committee.[5, 6]

Nelson summarizes the obstacles for implementing more traditional ethics committees in rural settings in a 2006 article in *The Journal of Rural Health*.[7] The obstacles are listed in Box 4.1.

BOX 4.1

OBSTACLES TO IMPLEMENTING A TRADITIONAL ETHICS COMMITTEE IN RURAL SETTINGS

- Lack of multidisciplinary professionals
- Limited time available for a small staff with multiple responsibilities, making regular meetings difficult or impossible to conduct
- Lack of ethics knowledge and skills
- Limited opportunities for relevant ethics training
- Lack of effective training materials that focus on rural ethics conflicts
- Lack of regulatory incentive: rural hospitals are less likely to be reviewed by the Joint Commission on Accreditation of Health care Organizations, which requires an ethics "mechanism" to address ethics conflicts
- Overlapping relationships among patients, clinicians, administrators, and ethics committees; this raises challenges rarely seen in non-rural facilities

MECHANISMS FOR ETHICS DELIBERATION IN RURAL FACILITIES
In spite of the many challenges, being able to access ethics resources in rural facilities is important to administrators and to clinicians. No less than their urban counterparts, rural administrators and clinicians face ethical challenges that can negatively impact the quality of care. Therefore, the need for ethics resources as a component of providing quality care is essential in all health care settings. The important thing for providers to remember is that the ethics resources must relate and be contextually grounded in the rural setting. Because of the diversity in rural settings, it is not possible to have one rural model fit all needs for effective ethics deliberation. Several models have been suggested in Box 4.2.

BOX 4.2

MECHANISMS FOR ETHICS DELIBERATION IN RURAL SETTINGS

- A designated ethics expert to develop a facility ethics committee
- Linked institutional ethics committees through a network or academic center
- A multi-facility ethics committee (MFEC)

Designated Ethics Expert
The first possibility in developing a local strategy for a health care facility ethics resource is to designate a person to become the "local expert" in ethics, who could then train and support local practitioners and members of the local ethics committees. That person would be designated and supported by their organization to attend ethics training courses, to develop relationships with helpful ethics resources available from universities and other centers, and to inform the health care facility on ethics. The development of one local expert's knowledge can be passed on members of an evolving ethics committee. This strategy might be more cost-effective for resource-strapped institutions, rather than sending an entire committee for ethics training.[7-9]

Ethics Network
A second possibility is for ethics committees to be linked through local and state-based networks. But to be maximally effective, the networks would have to be familiar with rural issues.[10] A network that only deals with the ethics issues that are seen in larger tertiary centers, focusing on highly technological treatments including transplantations or reproductive technologies, or where there are numerous ethical resources like ethics

consultants, may not be equipped to deal with questions and conflicts that involve ethics issues arising in critical access hospitals or small rural clinics. See the discussion of ethics networks in Chapter 16.

Multi-Facility Ethics Committee (MFEC)

Sometimes an institutional ethics committee is just not feasible in small rural or frontier facilities. In these cases, an ethics resource can be made possible when multiple facilities share an ethics committee, known in the literature as a multi-facility ethics committee (MFEC).[7] The MFEC would provide several of the basic functions of the traditional model by overcoming many of the obstacles mentioned above. A committee shared among facilities has the potential to be both efficient and effective, by sharing ethics expertise and financial support and by reducing possible duplication of effort.[7]

How would the MFEC work? One model is for each facility to identify one or two professionals who are well respected in their institutions, willing to participate in regular meetings, and committed to developing ethics knowledge and skills. These members would select a chair or co-chairs of the committee. Each participating institution would provide modest financial support for their representatives and for the operation of the committee. Because of geographical distances between facilities, meetings could be conducted by conference calls, or, where available, video-conferencing.

The MFEC could sponsor educational activities not only for its members, but also for staff at the participating institutions. A second function could be the proactive review of organizational practices. All too often, traditional ethics committees function in the reactive mode—consulting on individual cases as they come up. A MFEC document could be a procedure, policy, and/or educational plan. The activities of a MFEC are listed in Box 4.3.

BOX 4.3

MULTI-FACILITY ETHICS COMMITTEE ACTIVITIES

- Identify and prioritize common ethics conflicts
- Study the conflicts
- Review the ethically grounded alternatives to the conflict
- Select and document the appropriate response, such as a better procedure, policy, or educational plan

Each institution would review the multi-facility ethics document for potential implementation. Such a process could promote well-reasoned ethical practices without burdening any one facility. Once the multi-facility committee is established and respected at each facility, the third function of real-time case consultation can be implemented.

The development of an MFEC requires much trust among various institutions, which are often in competition with each other. Institutions might prefer not to air institutional "dirty laundry," and confidentiality is of particular concern. The MFEC model is particularly plausible where there is an existing relationship among institutions. My own experience in central West Virginia is that it can be done, even without such an existing relationship. I participated in an effort in which three counties worked closely together to start an ethics committee that would serve two small rural hospitals and a number of long-term care institutions. Key factors included the resources available from the Center for Health Care Ethics and Law at West Virginia University, and the willingness of the top administration at each institution to support the plan.

A MODEL PROCESS FOR ETHICS DELIBERATION

Even though ethics is part of everyday clinical decision-making, sometimes a more formal mechanism for ethics deliberation is necessary. In a model ethics deliberation process, the provider steps back from the situation and applies a decision template to determine and review the various stakeholders' values that may be competing with one another. The process also pushes the decision-maker to carefully identify and review all potential options for addressing the ethics conflict. The goals of this deliberative ethics process are to make sure that all ethics issues are adequately articulated and understood; that the perspectives of all relevant stakeholders are heard; and that ultimately, a course of action that is ethically justifiable is chosen. Several models for ethics decision-making are available in the literature, but all share some of the basic components or steps that are highlighted below:[11-14]

Process for Ethics Decision-Making

Step 1: What are the ethics questions? (These are the "should" questions)

Step 2: What is your first reaction to this case? What is your "gut" telling you to do on an emotive level? Why do you think you are reacting this way?

Step 3: What are the relevant facts, including both the facts that you know currently, and the facts that you need to gather?

Step 4: What are the values at stake for all the relevant parties? What is/are the conflict(s) among values?

Step 5: What can you do to address the ethics question; what are your options?

Step 6: What should you do? Make a choice. Include a discussion of the implementation process; describe how it actually would be done.

Step 7: Justify your choice. Give the reasons to support your choice—referring to the values in Step 4. Anticipate and respond to objections to your reasons. Are there any options that shouldn't be done? What are the relevant ethical guidelines, like relevant code(s) of ethics that speak to this issue?

Step 8: How could this ethics issue have been prevented? Would any policies/guidelines/practices be useful in changing any systemic problems?

APPLYING THE MODEL PROCESS TO A CASE

Case Summary 4.1

BALANCING PROFESSIONAL AND PATIENT VALUES[15]

Dr. Olsen is a primary care physician who has been taking care of the O'Mara family since coming to a rural community five years ago. Mr. O'Mara is a rancher who presents to Dr. Olsen with symptoms of coronary artery disease. Mr. O'Mara doesn't want to go to a large, distant medical center for further assessment and tests, and without savings or medical insurance, Mr. O'Mara does not want to 'ransom his place' and possibly leave his family destitute to pay for medical care, when he may die anyway. Mr. O'Mara wants Dr. Olsen to keep the information only between the two of them.

Note: This case is adapted from reference #15, but the following discussion was uniquely developed and written by this chapter's author.

The O'Mara family has ranched in the Sweetwater Valley since the 1850s. "It's what my grandfather left us," says Sam O'Mara, "and I don't plan to let him down." There's nothing easy about this life—too much snow in the winter, not enough rain in the summer. On eight sections of land, Mr. O'Mara and his sons put their cattle out to graze, grow hay, and if they're lucky and get the moisture, harvest some wheat. "In a good year, we make a buck, and in a bad year, we lose two, but we're here and we're not going anywhere else," says Mr. O'Mara. The little hilltop cemetery on the edge of his property quietly underscores his statement. Fenced with barbed wire, it's the resting place for Mr. O'Mara's grandparents, his parents, his uncles and others who worked this land during the past one hundred and fifty years.

When Dr. Olsen moved to this ranching community about five years ago, Sam O'Mara was one of the first people he met. Since then, Dr. Olsen has provided medical care to Mr. O'Mara and his wife and sons. He attended the festivities at the ranch when Sam O'Mara's son was married, and just last year, he delivered the rancher's first grandchild.

When Mr. O'Mara arrives for his appointment, he admits to "being a little slow this spring." But it's been a cold spring, he explains, and long hours have been spent protecting the new calves. He'd be grateful, though, if he could get something for his chest pain and his shortness of breath. The "funny, sick feeling" he's had for the past few weeks doesn't seem to be passing.

Dr. Olsen examines Mr. O'Mara and is frankly concerned. He suspects coronary artery disease, and explains to the rancher the need for more tests. "You need to go to the city," says Dr. Olsen. He carefully explains the tests that will be conducted, and the procedures that might be done. "I've heard of those by-passes," says Sam O'Mara. "And I know Pete, my neighbor, had an angioplasty; that was the beginning of his troubles. He died anyway, but not before he had more surgery and a lot more bills." Mr. O'Mara says he'll go home and think about the whole situation. He and his wife don't have health insurance, and there's nothing they can sell right now to pay for a lot of medical care. "The boys can take care of the ranch," he says. "And they'll take care of their mother and she'll have a home. My grandson can grow up knowing he has a place. But if I ransom this place to pay for a heart, well, there won't be much left for anyone to live for."

"I expect that we can keep this between us," says Sam O'Mara. "My wife is just glad I made the appointment. I'm not going to have her choose between life for me or life for her boys." The rancher does not indicate exactly what he will tell his wife, their sons, and his friends. Dr. Olsen is pretty sure that Mr. O'Mara will just attribute his difficulties to hard work— and nothing that a little rest can't cure. Mr O'Mara expects that Dr. Olsen will go along with the story .

Step 1:   What are the ethics questions?

What are Dr. Olsen's ethical obligations to Mr. O'Mara? What should he tell him? What are Dr. Olsen's obligations to Mr. O'Mara's family? If they ask Dr. Olsen, what should he tell them? What are Dr. Olsen's obligations to the community?

Step 2:   What is your gut reaction as a provider?

"Gut" reactions range from wanting to get Mr. O'Mara the tests and possible treatment (access to health care just like anyone else) to wanting to respect his courage to spare his wife and family a choice between his health and his family's financial security.

Step 3:   What are the relevant facts?

Sam O'Mara's ranch has been in his family since the 1850s; Dr. Olsen moved to this ranching community about five years ago; Mr. O'Mara was one of Dr. Olsen's first patients; Mr. O'Mara's wife and sons are also Dr. Olsen's patients; Mr. O'Mara has been experiencing chest pain and shortness of breath since the spring; Dr. Olsen suspects coronary artery disease after the rancher's physical examination; Dr. Olsen recommends that Mr. O'Mara "go to the city" for more tests; Dr. Olsen carefully explains the tests and possible procedures; Mr. O'Mara says that he will go home "and think about the whole situation;" He and his wife don't have health insurance; there is nothing that they can sell to pay for medical care; Mr. O'Mara's friend had angioplasty and "that was the beginning of his troubles. He died anyway…. with more surgery and a lot more bills;" Mr. O'Mara asks Dr. Olsen to keep this information between them—not to tell his wife; The rancher is concerned that his wife not have to choose between "life for her husband or life for the boys;" Mr. O'Mara doesn't say exactly what he will tell his wife, sons and friends; Dr. Olsen suspects that the rancher will attribute his difficulties to hard work—"nothing that a little rest can't cure."

The facts that need to be gathered: How long has Mr. O'Mara been experiencing his symptoms? How urgent is his need for further evaluation and treatment? How far away is "the city?" Are there any alternative clinics where he could get tests at reduced costs? What does Mr. O'Mara expect Dr. Olsen to say if his family asks about his health status? How does this family usually make tough decisions that impact everyone in the family? Are there other sources of support, i.e., other relatives, neighbors, and/or a faith community?

Step 4:   What are the values at stake for all the relevant parties?

Mr. O'Mara's values center around his family's well-being—he wants to preserve the family ranch and not incur large medical bills that could put the financial viability of the ranch at risk for his wife, sons and grandchildren. He is concerned enough about his health to visit the doctor. But perhaps he is more concerned about his relationship with his wife—because he has come to see the doctor at her request. Sam O'Mara also values privacy—even from his family. He wants Dr. Olsen to keep their conversation confidential.

Dr. Olsen's professional values include promoting Mr. O'Mara's well-being by offering him the standard of care in pursuing further evaluation and treatment of his suspected coronary artery disease. Other values include truth-telling—making sure that Mr. O'Mara has enough information to make a reasoned decision to refuse further testing—and not lying to Mr. O'Mara's family if he is asked direct questions. It may also be a form of lying by omission if he accepts Mr. O'Mara telling his family something that is not true, and Dr. Olsen does not correct the misinformation. Trust is at stake for the doctor's relationship with Mr. O'Mara, but also for his relationship with the rancher's family—who are also his patients. Dr. Olsen wants to respect Mr. O'Mara's decisions (respect his autonomy), but not at the expense of being untruthful and unfair to his family. Mr. O'Mara will need a lot of support during his illness, if he seeks treatment, but especially if he doesn't. It is not guaranteed that Mr. O'Mara will die suddenly of a heart attack. Is that what the rancher is assuming? Dr. Olsen should discuss alternative futures with Mr. O'Mara so he clearly understands what's at stake by refusing further testing. He may have a progressive decline, and if so, may need a lot of supportive care. Is it fair to his family to keep them uninformed and unable to prepare to help Mr. O'Mara? The rancher is sparing his wife a decision that he thinks she shouldn't have to make. But is that fair to her? Also at stake is the trust of this rural community. If people believe that Dr. Olsen failed to diagnose Mr. O'Mara's problems, will they still trust Dr. Olsen to provide their care? Justice is also a value of Dr. Olsen's. He is treating Mr. O'Mara, even though the rancher doesn't have insurance, and the doctor wants to offer the same level of care to Mr. O'Mara as to his other patients who do have insurance. The doctor has compassion for Mr. O'Mara and his predicament—he wants to be able to get Mr. O'Mara any needed services without sacrificing the family ranch.

We can assume that Mr. O'Mara's wife values her husband's health and well-being. She is the one encouraging her husband to see Dr. Olsen. We don't know anything about how this family makes important decisions, but it doesn't seem like shared decision-making and openness are priorities—at least for Mr. O'Mara, since he is asking to make this decision alone and wants to keep the information from his wife. But learning how this family usually makes tough decisions would be important information to aid the professional in solving the ethics issues.

The conflict arises between the clinician's desire for truth-telling among the family, and promoting the well-being of Mr. O'Mara by securing further tests and possible treatment—versus respecting Mr. O'Mara's desire to make this decision alone (autonomy/privacy/confidentiality) and to not spend money on tests (to protect the family's financial well-being).

Step 5: What can a provider do to address the ethics question; what are the options?

1. Dr. Olsen could do as Mr. O'Mara requests, but with one caveat: he could tell Mr. O'Mara that if his family asks, he will direct them to talk with Mr. O'Mara. Dr. Olsen will not lie to Mr. O'Mara's family.
2. The doctor could call Mr. O'Mara's wife and recruit her to help convince Mr. O'Mara to pursue the tests.
3. Dr. Olsen could try to try to persuade Mr. O'Mara to allow a discussion about options between the doctor, Mr. O'Mara and Mr. O'Mara's wife.

4. Dr. Olsen could try to coerce Mr. O'Mara into getting further tests by means other than recruiting Mr. O'Mara's wife.
5. Dr. Olsen could discharge Mr. O'Mara from his practice, if the patient is not willing to get more tests.

Step 6: What should the provider do?

Dr. Olsen should try to persuade Mr. O'Mara to allow a discussion about his situation and various options with Mr. O'Mara and his wife (option 3). Then, Dr. Olsen could do as Mr. O'Mara requests on one condition: he could tell Mr. O'Mara that if his family asks questions about his health situation, he will direct them to talk with Mr. O'Mara. Dr. Olsen will not lie to Mr. O'Mara's family (option 1).

Step 7: The provider justifying his or her choice

Unless Dr. Olsen knew Mr. O'Mara and his family very well, options 2 and 4 are unacceptable violations of Mr. O'Mara's trust, and could result in more harm than good. Option 3 is much better, because it honors Mr. O'Mara's wishes and also tries to help Mr. O'Mara bring his family in for assistance. This option maximizes trust, openness, truthfulness, and a shared understanding of everyone's well-being. But if Mr. O'Mara cannot be persuaded to have his wife join a discussion of options with Dr. Olsen, option 1 seems like the next best course of action. Option 5 seems out of the bounds of moral acceptability, as it both violates Dr. Olsen's obligations to provide care, and the trust that he has built with Mr. O'Mara, the patient's family and the community. Where would Mr. O'Mara find care if Dr. Olsen did not provide it? Although Dr. Olsen does not have an unqualified obligation to provide care, this disagreement about care would not seem an adequate justification for risking the abandonment of Mr. O'Mara, given the rural difficulties in finding other health care providers. With option 1, Dr. Olsen could set some limits around what he's not willing to do (i.e., not willing to lie to Mr. O'Mara's family) and still honor Mr. O'Mara's preferences for care. This seems like a better balance of obligations.

The major difficulty with option 1 is that it potentially leaves Dr. Olsen providing less than the standard of care, and also potentially deceives Mr. O'Mara's family (if they never ask for more information). It would be very hard for Dr. Olsen to see Mr. O'Mara and his family at appointments, and otherwise around town, with this secret between them. But rather than taking matters into his own hands, and approaching the family independently of Mr. O'Mara, Dr. Olsen could keep asking Mr. O'Mara to involve the rest of the family or maybe a trusted spiritual leader. Maybe over time, Mr. O'Mara would be willing to see the possible benefits of being more open with his family—and the harms associated with keeping the current secrets.

Step 8:   How could this ethics issue have been prevented?

One possible prevention strategy is for providers to have conversations with all patients about the scope and limits of confidentiality, including between family members. It might be easier for Dr. Olsen to keep Mr. O'Mara's wishes private if he had previously had a conversation with Mr. O'Mara's wife, and she had understood that sometimes Dr. Olsen would not share things with her about Mr. O'Mara's care.

CONSENSUS AND CONSCIENCE IN ETHICS DELIBERATION
Providers and administrators reading this discussion may disagree with my analysis of this case. Such disagreement is not a bad thing. In fact, it is a necessary part of ethics analysis. Confronting counter-arguments and responding to them makes an accepted reasoning stronger. Good reasoning is based on sound information, and is supported by respect for differing values, the ranking of competing values, and/or by the least infringement of key values. It is important to identify the possible sources of disagreement. Disagreement about how to balance differing values is the most difficult issue to resolve. Resolution requires the skills of respectful attention, patience, and open inquiry.

Although a comprehensive and careful process of ethical decision-making usually results in consensus, deep disagreement can still exist. A provider's responsibility is to be thorough and clear-thinking, to challenge assumptions, to figure out where disagreements lie, and to strive to resolve them.

CONCLUSION
Ethical values are a part of everyday clinical decision-making, whether they occur in small clinic practices or critical access hospitals. But sometimes value conflicts arise, and need to be resolved before a plan of care can go

forward. It is important for rural administrators and health care professionals to be able to identify ethics issues and work to resolve them. Using a deliberative process to address ethics conflicts, such as the one I have proposed, can be a useful tool to ensure that there is good reasoning and thoughtful consideration of all competing values. The facility's ethics committee or other ethics mechanism can employ such a deliberative process. Even though such a process can be used by any person or group of health care professionals, having an effective and competent ethics committee or mechanism available is a valuable resource to clinicians and facility administrators, because disagreement is part of the moral life.

REFERENCES

1. Gert B. *Common Morality: Deciding What to Do.* New York, NY: Oxford University Press; 2004.

2. Ross JW, Glaser JW, Rasinski-Gregory D, Gibson JM, Bayley C. *Health Care Ethics Committees: The Next Generation.* Chicago, IL: American Hospital Publisher; 1993.

3. Ethics committees and ethics consultation. University of Washington School of Medicine. http://depts.washington.edu/bioethx/topics/ethics.html. Accessed Feb. 5, 2009.

4. Mills AE, Rorty MV, Spencer EM. Introduction: ethics committees and failure to thrive. *HEC Forum.* Dec 2006;18(4):279-286.

5. Cook AF, Hoas H, Guttmannova K. Bioethics activities in rural hospitals. *Camb Q Healthc Ethics.* Spring 2000;9(2):230-238.

6. Cook AF, Hoas H. Where the rubber hits the road: implications for organizational and clinical ethics in rural healthcare settings. *HEC Forum.* Dec 2000;12(4):331-340.

7. Nelson W. Where is the evidence: a need to assess rural ethics committee models. *J Rural Health.* Summer 2006;22(3):193-195.

8. Niemira DA. Grassroots grappling: ethics committees at rural hospitals. *Ann Intern Med.* Dec 15 1988;109(12):981-983.

9. Niemira DA, Meece KS, Reiquam CW. Multi-institutional ethics committees. *HEC Forum.* 1989;1(2):77-81.

10. Cook AF, Hoas H. Voices from the margins: a context for developing bioethics-related resources in rural areas. *Am J Bioeth.* Fall 2001;1(4):W12.

11. Purtilo R. *Ethical Dimensions in the Health Professions.* 4th ed. Philadelphia, PA: Saunders; 2005:15-16.

12. Lo B. *Resolving Ethical Dilemmas: A Guide for Clinicians.* 2nd ed. Philadelphia, PA: Lippincott Williams & Wilkins; 2000.

13. Jonsen AR, Siegler M, Winslade WJ. *Clinical Ethics: A Practical Approach to Ethical Decisions in Clinical Medicine.* New York, NY: McGraw Hill, Medical Pub. Division; 2002.

14. Glover JJ. Ethical decision-making guidelines and tools. In: Harman LB, ed. *Ethical Challenges in the Management of Health Information.* 2nd ed. Sudbury, MA: Jones and Bartlett; 2006.

15. Decisions and obligations: "It's a matter of priorities". National Rural Bioethics Project, University of Montana. http://www.umt.edu/bioethics/health care/resources/educational/casestudies/ruralfocus/decisions.aspx. Accessed July 2, 2009.

Common Ethics Issues in Rural Communities

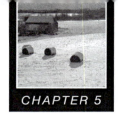

CHAPTER 5

Ethics Conflicts in Rural Communities:
Patient-Provider Relationships

Rachel Davis, Laura Weiss Roberts

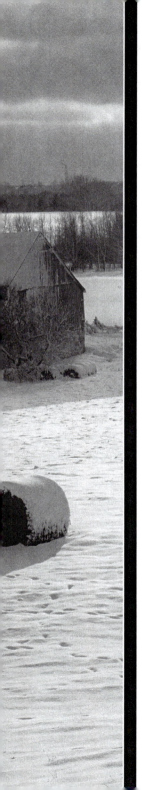

Ethics Conflicts in Rural Communities: Patient-Provider Relationships

Rachel Davis, Laura Weiss Roberts

ABSTRACT

The patient-provider relationship is privileged and complex. Those who practice in rural areas encounter additional layers of complexity due to the commonality of overlapping roles, increased patient and provider visibility, and limited sources of ethics support. The core ethical principles of beneficence, nonmaleficence, patient autonomy, and justice have unique considerations in rural areas, and are the foundation for the patient-provider relationship. Rural ethics conflicts commonly involve concerns such as privacy, confidentiality, trust, professional duties, and boundaries. These conflicts may differ in nature and frequency from those encountered in urban areas. At times, the nature of the rural patient-provider relationship may lead to more effective and rewarding interactions. At other times, the complex interpersonal dynamics may be stressful and difficult to tolerate. This chapter will explore potential ethics issues in the rural patient-provider relationship, as well as approaches and methods for resolving them. Two case studies will highlight some of the ethics conflicts and ways in which rural communities might respond. This chapter will also recommend steps that rural health care providers can take to anticipate and prepare for ethics conflicts.

CASE STUDIES

CASE 5.1 | Provider stress and burnout

Dr. Alan Morrison has been the only physician in a small community of 1,500 people for about 20 years, and is known as the "Town Doc." When he first came to town, he quickly became involved in the community. The longer he practiced, the more awkward his social life became. Dr. Morrison volunteered as the school baseball coach, but he also treated one of the boys on the baseball team for chlamydia. The boy stopped coming to practice. Dr. Morrison did not sign up to coach the following year. As more and more acquaintances have become his patients, he has begun to turn down social invitations. As the years have passed, he has felt increasingly burdened and overworked, but unable to decrease his workload. He has attended to numerous horrific farm accidents and motor vehicle crashes, often as the only provider for multiple patients. He feels indebted to the community, but is beginning to feel resentful. Where he once took pride in the fact that people looked to him for support, he now feels overwhelmed and useless. Dr. Morrison recognizes that he is depressed, but has no idea where to turn for help. His patients have begun to notice that he seems tired and irritable. At the critical access hospital where Dr. Morrison is on staff, colleagues and administrators are increasingly concerned about his ability to practice, and they fear that their colleague might resign.

CASE 5.2 | Confidentiality in the context of dual relationships

Joanne Baker, NP, prescribes clonidine and lorazepam for a young man, Brian Murphy, for treatment of prescription opiate withdrawal. The young Mr. Murphy is outgoing and talented, and he plays on the same soccer team as nurse Baker's son. Three weeks later, Mr. Murphy is found unresponsive and requires intubation and medical evacuation to a city three hours away. The young man recovers, but does not want others in the community to discover that he has attempted suicide. He begins to spread rumors that his nurse practitioner, Ms. Baker, is incompetent and has prescribed medications that she does not know how to use. Another patient brings up these rumors during his own appointment with nurse practitioner Baker. She wishes she could set the record straight, and let people know that Mr. Murphy had obtained opiates from a provider in a neighboring town, and had taken these in large quantities in a suicide attempt. The nurse is unsure how to address the situation without breaching her patient's confidentially.

OVERVIEW OF ETHICS ISSUES

An ethical patient-provider relationship is based on trust, honesty, confidentiality, privacy, advocacy for patient interests, and the shared desire for quality care.[1, 2] The American College of Physicians Ethics Manual states that the physician must be professionally competent, act responsibly, and treat the patient with compassion and respect.[3] Loewy and Loewy noted that the patient-provider relationship has at least three roots which are defined in Box 5.1.[4]

BOX 5.1

ROOTS OF THE PATIENT-PROVIDER RELATIONSHIP

Social Contract:	relying upon a mutual perception of interpersonal obligations as well as upon profession
Historical Tradition:	of society and profession
Personal Root:	deriving strength from the unique relationship produced by an interaction of the various professionals, patients as well as the differing personalities of members of the health care team

The American Medical Association Code of Medical Ethics notes that physicians can strengthen the patient-provider relationship by advocating for their patients and protecting basic patient rights.[2] In this relationship, commitment to quality patient care is paramount. Patient rights are outlined in Box 5.2.

The foundation for a patient-provider relationship is also reflected in personal behaviors. A 2006 Mayo Clinic study identified seven "ideal physician behaviors" via patient interviews,[5] and it may be useful for providers to consider these ideals. Ideal physician behaviors are listed in Box 5.3.

BOX 5.2

PATIENT RIGHTS

- The right to accurate information
- The right to make decisions
- The right to "courtesy, respect, dignity, responsiveness, and timely attention to (the patient's) needs"
- The right to confidentiality
- The right to continuity of care
- The right to the availability of adequate health care

BOX 5.3

IDEAL PHYSICIAN BEHAVIORS

▪ Confident	▪ Personal	▪ Respectful
▪ Empathetic	▪ Forthright	▪ Thorough
▪ Humane		

The patient-provider relationship, by its very nature, engenders complexities that are often difficult to navigate. For example, the patient-provider relationship is characterized by an inherent power differential, and providers must be careful to maximize patient autonomy. Patients and providers may not share similar value systems, and may originate from very different cultures. So it is important that patients know that their values will be respected and considered, even when such values differ from those of their provider.[6] The degree of trust necessary for a successful patient-provider relationship exceeds the level of trust found in most other relationships, and these dynamics often occur in a context in which both participants know relatively little about each other. For these reasons, society requires a higher moral standard in the behavior and conduct of professionals.[7]

The patient-provider relationship has come under increased scrutiny in recent years, and determining what constitutes ethical patient-provider interactions has been complicated by evolving legal and ethical standards.[8] Those who practice in rural areas encounter additional layers of complexity, due to the commonality of dual roles. The local pastor is likely to be a patient of the rural provider, as are the town mechanic and postal carrier. These dual relationships can create awkward and ethically challenging situations.

Health care providers may find it useful to familiarize themselves with the four core ethical principles presented by Beauchamp and Childress: beneficence, nonmaleficence, respect for autonomy, and justice.[9] The principle of beneficence refers to the obligation to contribute to the well-being of others. The principle of nonmaleficence relates closely to the adage, *"Primum non nocere"* (First, do no harm).[9] The principle of respect for autonomy maintains that providers should strive to include individuals in health care decisions and involves the aspects of informed consent and refusal of treatment. The principle of justice refers to the attempt to delineate the fair allocation of health care resources. These and other related principles are described further in Chapter 3 of this *Handbook*.

Ethics conflicts occur as the result of competing ethical principles, or when a provider considers violating one of the principles; for example, when a provider ponders whether it is morally justifiable to breach confidentiality. Therefore, it is important for rural health care providers, when addressing conflict situations, to be aware not only of the basic principles, but also to understand how they may interact within a coherent system of ethics reasoning.

Beneficence and Nonmaleficence
Several factors unique to rural areas complicate the task of balancing the benefits and risks involved in medical treatment. In particular, the commonality of dual relationships contributes to this difficulty. Providers may feel compelled to practice outside their areas of expertise in order to provide necessary care to a patient who is an acquaintance or friend. A health care provider may be less impartial in balancing the presentation of benefits against risks regarding a recommended treatment if the provider believes he or she knows the values and health goals because the patient is also a neighbor. These situations increase both the potential for benefit and the risk for harm.

Similarly, because patients may have a personal relationship with the provider, it is possible that patients will not view the patient-clinician relationship as private and confidential. They may fear sharing potentially embarrassing information. Despite the obligation that patients have to be honest and open about health-related issues and behaviors, patients may withhold information on problems such as substance abuse, psychiatric illnesses, sexually transmitted diseases or other stigmatized illnesses; thereby limiting the provider's ability to give necessary assessment and treatment. As a result, patients may be at increased risk for harm. For example, a patient with secondary syphilis who presents with fatigue, fevers, and malaise, but fails to disclose that he has had sexual intercourse with prostitutes, and had some genital lesions a few months ago, risks unnecessary medical testing and further progression of his illness.

Yet another area of concern is the risk that a rural community may tolerate substandard care or unethical behavior for fear of losing their health care provider. The belief that "some care is better than no care" may lead clinic administrators and other rural community members to avoid addressing issues like provider substance abuse, burnout, or illness. Health care providers with an understanding of the principles of beneficence and nonmaleficence will be better equipped to recognize and address conflicts among professional duty, trust, and confidentiality.

Respect for Patient Autonomy
Unlike the typical urban patient-provider relationship, it is common for rural providers to have "everyday" casual community contact or relationships with the same individuals they see in the privileged, professional patient-provider relationship. Health care providers may have children in the same class as their patients, or the local grocer or pharmacist may be their patient. They may even end up caring for their own family members. As a result, providers have increased knowledge of their patients' lives, behavior, and activities that may potentially influence their perception of those patients. For example, a provider has only to drive by the local bar to recognize the car of a patient who had adamantly stated that he or she no longer drinks. When providers know their patients[6, 10] outside of the clinical setting, they may be tempted to make assumptions about a patient's preferred treatment or be more apt to cave to a patient's request to, "just do what you think is best, 'doc'." Knowing patients in non-professional settings can also lead health care providers to be less thorough with history-taking, because they assume they know the whole story. Health care providers must take care to maximize patient autonomy and to treat all patients with respect and dignity, while carefully considering how their own assumptions might influence the situation.

Justice
Rural health care providers are often acutely aware of the competition between justice and beneficence. What is in the best interest of an

individual patient may be detrimental to the community in general. For example, a provider may feel that it is in a patient's best interest to have a procedure in a nearby city rather than at the local surgery center. However, this would deprive the community's health care system of income that helps sustain the local health facilities. Only 8% of physicians practice in rural areas, while 20% of the population resides there.[11] Due to the high levels of uninsured patients in rural areas, providers or health care organizations may provide a large amount of uncompensated health care. This may occur to the extent of endangering the ability of such institutions to continue to provide care.[12, 13] Providers (who often do not have backup or "on call" coverage as they might in a larger hospital or private practice with more partners) may feel obligated to provide necessary treatment to patients at all hours of the day, therefore risking exhaustion and burnout. Because a rural community may only be able to support one health care provider, getting coverage for the provider to have time off can be a challenge. J.C. Hadley, a rural physician, noted in conversation that there were times when he had to leave town during which no medical coverage was available (Personal communication, Hadley JC, September 2007). While this situation would certainly be unethical in an urban area, it is less clear in rural areas.

All of these issues complicate and challenge the traditional, ethically grounded patient-provider relationship. Therefore, patient-provider ethics issues must be understood within the broader context of the community in which the provider and the patient reside.[6, 10]

CASE DISCUSSION
The following case discussions are based on the analysis method discussed in Chapter 4.

CASE 5.1 | Provider stress and burnout

This case highlights the ethical principles of beneficence, justice, and nonmaleficence, particularly in the areas related to self-care, as well as the community's tolerance of deviant behavior or substandard care by providers. This case also examines the issues of confidentiality and privacy.

Dr. Morrison was initially eager and involved in the community. As he has begun to encounter the numerous layers of complexity in patient relationships, he has come to feel isolated. The concerns of confidentiality and privacy are particularly awkward, such as the sexually transmitted disease situation mentioned. Dr. Morrison deals with these situations by pulling away from the community.

J.C. Hadley described his own personal experience as a country doctor as one of avoidance. "Only go to the post office after hours, when nobody else is there. Be wary of going into businesses where there is only one entrance and exit... no good escape route... easy to get cornered. Check out who might be in the place before you enter" (Personal Communication, Hadley JC, September 2007). It is important that providers consider alternate means of interaction, so that they do not find themselves isolated from their communities.

Dr. Morrison has become exhausted, resentful, and impolite. The community fears losing him, so they tolerate his behavior. This creates a perilous situation. The community will suffer if they lose their physician. If Dr. Morrison stays, he will likely continue to decompensate until change is forced, be it by a serious medical mistake, substance dependence, suicide, or any other number of possible negative outcomes.[14-16]

Some of these difficulties stem from the tendency of society to hold health care providers to a higher standard than those in most other professions.[8] A rural provider may not be able to go home at night, even if exhausted, because there is no one else to provide needed care for the victims of a motor-vehicle accident. A provider may try to uphold the most rigorous set of professional responsibilities and values, and yet be regularly challenged to fulfill either his or her own expectations and/or those of the community.

There is often some inherent conflict in ranking the needs of a provider and the needs of a community. There may also be conflict between beneficence that a provider directs toward the entire community (via the community having a healthy physician to care for its members) and the beneficence she directs toward an individual patient (for example, if the provider sees patients every weekend because no one else is available). Rural health care providers face unique challenges as they seek to balance their personal values with the community's needs, while maintaining professionalism within each patient-provider relationship.

Another aspect highlighted by the case above is the degree of trauma encountered in rural areas—a reality that intensifies the stress faced by Dr. Morrison. This can have a strong impact on rural health care providers, more so than in urban areas, for several reasons which are outlined in Box 5.4.

BOX 5.4

REASONS FOR INTENSIFIED TRAUMA IMPACT ON RURAL PROVIDERS[15-17]

- Lack of colleague support
- Lack of resources
- Technological limitations
- Delays in advanced treatment
- Need for medical care beyond one's own expertise
- Greater sense of responsibility and duty
- Increased frequency of death related to severe trauma
- More familiarity with the victims of these tragedies and traumas

CASE 5.2 | Confidentiality in the context of dual relationships

The case of nurse practitioner Joanne Baker focuses on the ethical issues of trust and confidentiality within dual relationships. Dual relationships may be difficult, if not impossible to avoid in rural areas.[6, 10] Dual relationships may have many benefits, including allowing the provider a greater awareness of a patient's entire life, fostering a deeper sense of trust, or encouraging a stronger sense of duty. However, dual relationships, as illustrated in this case, also complicate the patient-provider interaction. Ms. Baker knows Brian Murphy as a member of her son's soccer team. Her knowledge of him may have prevented her from asking important questions about his mental health. Likewise, Brian Murphy may have been hesitant to disclose the extent of his problems due to his knowledge of Joanne Baker not only as his provider, but also mainly as "Jason's mom."

Many patients will talk, gossip, and spread rumors while providers are professionally and ethically bound to maintain confidence.[18, 19] When the second young man comes in and confronts her with the rumors spread by Mr. Murphy, Ms. Baker is caught between reassuring her new patient of her knowledge and expertise, and violating the first young man's patient confidentiality. Not only is her reputation perhaps marred by Brian Murphy's rumors, but other patients are beginning to have more difficulty trusting her. Trust is an essential component of the patient-provider relationship. Whereas patients in urban areas must base their trust in physicians on experience related to their medical care and treatment interaction alone, those in rural areas may base their trust on their broader understanding of the provider as a member of the community and as a human being. At times, this may be beneficial and serve to foster trust. At other times, as in the case with Brian Murphy, patients may be more wary and distrustful.

Ms. Baker would be breaching confidentiality and privacy requirements if she were to disclose to other patients the factual circumstances. She would be violating Mr. Murphy's confidentiality, which would likely harm him. The principle of justice competes with the principle of nonmaleficence in this scenario. One would hope community members would judge Ms. Baker based on the sum of her care, not just one patient's rumors. But that is not always the situation. Despite being unfair, members of the community can hold to the false belief that their health care provider is incompetent. They may wait longer before seeking necessary treatment, or they may disregard important treatment options. Does she uphold the principle of nonmaleficence, by not violating Brian Murphy's confidentiality, despite the reality that, as a result of his gossip, some patients may hold false beliefs regarding their safety and the medical care they receive from her? Would it be morally justifiable for her to simply mention to her patients that they had been misinformed about the circumstances surrounding her patient Mr. Murphy?

RESPONDING TO PATIENT-PROVIDER ETHICS CONFLICTS

CASE 5.1 | Provider stress and burnout

Dr. Morrison faces a problem that is common to health care professionals in small, rural towns. In cases of provider stress or burnout, both the provider and the clinic administration have ethical obligations. The provider, once he recognizes that stress is interfering with his ability to provide care, must address his limitations and seek help.[20] Most states have confidential resources for health care providers. For example, the Colorado Physicians' Health Program offers confidential evaluation and referral for medical, mental health, and substance use disorders.[21] If the physician in this case fails to acknowledge the situation, then his professional colleagues and/or hospital administration should respectfully confront him and assist him in problem-solving. It will not benefit the physician, his individual patients, or the community in general to ignore the signs of burnout. Likewise, it is of no benefit to address the situation in a punitive, disrespectful manner.

In circumstances in which patients have actually been harmed, the provider is obligated to report himself to his professional organization to obtain the necessary help. Those aware of this provider's difficulties have an ethical obligation to address his performance, rather than ignore it because they fear losing the physician.[21] Administrators can often provide help and support to providers, without needing to alienate them, or terminate them in the more extreme case. Management may provide medical leave, suggest treatment resources, limit the provider's hours, or allow time for continuing medical education.

In the case of Dr. Morrison, following a careful review of the situation with clinicians and administrators from the nearby critical access hospital, local administrators decided to discuss Dr. Morrison's behavior with him. The clinicians and management decided that two colleagues with whom Dr. Morrison had good relationships, a fellow physician and a nurse, would privately approach him to discuss changes in his behavior and attitude. Initially, he was angry, and gave his resignation to the hospital. The hospital administrator worked with Dr. Morrison and other clinicians to negotiate a lighter schedule and provide coverage through a *locum tenens* agency. In addition, the administrator referred Dr. Morrison to the local physician's health program. Dr. Morrison began seeing a therapist in a city two hours away, and took some vacation time. He also obtained a mentor through the physician's health program, and continued to work a lighter schedule. The hospital had to rely on *locum tenens* coverage for almost a year until they were able to recruit another physician to help fill the schedule.

CASE 5.2 | Confidentiality in the context of dual relationships

The case of Joanne Baker, the nurse practitioner, highlights the difficulties that are common in dual relationships. Providers must be especially careful not to overlook important aspects of a patient's history due to assumed familiarity. For example, Ms. Baker had known Brian Murphy as an outgoing and talented young man, not one who was, to her knowledge, suicidal and drug-addicted. She should openly discuss with Mr. Murphy the difficulties that their dual relationship poses, and offer a referral to another provider if this patient does not feel comfortable working with her. Patients who have believed Brian Murphy's slandering comments about this nurse may have to weigh the difficulties and benefits of continuing to work with Ms. Baker, compared to the inconvenience of traveling.

Another unfortunate, yet common, problem is that people often gossip in rural areas because of the close-knit living environment, and the fact that residents tend to be so familiar with their neighbors' and friends' activities.

In many rural areas, a large fraction of the inhabitants are related to each other, after decades or centuries of their extended families living in the area with the core families intermarrying.

Despite the negative impact on Ms. Baker's professional image, she must maintain Brian Murphy's confidentiality. There may be some people left with inaccurate perceptions of her abilities, but Ms. Baker cannot comment to one patient about another patient. It is not possible to control what people choose to say or believe. This is the responsibility of each individual, not the provider. J.C. Hadley noted, "Gossip will always occur, and it will always be hurtful and potentially damaging to you professionally . . . Unfortunately I have no defense against those patients who . . . tell any story that might be far from truthful... you just have to continue to prove yourself to others through good health care" (personal communication, Hadley JC, September 2007).

ANTICIPATING PATIENT-PROVIDER ETHICS CONFLICTS
Health care providers can anticipate potential patient-provider ethics conflicts in order to prevent or minimize them, as opposed to only addressing conflicts as they arise. Both individual health care providers and administrators can play a role in anticipating potential ethical conflicts as noted in Box 5.5.

BOX 5.5

ANTICIPATING PATIENT-PROVIDER ETHICS CONFLICTS

- Be aware of local culture, customs, and resources
- Identify a professional mentor
- Develop a support network
- Set and communicate professional boundaries and limits
- Develop skills in analyzing boundary crossings
- Actively address potential conflicts in dual relationships
- Emphasize confidentiality to patients and colleagues
- Be proactive about self-care

Enhance Understanding of Local Culture, Customs, and Resources
Lisa Cooper-Patrick, *et al.* note that improved cross-cultural communication results in improved patient care, satisfaction, and outcomes.[22] When taking a new position in a rural setting, providers should seek venues to understand the local culture. For example, if the situation

allows, health care providers may consider moving to the area in which they will be practicing prior to actually beginning work. This allows them the time to become familiar with the local culture and customs.[23] Providers can begin this process by reviewing the cultural diversity literature and other resources. Administrators of rural facilities should consider providing both time and financial support so that new health care providers can familiarize themselves with the local culture and customs. To maximize new providers' efficiency and to ease their orientation, administrators of small rural hospitals should also supply a directory of local resources and referral sources. Providers may find it useful to meet with community leaders, such as clergy or law enforcement officers, to discuss the community's culture and explore how such community leaders handle issues like confidentiality and dual relationships. It is equally important that providers be aware of the mechanism for obtaining medical or mental health help for themselves, which could also be introduced by administrators at orientation time.

Identify a Professional Mentor

Providers should identify professional mentors throughout their careers. Since rural providers often reside in remote areas, a mentor may be someone who lives at a distance, but is available via phone or e-mail when doubts or conflicts arise. For example, a mentor may be a professional who has previously practiced in the community, or the mentor might be a provider in another rural community. It would have potentially been very helpful for both Dr. Morrison and Ms. Baker to have had a relationship with a trusted, supportive, rural provider, with whom to discuss problems.

Develop a Support Network

Health care providers should also develop relationships with members of the local health care community, including a mix of mental health professionals, doctors and nursing staff, hospital technologists, and alternative providers, as well as health professionals in neighboring communities. It is also important to develop local ethics resources and mechanisms for addressing ethics conflicts, as discussed in Section III of this *Handbook*. These mechanisms provide confidential resources for providers to consult when conflicts arise. In the first case presented, Dr. Morrison would have benefited from having a support network to help him deal with difficult patient interactions, to prevent him from becoming overwhelmed, and to support him when he began feeling depressed. Such a support network might also, in general, develop coverage arrangements, so that each provider might have time off when necessary, and could have backup medical and technical support when traumatic events require additional help.

Set Boundaries and Limits

Rural providers may frequently be afraid to set limits on their work time or skill set for fear of alienating members of the community. Some find it useful to be direct, clear, and concise with patients about their professional-personal limits. It is a challenging balance to completely separate professional responsibilities from a personal life, and may result in awkwardness and resentment for both the provider and the patient. Proactive, open communication is essential to clarifying an understanding between the provider and the community. Once the understanding is communicated, providers should adhere to the boundaries based on their own needs, values, and personalities.

Providers should also be prepared for queries about their personal lives. Different individuals will have different comfort levels. Some may find it most useful to be direct and concise when asked about a personal experience while others may find it more comfortable to provide some level of detail. Providers should not be surprised by these inquiries (often they are made out of sincere, friendly interest or even small talk on the part of a patient—especially during an encounter that could occur outside of the clinic—say, at the grocery store or golf course) and should think about how much they want to share prior to such inquiries.

Develop Skills in Analyzing Boundary Crossings

It is important to be aware of potential conflicts in dual relationships. Dr. Martinez refers to a graded-risk model for boundary crossings and speaks of four types of boundary crossings as listed in Box 5.6.[24]

Dr. Martinez further writes that six ethical guidelines should be considered when analyzing potential boundary crossings.[24] These guidelines are found in Box 5.7.

Actively Address Potential Conflicts in Dual Relationships

Health care providers should be careful not to make assumptions, even though they may be aware of patients' lives outside the treatment setting. Providers and patients should explore health care options and treatment possibilities, even when value-based differences may exist. If a patient is aware that her provider's value system is different from her own, and could influence the treatment, both the provider and patient should openly discuss any potential conflict. For example, if a patient is interested in discussing birth-control options, but knows that her provider attends a conservative Catholic church, the patient should still be able to openly

BOX 5.6

TYPES OF BOUNDARY CROSSINGS

Type I

Type I boundary crossings are discouraged and/or prohibited. They include behaviors that are liable to criminal and civil litigation. Examples include physically abusing a patient or conspiring to commit a crime with a patient.

Type II

Type II boundary crossings involve a high risk of harm and low risk of benefit to the patient or the patient-provider relationship. Examples include a provider falsifying an insurance form for a patient, or trading psychotherapy for housecleaning services.

Type III

Type III boundary crossings involve a low-to-medium risk of harm and a medium-to-high opportunity for benefit. Examples include attending a patient's wedding or disclosing significant personal information. Use of professional judgment and consideration of cultural context are very important in Type III.

Type IV

Type IV boundary crossings involve either a low risk of harm or no risk of harm, and a medium-to-high opportunity for patient benefit. These boundary crossings will often have a positive effect on the provider-patient relationship. Examples include using sliding-scale fees, making a home visit to a terminally ill patient, or making a cup of tea for a patient.

discuss the various medical options. When a provider feels that her personal values may impede her ability to support patient autonomy—for example, if a patient requests the morning-after pill and the provider is uncomfortable giving it—the professional should offer appropriate referrals to address the patient's need.

In rural communities, it's not always possible for providers' friends to see different providers. When patients are also friends, providers should talk openly about the difficulties in a dual relationship. There may be situations in which the patient needs to be referred to a different provider, even if it creates hardships such as driving a certain distance away. During

BOX 5.7

POTENTIAL BOUNDARY CROSSINGS

- Actions under consideration should involve a low-to-medium risk of harm to the patient and to the patient-provider relationship
- Coercive and exploitative elements should be absent on both sides
- There should be some potential benefit to the patient or to the patient-provider relationship
- Patient interests should be greater than professional self-interests
- The provider should aspire to maintain professional ideals
- The context of potential boundary crossings should always be considered

patient-provider interactions, providers should initiate conversations about stigmatized issues such as sexual health, mental health, substance dependence, and domestic violence, so friends are aware that they can ask for referrals if needed.[25] As in the second case, Ms. Baker should have discussed with Mr. Murphy their relationship outside the clinic and made sure he was comfortable discussing sensitive issues with her before proceeding with treatment.

J.C. Hadley commented on the difficulties with friendships in rural areas, stating that, "Anybody can get upset with the health care provider for any number of reasons, such as access, cost, and unsatisfying outcomes, which can affect a relationship of any type. Realizing this reality helps you to prepare. I deal with this by being true to my professional ethical standards first, (and) doing what is best for them as a patient; true friendship will survive professional glitches" (Personal Communication, J. C. Hadley M.D., September 2007).

Emphasize Confidentiality

Health care providers need to reassure patients of the importance of confidentiality. Medical professionals are repeatedly reminded of its significance, but patients may not be aware of its value or the role it plays in the patient-provider relationship. Remind office staff of the importance of confidentiality, and develop strategies for assuring it is maintained. Clinicians and administrators need to collaborate to enforce consequences when confidentiality is breached. When other patients confronted Ms. Baker with questions about Brian Murphy, she could have used the opportunity to explain the patient confidentiality rules and the value of privacy, rather than being tempted to defend herself or her actions as a clinician.

Be Proactive About Self-Care

It is critical that providers maintain their own health to maximize their ability to maintain an ethically grounded patient-provider relationship. Physicians who are experiencing burnout are more likely to provide sub-optimal care.[26, 27] A list of suggestions for rural providers is supplied in Box 5.8.

BOX 5.8

PROVIDER SELF-CARE

- Develop a support network
- Network with community officials and leaders
- Spend time alone (and with friends and family)
- Maintain physical and mental health care, including having one's own health care provider(s)
- Exercise, get regular sleep, and maintain healthy nutrition
- Set limits with staff to maintain professional boundaries
- Anticipate and allow for the grieving process that providers may experience following a patient's death, particularly if there had been a close friendship or relationship
- Expect criticism, learn to tolerate it, and be comfortable changing or not changing in response
- Take time off
- Work with colleagues or administration to address unreasonable or unmanageable workloads

Rural providers may need to be creative to develop a support network; some examples might include obtaining a therapist in a different community, or joining a hiking club in a nearby city. It may be especially useful for providers to maintain contact with other community officials or leaders to help decrease a sense of isolation. Health care providers with mutual patients may offer support to each other during difficult times. Health care professionals such as physicians, nurses, and administrators can offer support by attending funerals and contacting each other following difficult situations, such as patient deaths or particularly horrific accidents.

It is important to be in contact with people who can offer a realistic perspective, since providers are often idealized or criticized unrealistically.

There are few places like small, rural towns where your faults are quite so obvious and open to public scrutiny. Likewise, there are few places where people may so readily construct "faults" in response to perceived injustice or differences in belief systems. When faced with negative perceptions, providers must be prepared to sort areas for improvement from those that they are not compelled to change.

Health care providers are trained to take care of others and often neglect self-care.[28] Despite time constraints or geographic barriers, rural health care providers should have their own medical and mental health providers available to address personal health issues. In general, people frequently need time to be alone[28] and providers may find that continuing or developing a hobby or exercise routine is relaxing and enjoyable. Time alone may also be an opportunity for meditation or prayer.

It may be difficult to set professional limits with staff when they are friends or acquaintances, but doing so is critical. One necessary limit is the amount of time providers are willing to work. Providers need to take time off, even if they are the only local health care provider, and they shouldn't take work along on vacation.[28] If the workload is unreasonable and unmanageable, this should be addressed by working with colleagues or clinic administration.[28] Hospital administrators will likely prefer having you work fewer hours, rather than having you resign in frustration and then having no health care provider at all. If the unreasonable workload is not addressed, providers might consider moving to an area with more support.

CONCLUSION

The unique nature of the rural patient-provider relationship presents both rewards and challenges. Rural health care providers and patients enjoy a broad understanding of each other, as members of a community and as human beings. This closeness often enriches relationships, fosters trust, and deepens understanding. It also presents many challenges and potential ethics conflicts. These conflicts can be overwhelming and frustrating to a provider, if they are addressed blindly and without support. However, providers who develop an understanding of the core ethical principles and how these principles interact in rural patient-provider relationships can be proactive about addressing these conflicts.

Health care providers are obligated to provide care that is beneficial to patients and to minimize interventions or actions that are likely to be harmful. They should seek to maximize patient autonomy, by regularly and non-selectively practicing thorough history-taking, and by including their patients in discussions and decisions about the risks and benefits of medical treatment. Because rural health care resources are often scarce, rural providers must routinely consider the ethical principle of justice in their daily decisions. Most importantly, rural health care providers must insure that their own mental, emotional, and physical needs are met so that they are able to provide excellent, ethically grounded health care.

REFERENCES

1. Balint J, Shelton W. Regaining the initiative. Forging a new model of the patient-physician relationship. *JAMA*. Mar 20 1996;275(11):887-891.

2. American Medical Association, Council on Ethical and Judicial Affairs. *Opinions on the patient-physician relationship. Code of Medical Ethics*. http://www.ama-assn.org/ama/pub/physician-resources/medical-ethics/code-medical-ethics/opinion1001.shtml. Accessed April 5, 2009.

3. Ethics manual. Fourth edition. American College of Physicians. *Ann Intern Med*. Apr 1 1998;128(7):576-594.

4. Loewy E, Loewy R. Patients, society and healthcare professionals. IN: *Textbook of Health care Ethics*. 2nd ed. Boston, MA: Kluwer Academic Publishers; 2004:97-140.

5. Bendapudi NM, Berry LL, Frey KA, Parish JT, Rayburn WL. Patients' perspectives on ideal physician behaviors. *Mayo Clin Proc*. Mar 2006;81(3):338-344.

6. Roberts LW, Battaglia J, Smithpeter M, Epstein RS. An office on Main Street. Health care dilemmas in small communities. *Hastings Cent Rep*. Jul-Aug 1999;29(4):28-37.

7. Martinez R. Professional role in health care institutions: towards an ethics of authenticity. In: Wear D, Bickel J, eds. *Educating for Professionalism: Creating a Culture of Humanism in Medical Education*. Iowa City, IA: University of Iowa Press; 2000:35-48.

8. Henry MS. Uncertainty, responsibility, and the evolution of the physician/patient relationship. *J Med Ethics*. Jun 2006;32(6):321-323.

9. Beauchamp TL, Childress JF. *Principles of Biomedical Ethics*. 5th ed. New York, NY: Oxford University Press; 2001:57-282.

10. Nelson W. Addressing rural ethics issues. The characteristics of rural healthcare settings pose unique ethical challenges. *Healthc Exec*. Jul-Aug 2004;19(4):36-37.

11. Rural health fact sheet. Health Resources and Services Administration, US Dept of Health and Human Services. Available from: http://www.hrsa.gov/about/factsheets/orhp.htm. Accessed Jan. 19, 2009.

12. Rowley T. The rural uninsured: highlights from recent research. Office of Rural Health Policy, US Dept of Health and Human Services. http://ruralhealth.hrsa.gov/policy/UninsuredSummary.htm. Accessed Feb. 23, 2009.

13. Bailey J. Health care in rural America: a series of features from the Center for Rural Affairs Newsletter. Center for Rural Affairs; 2004. http://www.cfra.org/pdf/Health_Care_in_Rural_America.pdf. Accessed Feb. 23, 2009.

14. Warner TD, Monaghan-Geernaert P, Battaglia J, Brems C, Johnson ME, Roberts LW. Ethical considerations in rural health care: a pilot study of clinicians in Alaska and New Mexico. *Community Ment Health J*. 2005;41(1):21-33.

15. Moszczynski AB, Haney CJ. Stress and coping of Canadian rural nurses caring for trauma patients who are transferred out. *J Emerg Nurs*. Dec 2002;28(6):496-504.

16. Levin A. Stress of practicing in rural area takes toll on psychiatrist *Psychiatric News*. Dec. 13, 2008 2006;41(9):4.

17. Rogers FB, Shackford SR, Hoyt DB, et al. Trauma deaths in a mature urban vs rural trauma system. A comparison. *Arch Surg*. Apr 1997;132(4):376-381; discussion 381-372.

18. American Medical Association, Council on Ethical and Judicial Affairs. *Opinions on confidentiality, advertising, and communications media relations. Code of Medical Ethics*. http://www.ama-assn.org/ama/pub/physician-resources/medical-ethics/code-medical-ethics.shtml. Accessed April 5, 2009.

19. Confidentiality. Colorado Physician Health Program. http://cphp.org/confidentiality.html. Accessed Dec 5, 2008.

20. Schneck SA. "Doctoring" doctors and their families. *JAMA*. Dec 16 1998;280(23):2039-2042.

21. American Medical Association, Council on Ethical and Judicial Affairs. *Reporting impaired, incompetent, and unethical colleagues, Opinion 9.031. Code of Medical Ethics*. http://www.ama-assn.org/ama/pub/physician-resources/medical-ethics/code-medical-ethics/opinion9031.shtml. Accessed April 5, 2009.

22. Cooper-Patrick L, Gallo JJ, Gonzales JJ, et al. Race, gender, and partnership in the patient-physician relationship. *JAMA*. Aug 11 1999;282(6):583-589.

23. Han GS, Humphreys JS. Overseas-trained doctors in Australia: community integration and their intention to stay in a rural community. *Aust J Rural Health*. Aug 2005;13(4):236-241.

24. Martinez R. A model for boundary dilemmas: ethical decision-making in the patient-professional relationship. *Ethical Hum Sci Serv*. Spring 2000;2(1):43-61.

25. Rourke LL, Rourke JT. Close friends as patients in rural practice. *Can Fam Physician*. Jun 1998;44:1208-1210, 1219-1222.

26. Maslach C, Jackson SE, Leiter MP. *Maslach Burnout Inventory Manual*. Palo Alto, CA: Consulting Psychologists Press; 1996.

27. Shanafelt TD, Bradley KA, Wipf JE, Back AL. Burnout and self-reported patient care in an internal medicine residency program. *Ann Intern Med*. 2002;136(5):358-367.

28. Gendel M. Physician work stress. Colorado Physician Health Program; 2007. http://cphp.org/list-of-informative-articles.html. Accessed Mar 4, 2009.

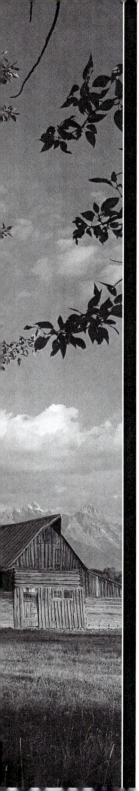

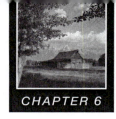

Ethics Conflicts in Rural Communities:
Overlapping Roles

Andrew Pomerantz

Ethics Conflicts in Rural Communities: Overlapping Roles

Andrew Pomerantz

ABSTRACT

Health professionals who live and work within rural communities are more likely to interact with patients in multiple settings than are their urban peers. Outside the office or hospital, health care professionals may be their patients' friends, customers, parishioners, employees, or employers. The boundary that exists between patient and provider can become unclear in these contexts, potentially leading to ethics conflicts that are both personal and professional in nature. Knowledge obtained in the clinical arena may have significant relevance for the clinician in his or her community role(s). This chapter presents three situations that illustrate some of the ethics conflicts that can develop in rural contexts, when personal and professional responsibilities are challenged by blurred boundaries. These cases demonstrate professional responsibility conflicts that can develop for health care providers regarding the traditional patient-clinician relationship. In an urban area, lack of incidental patient contact outside the professional realm makes cases like these quite rare, whereas in rural settings they are the norm. The key to prevention and resolution of ethics conflicts is for the health care professional to prepare and anticipate such conflicts, and to develop appropriate management strategies.

CASE STUDIES

CASE 6.1 | A physician's family gaining an unfair advantage

Dr. Dallace, a family practitioner, attends a local farm auction with his wife. The young auctioneer, a grateful patient whom Dr. Dallace is treating for narcotic dependence, observes the doctor's wife examining and admiring a chair. When the bidding opens, the auctioneer makes reference to the chair needing a great deal of repair. Though she knows it needs no work, Mrs. Dallace offers a low bid that is accepted, thus allowing her to purchase the chair at a remarkably reduced cost.

CASE 6.2 | Choosing between loyalty to the hospital and loyalty to the patient

Dr. Boardman is a surgeon at a small rural hospital. The hospital is struggling to stay afloat in the face of competition from larger hospitals. All physicians at the hospital are being pressured to keep the beds full. While in the emergency room, Dr. Boardman is faced with a complicated case that he has not seen since he was in training years ago. He realizes that the patient may receive better care at one of the larger tertiary hospitals, but that would mean lost revenue as well as the lost opportunity to care for an interesting, complicated case. Faced with the choice, he elects to keep the patient in his hospital. Following admission, the patient asks her nurse, Linda Robinson, who is also a friend, if she ought to ask to be transferred to the large tertiary care center a hundred miles away because she is aware that they have more specialists. Ms. Robinson is aware of what Dr. Boardman said; she is uncertain how to respond.

CASE 6.3 | Breaching patient confidentiality to prevent possible harm

Andy Cox is a nurse in a physician's office some 30 miles from his hometown. He is also a member of his town's school board. One day Mr. Richards, a teacher from the school, visits the physician for a check-up. Mr. Cox thinks it odd that Mr. Richards has traveled so far to see the doctor, since most people in his hometown see a family physician in the town. Andy Cox says hello, but has little contact with the patient. A few days later, Nurse Cox is retrieving lab information and learns that the teacher has tested positive for several drugs, suggesting substance abuse. The nurse wonders if he could or should warn school administrators or fellow school board members about the teacher's drug use.

OVERVIEW OF ETHICS ISSUES

Working in rural health care sets the stage for many overlapping relationships and responsibilities, since health care workers are also parents, siblings, friends and community members. In densely populated areas with multiple, separate neighborhoods and suburbs, these many responsibilities are less apparent to the provider's patients because their lives are less likely to intersect outside the office. Rural residents frequently live within the same community as their provider and, unless the provider avoids all community contacts, interactions with patients outside of the professional relationship are likely to occur on a regular basis. In many communities, physicians, nurses and other medical professionals enjoy a special status among the community's population, further enhancing the likelihood that they will be in public positions and thus interact with patients in multiple settings outside of the clinic or hospital. Rural clinicians are frequently challenged to keep their personal responsibilities from coloring their interactions with patients within the clinical arena.

Overlapping relationships can create ethics challenges between clinician and patient, because they are inherently unequal parties, at least in the medical relationship; clinicians are typically in a position of power, and patients may feel vulnerable or dependant. Patients put their trust in their health care provider(s); they must trust enough to provide very personal and often embarrassing information that is necessary for accurate diagnosis and effective treatment. Thus, it is particularly important for rural health care providers to clearly define their professional responsibilities, including roles and boundaries within the patient-clinician relationship.

Traditional ethical standards for the patient-provider relationship are based on respect, honesty, trust, confidentiality, promotion of the patient's well-being, and avoidance of self-interest. This basic understanding is grounded in the principles of nonmaleficence, beneficence, respect for patient autonomy, professionalism, and justice, discussed in Chapter 3 of this *Handbook*.[1] Furthermore, Gert's *Common Morality* emphasizes the moral rule of "do your duty."[2] "Duty" in this case refers to the responsibilities established by one's profession. For medical providers, this means that the physician's, nurse's or other clinician's behavior and actions are to reflect the ethical standards of the patient-clinician relationship. These principles guide the care of individual patients the clinician's obligation to society.

The American College of Physicians' *Code of Medical Ethics* states that, "The relationship between patient and physician is based on trust, and gives rise to physicians' ethical obligations to place patients' welfare above their own self-interest and above obligations to other groups, and to advocate for their patients' welfare..."[3] The physician should not reveal confidential communications or information without the consent of the patient, unless provided for by law or by the need to protect the welfare of the individual or the public interest.[3] The appropriate patient-clinician relationship stems from adherence to ethically grounded professional responsibilities, which include informed consent, shared decision-making, respect for privacy and confidentiality. Providers are also responsible for doing what is best for the patient, avoiding exploitation and harm, as well as for treating and distributing care equitably, without bias.

An ethics conflict typically arises when the above responsibilities compete with others, or when they are being violated. For example, a conflict arises when a provider treats a competent patient who does not wish to pursue a treatment, even one that the provider knows will clearly be helpful. In that instance, the conflict lies between the provider's responsibility to respect patient autonomy and the provider's desire to encourage what is best for the patient's health.

Professional responsibility conflicts may also arise when information pro- vided by patients has health care implications for the community or society at large. The ethical clinician must balance the needs of an individual pa- tient with the needs of the community, professional ethical standards, and his or her own personal values. In some instances, the balance of these various perspectives is incorporated into laws. For example, all states have mandatory reporting of certain diseases (e.g., HIV/AIDS) in order to assure that the community at large is protected. A similar standard exists when a psychologist is bound to report cases of child abuse or threats of violence to authorities. In such instances, confidentiality for the individual patient becomes secondary to the good of society. In other cases, providers are burdened when they have information that could protect the health of oth- ers, but cannot breach patient confidentiality, as in the case of a sexually transmitted infection, where the infected party is refusing to inform his or her partners. In both situations, commitment to one's professional responsibility is key to resolving ethics conflicts. However, in other situations, there may be a moral justification to breach the responsibility, as with legally required mandatory reporting.

The law generally reflects accepted ethical standards such as the criteria for informed consent. However, clinicians sometimes find themselves confronted with a very difficult choice between what the law requires and what is best for their individual patient. A common example is the temptation of a clinician, faced with a patient lacking adequate financial resources, to enter a false diagnosis code in order to ensure that the patient's insurance company pays the claim. Regardless of the potential ethical justification for such an action, physicians and other providers still face the legal consequences and ethical repercussions of their actions, such as a formal ethics grievance brought to the attention of a medical society.[4] It is the clinician's professional responsibility to do his or her best for the patient under the parameters of the law.

Many patient-provider role and boundary ethics conflicts arise in rural settings when there are personal and professional relationships with patients. Conflicts also can arise between the provider's obligations to individual patients and to the broader community, as is the case where the nurse worries about the impact of the teacher's potential drug abuse on his students. Providers struggle to balance or rank their obligations to both individual patients and society as a whole. Overall, the provider's obligation is first to the patient. The provider must offer respect, must avoid deception and disclosure of pertinent information, must maintain confidentiality, must keep promises, must act in the best interest of the patient, and must allocate resources justly. Providers should review exceptions to these duties and/or consult a third party ethics resource, as needed, to help assess any ethics conflicts.[5, 6]

CASE DISCUSSIONS

The discussion of the following cases is based on the analysis method presented in Chapter 4.

CASE 6.1 | A physician's family gaining an unfair advantage

Dr. Dallace's dilemma merits careful reflection, including an understanding of the values of the various stakeholders. He, his patient, his wife, and the person harmed by his wife's purchase of a chair at reduced cost all have important roles. It appears that Dr. Dallace's wife has gotten the chair only by virtue of her husband's professional relationship with the auctioneer. Does her acceptance of the falsely low purchase price constitute patient exploitation by her husband, the doctor? Perhaps the auctioneer may now want more favorable attention and treatment. Will Dr. Dallace be likely to give him "favored" status at the expense of other patients?

There are also ethics questions regarding the relationship between Dr. Dallace and the chair's original owner, other patients, and other health care providers in the community. If Dr. Dallace's wife buys the chair at the reduced cost, the original owner of the chair will receive less reimbursement. The auctioneer's lying about the chair has also misled other potential buyers. If other patients or health care providers find out about this special behavior, how will they be impacted or influenced?

Dr. Dallace feels that the chair "deal" is wrong, but is unsure about how to proceed. He fears exploiting the patient, but doesn't want to hurt his feelings by refusing the "gift." Dr. Dallace also is concerned about the chair's original owner receiving reduced reimbursement. Finally, Dr. Dallace does not want other patients to think that they will receive favored care if they give him gifts, and does not want his medical colleagues to think he favors or exploits patients. Though the offer for the chair is thoughtful, Dr. Dallace knows he and his wife should not accept it in its current form, if at all.

In large health care facilities there are often formal policies about accepting gifts. However, in clinics and small rural hospitals, such policies are rare, and are even more so in rural clinics.

CASE 6.2 | Choosing between loyalty to the hospital or to the patient

With their extensive medical knowledge, nurses in rural settings are often important community resources. This is particularly true when community members are looking for a second opinion. Such is the case for nurse Linda Robinson, who believes that Dr. Boardman has chosen a course of care that may be good for the hospital's bottom line, but may be potentially risky for his patient. Nurse Robinson believes that Dr. Boardman should instead foster the patient's autonomy, and support it through full disclosure and informed consent regarding the treatment options.

Dr. Boardman, like many providers in both rural and urban settings, feels a strong responsibility to his hospital. He believes that there may be a greater good to the community in preserving the hospital rather than providing the best care for one individual patient. This thinking is based on a utilitarian perspective, i.e., to do the greatest good for the greatest number of people.

Nurse Robinson has both a commitment to quality care and a strong allegiance to the hospital that provides her employment. If the hospital were to fail, she might not have a job, and the community would lose both an important source of health care, and a socioeconomic asset —the hospital being the major local employer. However, if the procedure were done at the hospital and a bad outcome resulted, negative word-of-mouth publicity might steer other patients away, and further threaten the hospital's viability. In this case, the patient is seeking Ms. Robinson's opinion as both a professional and a friend.

Nurse Robinson thinks the patient should be fully informed about the procedure, and worries that Dr. Boardman is inadvertently exploiting the patient for the hospital's gain. She feels that the patient should be given full disclosure and understanding of the treatment options—including the choice to stay or to go to the larger tertiary hospital, and the benefits and drawbacks of either choice. Ms. Robinson wants to inform the patient of her honest opinion, but is unsure how to do so without undermining the credibility of either the local hospital or Dr. Boardman himself.

CASE 6.3 | Breaching patient confidentiality
                     to prevent possible harm

Nurse Andy Cox's situation—personal knowledge of another individual's life—can be the norm in any health care environment, but is particularly problematic in rural areas.[7] Mr. Cox has two different professional roles that are intersecting: licensed medical nurse, and community leader. As a school board member, Mr. Cox is Mr. Richards' employer; the teacher's drug screen implies that he engages in illegal behavior that is prohibited by the school. Mr. Cox, as school board member, worries that the children in the school may be at risk, and wonders about the outside possibility Mr. Richards is selling drugs to students. Mr. Cox, as nurse, is aware that he has confidential information that could jeopardize Mr. Richards' employment in the school. Releasing the health care information would be a clear violation of both ethical and legal standards, regardless of how ethical Nurse Cox might believe the action to be. Does Mr. Cox have ethical justification to violate his professional responsibility of not breaching patient confidentiality?

Mr. Cox wants to prevent harm to the students, but is unsure about how to proceed without violating Mr. Richards' right to confidentiality. The nurse also would like to prevent harm to Mr. Richards by encouraging him to seek drug treatment. He wonders how he can balance his professional responsibility as a health care provider and as a community and school board member.

RESPONDING TO PROFESSIONAL RESPONSIBILITY ETHICS CONFLICTS

Adhering to appropriate professional boundaries is a critical part of maintaining professional responsibility in patient-clinician relationships. The physician, nurse, or other provider must identify and maintain his or her professional and personal roles in relation to those of the patient. When patients and providers have overlapping relationships, the resulting boundary conflicts can cause confusion and concern. Therefore, it is imperative for health care providers to clearly communicate to patients their professional responsibilities and limits, as well as their concerns about inevitable ethics conflicts caused by overlapping relationships.

In the past, boundary crossings have been viewed as the first step on a "slippery slope" that leads to increasing frequency and magnitude of such boundary conflicts. More recently, authors have argued that this is not inevitable, and that conflicts should be more closely examined for their merits and not universally categorized as "wrong."[6] What is applicable in one specialty may be contraindicated in another. For instance, the office setting is often where general physicians first meet people who eventually become friends or even romantic partners. For psychiatrists or psychologists, this is unacceptable; an ethically grounded therapeutic relationship forecloses such possibilities.

CASE 6.1 | A physician's family gaining an unfair advantage

After weighing several options, including returning the chair, Dr. Dallace decides to voluntarily pay a fair price for the chair. In doing so, he can clarify his reasoning. Though he feels better after making this decision, he then ponders how best to explain the decision his wife. If he tells her directly why he is paying more for the chair, he might be violating patient confidentiality. In his mind, the fact that he is treating the auctioneer for a narcotic dependence makes his role similar to that of a psychiatrist. He therefore believes that he should maintain a strict standard of confidentiality that applies to that specialty. If he fabricates a story to tell his wife, he will further escalate the situation by deceiving her. In the end, Dr. Dallace thanks the patient for his kind gesture, and communicates his concerns regarding the potential for conflict of interest and his commitment to professional ethics. Dr. Dallace determines the chair's fair value, contributes the money to the auction proceeds, and keeps the chair.

The ethical guidelines and practice standards of medical specialties preclude using patients to meet the personal needs of the physician.[3] However, in many instances, accepting a small gift from patients is an acceptable community expectation. As the clinician, ethicist Dr. Lo argues, "Indeed, patients would rightly feel insulted if physicians did not accept home-made cookies, toys at Christmas, or clothes for a new baby. Similarly, it would be unfeeling not to accept a small gift after the physician has devoted a great deal of effort in helping a patient recover from a difficult illness."[5] Providers must be aware, though, that some gifts are problematical, often because of monetary value. These gifts should not be accepted if doing so causes conflict with other health care providers or patients. In this case, Dr. Dallace is right to dispute the chair's value, because to accept it at the reduced cost would be detrimental to the chair's original owner and might also trouble Dr. Dallace's co-workers and community if they became aware of the situation. Likewise, Dr. Dallace gives proper thought to the role played by his own family when he considers how his actions might affect his spouse. In rural areas, family members are often very much a part of the professional's role conflicts, particularly regarding confidentiality.[8]

CASE 6.2 | Choosing between loyalty to the hospital or to the patient

Nurse Linda Robinson believes that an individual patient's quality of care should not be compromised to enhance her hospital's economic situation. She is concerned about the hospital's precarious economic situation and recognizes the important role that the hospital plays in the community. However, Ms. Robinson also feels that any patient should be aware of her health care options, including potential differences in the quality of care from one facility to another, because of the risk-benefit and volume-based sensitivity of many treatment procedures.

Ms. Robinson decides to discuss the situation and the patient's question with the director of nursing, who also chairs the newly formed ethics committee. They discuss the situation with Dr. Boardman. Dr. Boardman acknowledges that he wanted to give information selectively that would benefit the small hospital. The director clarifies that, while he and Ms. Robinson (like any employees, including even herself, the director) have a financial interest in the hospital's success, their first obligation should always be to the patient. Dr. Boardman and Ms. Robinson realize that if they did not fully inform the patient and the procedure were to result in a poor patient outcome, both Dr. Boardman and the hospital might suffer negative consequences, including poor public relations, and financial loss that might well include a lawsuit. Dr. Boardman admits that he would have shirked his professional responsibility and displayed a conflict of interest if he had put the hospital's success above the patient. Instead, he should communicate the strengths and weaknesses of both hospitals to the patient, and allow her to decide the most acceptable treatment site.

Following their meeting, Ms. Robinson and Dr. Boardman meet with the patient and review her treatment and facility options. The patient decides to be transferred to the large tertiary medical center. After the successful treatment, the patient returns to small rural facility for follow-up care. The case is later presented at a clinical staff meeting to discuss the scope of sharing decision-making and other ethics issues that were raised by the case.

CASE 6.3 | Breaching patient confidentiality
                      to prevent possible harm

Since he has always been careful to draw a clear line between his professional and personal lives, Andy Cox first wonders if he can simply ignore the laboratory results. This option leaves him feeling uncomfortable, because he doesn't know how the drug use might be affecting Mr. Richards' work or the teacher's interactions with students. Nurse Cox worries that Mr. Richards' drug use, even if not directly affecting his work, might impact his ability to participate in the required drug education by all teachers. As a school board member, Mr. Cox knows that drug use excludes individuals from teaching, and thinks he might be justified in divulging the privileged information.

Mr. Cox considers bringing the matter directly to his fellow school board members, but he knows that to do so would betray his professional relationship and responsibilities. Still, he believes that a potentially unsafe situation exists in the school and that he is obligated to do something. Mr. Cox wonders if the potential harms are great enough to justify disclosing the confidential information to others as part of the "duty to warn and protect." Alternatively, he considers confronting Mr. Richards directly with the information, exploring the situation and, if necessary, having Mr. Richards come forward to the school authorities regarding his drug problem.

Mr. Cox knows that he cannot safely breach patient confidentiality with a third party, without more information, so he begins by exploring ethical guideline literature on the Internet. He realizes that confidentiality is key to successful patient-clinician relationships because it helps to establish trust and protects patients from the stigmatization and discrimination that might be associated with their illness.[5] There are several generally accepted exceptions to confidentiality that require health care professionals to report certain behaviors, potential behaviors, and illnesses to various public officials as noted below.

However, rural caregivers and administrators should be aware of their state-specific reporting requirements. Despite the ethical obligation to respect patient confidentiality, as noted in Chapter 7, there are several morally justified exceptions to preserving confidentiality that may be permitted by law, depending on the particular jurisdiction.

In this situation, Mr. Cox believes that the risk to third parties (such as students) does not allow him to breach the patient's confidentiality, but he is still uncertain as to how to proceed.

Unable to confidently choose among his options, Nurse Cox contacts a nurse friend with whom he has gone to school. This nurse lives in another state and doesn't know any details of the situation or the person involved. Mr. Cox's friend suggests talking to the physician who has ordered the blood test. She also suggests contacting the local nursing board ethics representative for advice.

Nurse Cox takes the advice and talks with the physician, who confirms that the testing has been done as part of a routine insurance exam, and the patient has not yet been told of the results. After more discussion, the physician and Andy agree that the two of them should meet with Mr. Richards and review both the testing and Mr. Cox's difficult predicament. The teacher acknowledges that he has a drug problem, but denies that it is affecting his teaching. After talking with his physician, and having several sessions with a drug counselor through a telehealth network, the teacher speaks with school officials about his problem and takes a voluntary leave of absence to enter drug treatment, with the goal of being totally clean before returning to teaching.

ANTICIPATING PROFESSIONAL
RELATIONSHIPS ETHICS CONFLICTS

In each of the cases, it was very important that the clinicians step back to reflect on their overlapping professional and personal responsibility conflicts. Rarely is there only one reasonable action and some clinicians might have chosen courses different than those presented here. For example, even after considering his options, Mr. Cox still had no clear solution, so he sought counsel from other trusted sources. Ultimately, his solution came when he clarified his roles—with himself and with the patient in question.

The best approach to preventing ethics conflicts related to professional responsibility is through communication and planning. Rural providers who maintain clarity regarding their responsibilities in the lives of patients will help prevent ethics conflicts and the problems that arise from them. Preventing ethics conflicts can be aided by keys listed in Box 6.1.

BOX 6.1

KEYS TO ANTICIPATING AND PREVENTING ETHICS CONFLICTS

- Be aware of the ethical standards guiding the patient-clinician relationship
- Communicate with patients about professional responsibilities
- Expect ethics conflicts due to multiple roles
- Be able to recognize when boundaries are being crossed
- Recognize potential fallout from the professional realm to the interpersonal one
- Analyze ethics conflicts, and generate multiple potential responses—there is rarely only one solution
- Identify and use colleagues to discuss patient-clinician conflicts
- Identify and seek support from ethics resources regarding patient-clinician conflicts

Awareness of Ethical Standards

Maintaining awareness of the ethical aspects of professional responsibility is an important tool for the medical provider to use to successfully navigate the ethics challenges to patient-provider relationships in a rural community. Clinicians cannot assume that patients will fully understand all aspects of the ethical standards that guide the patient-provider relationship. Health care providers should be aware of those standards as part of their professional responsibilities, and communicate such standards to patients.

Communication with Patients

Although a clinician may be well aware of the difficulties caused by overlapping roles, such issues are generally unappreciated by patients unless made explicit. Patients may even see any personal relationship they have with the provider, outside of the clinic, as a positive influence on care and may thus emphasize it. It may sometimes be the case that an outside relationship would enhance care; however, any future conflicts may be prevented if the provider thoughtfully explains and discusses with patients how overlapping relationships might create problems.

Expect Ethics Conflicts

Role conflicts are the norm in rural health care. By expecting conflicts, providers are less likely to miss them or be surprised by their occurrence. The failure to recognize such conflicts will diminish the probability of successfully managing them.

Recognizing Boundary Crossings

At times, a provider may allow boundary crossings that do not harm patients, as when the provider accepts a friendly, small gift. At other times, such as when Dr. Dallace was offered the larger gift, boundary crossings could lead to harm, including patient exploitation. If boundary crossings are not recognized, proper analysis cannot occur. Patient-provider relationships and boundary crossings are discussed further in Chapter 5.

Fallout from Professional and Personal Overlapping Roles

Health care providers need to be aware that they may be susceptible to the influences of friendship on the professional relationship. A provider might, for example, fail to ask a friend (who is also a patient) an embarrassing personal question during an office visit. This omission could preclude the collection of medical data that might be vitally important to diagnosis and treatment.

Seeking Consultation

It can be difficult for the clinician to fully maintain objectivity if he or she has multiple relationships with a patient. If conflicts arise, such as the one Mr. Cox encountered, finding an uninvolved colleague for advice can be invaluable. Though often geographically and socially isolated from colleagues, the rural provider still has resources that include regional ethics networks, hospital ethics committees, and a growing number of Internet resources.

CONCLUSION

Providing health care in the rural setting poses many challenges for professionals that differentiate rural health care from medical practice in urban areas. The closeness of the rural setting makes it more likely that clinicians will interact with their patients in many situations outside of the professional office. In those situations, the professional will be in a very different role, perhaps friend, customer, or even employer. The three examples given illustrate some of the ethics conflicts related to professional responsibility that can develop in such contexts. Oftentimes, conflicts that arise have many potential solutions. Successful resolution requires that the provider undertake a great deal of thought and analysis, using ethical principles and resources, such as ethics committees and consultants. Methods of conflict anticipation and prevention, including open communication with patients, are essential steps that the provider can take toward minimizing and/or solving such conflicts.

ical Dilemmas: A Guide for Clinicians. 2nd ed. Philadelphia, PA: Lippincott Williams & Wilkins; 2000.

6. Martinez R. A model for boundary dilemmas: ethical decision-making in the patient-professional relationship. *Ethical Hum Sci Serv.* Spring 2000;2(1):43-61.

7. Nelson WA, Schmidek JM. Rural healthcare ethics. In: Singer PA, Viens AM, eds. *The Cambridge Textbook of Bioethics.* New York, NY: Cambridge University Press; 2008:289-298.

8. Slowther A, Kleinman I. Confidentiality. In: Singer PA, Viens AM, eds. *The Cambridge Textbook of Bioethics.* New York, NY: Cambridge University Press; 2008:43-48.

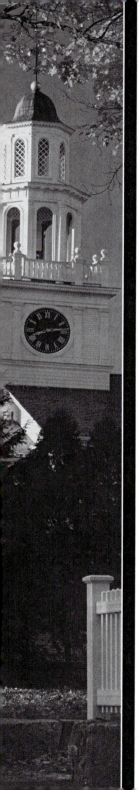

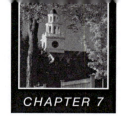

Ethics Conflicts in Rural Communities:
Privacy and Confidentiality

Tom Townsend

Ethics Conflicts in Rural Communities: Privacy and Confidentiality

Tom Townsend

ABSTRACT

This chapter explores the ethical challenges involving privacy and confidentiality in rural health care relationships, due to overlapping relationships and familiarity with patients and communities. In a rural setting, the professional relationship between a health care provider and a patient is frequently a long-term, personal relationship that involves friendship as well as professional responsibilities. In small communities, this is not limited to one-on-one relationship; it involves a family and mutual friends. In contrast, the health care relationships in urban or suburban settings are often like "strangers at the bedside," facilitated in large institution-style settings with care given by clinicians whom patients seldom know or see outside of the hospital or clinic setting. The intimacy of rural life is a key factor to many aspects of rural health care ethics discussions. An ethical relationship with strangers is different from the ethics of close-knit relationships. The ethics issues within the patient-provider relationship change when strangers, rather than friends, neighbors, or acquaintances, are involved. This distinction is key to many of the differences between urban and rural health care ethics. The reality of rural health care, and the ideals of the health care professional, can be at odds with professional standards of practice, because confidentiality, as a model, simply works differently in rural and urban settings. Trusting relationships in rural health care settings are enhanced by the familiarity common in rural living. In rural communities, residents know many of the details of each other's lives, which can lead to confidentiality issues.

CASE STUDIES

CASE 7.1 | A patient refusing needed care

Bob Jones is seeing Dr. Sampson for the first time. Dr. Sampson knows Mr. Jones slightly from the local gas station where Mr. Jones works. Mr. Jones' wife is also Dr. Sampson's patient, and the family has an infant son. Mr. Jones tells Dr. Sampson that he has gained approximately 75 pounds in the past year, after quitting smoking. He denies any significant symptoms, but does admit to shortness of breath when walking up an incline. He says he would not be here if it were not for his wife, who "does not like his color." Mr. Jones is 40 years old, weighs 310 pounds, and is slightly pale. He is quiet, intelligent, and friendly. An exam reveals massive edema and anasarca; frothy urine shows 2000 mg protein. Dr. Sampson is quite sure that Mr. Jones has nephrotic syndrome, and may have had it for some time, although a renal biopsy will be required to make a definitive diagnosis. There is an outside concern that an underlying malignancy may exist. Dr. Sampson informs Mr. Jones of his probable diagnosis. The patient tells Dr. Sampson that he does not wish to pursue assessment, and isn't troubled except for the tight clothes. He has no insurance, doesn't think his wife and son should have to shoulder the cost of his illness, and he's "not fixin' to be a charity case." Mr. Jones refuses to let Dr. Sampson talk to his wife, and says that he will tell her, "The doctor said to lose weight and to exercise."

CASE 7.2 | Disclosing health care information to family

Tammy Andrews, age 17, visits Dr. Cohen's office for a viral upper respiratory illness. During the course of the exam, she mentions that she is taking oral contraceptives that she obtained from a distant family planning clinic. Ms. Andrews states that her parents think the pill is being taken to regulate her periods, but she uses it for birth control, and has been sexually active for more than a year. After the exam for her upper respiratory complaint, she asks about painful blisters on her genitalia. A pelvic exam reveals typical genital herpes. After Dr. Cohen explains genital herpes, along with the risks of other sexually transmitted diseases (STDs), Ms. Andrews cries uncontrollably. She is devastated by the potential chronic infection, along with the guilt of sexual activity and its other risks. She is concerned that her father, a Baptist preacher, respected community leader and friend of Dr. Cohen, will discover her sexual activity and related disease, despite Dr. Cohen's assurance that her health information will not be disclosed. The lesions are less painful and prominent on the teenager's subsequent follow-up visit. Ms. Andrews appears to be depressed, worried about the impact of herpes on her future relationships. She does not want to tell her present partner about her STD. Her parents are concerned about her mood swings and anxiety, and want to know why their daughter seems so upset. The teenager has told them that she is tired due to a viral illness. Rev. Andrews leaves a message at Dr. Cohen's home, seeking information about his daughter. He asserts that he has a right to know and he believes that "a viral illness would not upset her like this." Rev. Andrews is afraid that his daughter is concealing a serious illness.

OVERVIEW OF ETHICS ISSUES

For many, the professional relationship between a rural physician and a patient represents an ideal long-term, close personal relationship that involves friendship as well as professional responsibility. In small rural communities, this relationship is frequently not just a private bond, but also one that involves family and mutual friends. Such a relationship appears quite different from those one might encounter in non-rural settings, where health care professionals are "strangers at the bedside" and health care is provided in large, institution-style settings by professionals that patients seldom know or see outside of the hospital or clinic setting. The relative intimacy of rural life is woven into the clinical and ethical management of health care ethics discussions. An ethical relationship with strangers is different from the ethics of intimate relationships. This distinction is key to many differences between urban and rural health care ethics.

Confidentiality and privacy are essential to all trusting relationships, especially in the professional setting. In various businesses, leaks of boardroom decisions make periodic headlines that prompt resignations and firings of corporate leaders. In health care, respecting confidentiality and privacy is not only a legal mandate but also a key to the trust that underpins the patient-clinician relationship. Confidentiality is a fundamental component of the American Medical Association's Code of Medical Ethics, "The information disclosed to a physician by a patient should be held in confidence."[1] Like the teen girl in Case Study 2, "The patient should feel free to make a full disclosure of information to the physician in order that the physician may most effectively provide needed services. The patient should be able to make this disclosure with the knowledge that the physician will respect the confidential nature of the communication."[1] Seeking to maintain confidential knowledge also adds to the value and meaning that sustain the long-term trusting relationship between a health care professional and his or her patient.

A foundation of confidentiality dates to the Oath of Hippocrates,[2] a pledge taken by many physicians to reflect their professional status, to inform society that physicians comprehend and value the importance of their calling, and to publicly promise their competence to the service of the sick. Specifically, the Oath's seventh paragraph is devoted to the special relationship of the healer to the patient when keeping each encounter private, or a shared secret only with the patient; "What I may see or hear in the course of the treatment, or even outside of the treatment in regard to the life of men, which on no account one must spread abroad, I will keep to myself holding such things shameful to be spoken about."[2]

The importance of confidentiality to the patient-provider relationship continues to be reinforced in modern codes of ethics and ethical standards of practice adopted by various health care professions. Additionally, the ethical concept of confidentiality as well as the legal obligation to maintain it is typically captured in health care organizations' policies and procedures.

Though health care providers may be dedicated to their various professional roles and diligent about fulfilling their ethical and legal obligations, modern medicine continues to present challenges.[3] Despite challenges to confidentiality, it is a fundamental tenet of the patient-clinician relationship.

Individual states have their own laws regarding the confidentiality of medical information. The Health Insurance Portability and Accountability Act (HIPAA) of 1996 addressed a variety of topics, but it is well known among health care professionals for the new federal privacy regulations that resulted, often referred to as a HIPAA Privacy rules. It is important for rural health care providers to be proactive in learning accurate information about what the law requires of them and their staff members with respect to sharing information, as well as what it permits.[4]

In rural communities, maintaining confidentiality is challenging, simply because residents are privy to each other's activities and lives. There continue to be some communities where local radio stations update listeners about current hospitalizations, and clergy offer public prayers to help guide a named physician in the diagnosis of a certain patient. This may seem quaint to an urban audience, but it is part of normal networking in some small communities. Imposition of outside standards on such practices often does not sit well with rural populations that practice a culturally important expectation of information sharing between neighbors, regardless of possible deleterious outcomes. Similarly, legislation or regulation may be viewed as an intrusive invasion of urban standards on the traditional way things are done—an officious imposition from the powerful "outsiders" who make most of the laws.

The dominant characteristic of familiarity in rural life and small communities creates clinical and ethical benefits for patients and health care professionals. For example, Mrs. Jones, in transit to a small hospital, is rarely described by age, symptoms, and vital signs by the volunteer rescue squads because the squads communicate with ER nurses who know people by their first names. The staff in the ER may know a lot about the incoming patient's disease and health care goals, if they know her personally. Care might be tailored for her even before the ambulance arrives if the hospital staff is familiar with her values, family, and outlook on life, as well as her preferences about health care. The depth of the staff's knowledge of "Mrs. Jones" as a patient can foster adherence to shared decision-making regarding the patient's choice of treatment. The example suggests that respecting confidentiality and privacy standards as well as the awareness and sharing of health care information can be beneficial to patient care.

CASE DISCUSSIONS

The previously presented cases are interpreted using the analysis method presented in Chapter 4 of this *Handbook*.

Both cases raise ethics issues related to sharing patient information with families in a rural community. Such challenges impact not only the patient and his or her family, but also the broader community.

CASE 7.1 | A patient refusing needed care

In this case, Dr. Sampson is faced with an ethics conflict involving his patient's confidentiality and autonomy. He is obviously concerned about Bob Jones' likely diagnosis of severe and chronically progressive kidney disease (nephrotic syndrome) as well as the need for further assessment and treatment. Mr. Jones tells Dr. Sampson that he does not want to pursue further evaluation or undergo any potentially helpful treatment. He tells Dr. Sampson that he has limited resources and lacks insurance, a common concern in rural communities. Mr. Jones emphasizes that he does not want to be a financial burden to his wife and son.

Dr. Sampson can understand Mr. Jones' desire not to create a financial burden for his family. However, the doctor strongly believes that his patient needs to better understand his illness and the possibility of treatment. All treatments seem difficult, time-consuming, and expensive to Mr. Jones. He appears to have little insight into the treatments' benefits, including the fact that treating his potential condition would likely allow him to enjoy a longer life with his family. Despite the clinical certainty of a serious renal disease, there are several potential related disease states. Even if a nonreversible disease process were to be found, renal dialysis or a transplant might be viable options offering Mr. Jones a longer life.

Complicating the health-related problems is Mr. Jones' apparent refusal to discuss the situation honestly with his wife. Dr. Sampson can respect Mr. Jones' autonomy and accept his decision not to pursue further work-up. As an alternative, the doctor could try to maintain regular medical contact, including screening for depression, to see how Mr. Jones' situation evolves. However, Dr. Sampson is clinically and ethically disturbed, because he believes this plan would postpone or eliminate the potential benefits of needed care. Dr. Sampson feels that sharing this health care information with Mr. Jones' wife is an important means to foster a more appropriate care plan.

Dr. Sampson discusses with Mr. Jones the nature of the syndrome, the need for further assessment, and the importance of sharing such information with his wife to gain her support, but Bob Jones continues to be adamant that he will have no treatment. However, Mr. Jones is willing to discuss the matter further in a follow-up appointment.

Dr. Sampson believes that Mr. Jones and his wife have a good relationship, but he is concerned that withholding the knowledge could help undermine the stability of that relationship. It is also hard to imagine how maintaining confidentiality could truly support a person's autonomy when that person doesn't have family and social support. A person with a new, serious diagnosis is not the same person emotionally as the person who did not have that diagnosis. Dr. Sampson believes that family and friends can actually help foster Mr. Jones' autonomy through communication and support.

CASE 7.2 | Disclosing health care information to family

In this case, Dr. Cohen struggles with several ethics issues, including patient autonomy, confidentiality, and privacy. Tammy Andrews' newly diagnosed genital herpes has created a problem that is not merely clinical—the guilt, anxiety, and chronic nature of a newly diagnosed sexual disease is psychologically distressing. The teen girl is overwhelmed, despite Dr. Cohen's reassurance that the illness can be monitored and controlled with medication. Tammy Andrews' health issue has also created a crisis within her family. Ms. Andrews has refused to let Dr. Cohen discuss the situation with her family. She has suggested that she is not planning on telling anyone, not even her sexual partner.

Dr. Cohen is placed in a difficult ethical position, because he is unable to reassure Ms. Andrews' father, Rev. Andrews, that her health problem is not life-threatening, without breaching confidentiality. Dr. Cohen realizes that Rev. Andrews' suspicions are understandable and may escalate. The situation also creates a broader challenge, because Rev. Andrews will potentially solicit the clinic's office staff for information regarding his daughter's illness. Such a situation raises concerns about maintaining patient privacy and confidentiality within the clinic as well as within the community.

Though Dr. Cohen believes it would serve the best interests of both his patient and her family if Ms. Andrews were to inform them of her situation, she refuses. Though he is committed to Ms. Andrews' right to confidentiality and privacy, Dr. Cohen is concerned that he and his staff will be not be able to pacify Rev. Andrews without her cooperation.

RESPONDING TO PRIVACY AND CONFIDENTIALITY CONFLICTS
Such scenarios are common for rural health care teams, because of the overlapping relationships found in small communities. Urban residents may dismiss these cases as simple issues settled long ago in ethics discussions and case analysis. However, when occurring in rural areas, these situations are never reducible to something occurring "anywhere," because the rural context is so unique.

CASE 7.1 | A patient refusing needed care

Dr. Sampson recognizes Bob Jones' need for further assessment to clarify the diagnosis and to determine any appropriate treatments. A traditional health care setting would likely respect Mr. Jones' autonomous decision to postpone treatment, after clinicians had undertaken a certain level of discussion to encourage him to pursue further testing at this time. But in this situation, Dr. Sampson knows the patient and his wife on many levels. He delivered their baby, and is aware of their desire to have a larger family. Knowing Mr. Jones' family, his values, and his medical and community contacts, Dr. Sampson believes that Mr. Jones' reasoning doesn't reflect his actual personal goals. Mr. Jones' reasoning may have been diminished in the face of the physical threat of serious illness. It is very difficult for Dr. Sampson to argue with Bob Jones about his decisions after such bad news, because Mr. Jones is not thinking about his life in the same manner as before.

Mr. Jones' desire for Dr. Sampson to maintain confidentiality by remaining mute, deflective, or maybe even lying in communication with Mr. Jones' wife, is ethically unacceptable to Dr. Sampson. Dr. Sampson also doubts that he could even "carry off" such deception in response to questions from Mr. Jones' wife. Questions will inevitably come from this patient's family and friends, because of the extent and obvious nature of Mr. Jones' symptoms. The doctor is not ethically allowed to lie or mislead his patient's wife, but he also may not breach his patient's confidentiality.

Dr. Sampson should emphasize to Mr. Jones the importance of seeking further assessment to better understand his illness and treatment options, including the benefits of treatments. Mr. Jones needs to be reminded of his stable, committed marriage, the importance of his wife's support, and the emotional weight for both of them in failing to communicate and share openly. The lack of communication with his family and friends will only foster more concerns, questions, and problems. Dr. Sampson should also explain the awkwardness he will feel when encountering Mr. Jones' wife, in both his office and in the community, if she remains uninformed.

Dr. Sampson's discussions with Mr. Jones will likely require multiple clinic visits and telephone contacts. In the meantime, the doctor needs to maintain confidentiality while actively encouraging Mr. Jones to honestly and openly disclose his condition to his wife.

CASE 7.2 | Disclosing health care information to family

Cases like the situation involving Tammy Andrews, the teen girl, do not only happen in rural areas; however, living in the rural setting does create a unique dynamic among Dr. Cohen, Ms. Andrews, and her parents. Despite rural-urban contextual differences in such cases, the appropriate response is similar.

As noted, there are many layers of concern for Dr. Cohen in the care of Tammy Andrews, which include clinical management of the disease, emotional support, and her family's needs. Despite Dr. Cohen's reassurance that the illness can be monitored and controlled with medication, his teen patient is overwhelmed and unwilling to share her troubles with anyone besides him, her doctor, at least at the present time. Dr. Cohen should strongly emphasize to Ms. Andrews the importance and value of sharing her health situation with her family, despite the disappointment they will likely demonstrate and the shame she already feels.

Tammy Andrews is very concerned that her family, especially her father, will not be able or willing to accept and support her in this situation. She thinks that her father will not be able to contain his anger regarding her sexual activity and resulting venereal disease. Dr. Cohen should offer to help her to share the health information as part of a family meeting. Ms. Andrews needs to understand that being deceptive with her family will foster further problems. Any deception will be difficult to maintain because of the need for regular medication for herpes. Dr. Cohen should reinforce the fact that if she refuses to share the health information and refuses to allow him to share the information, he will respect her decision. However, he will not suggest to the family that she has some other health problem. He will refer the family to speak with their daughter directly.

There are also concerns that Dr. Cohen's staff, who may also be members of the Reverend's congregation, will be pressured to reveal the clinical situation as they understand it, regardless of the accuracy. It is unlikely that personal contact between the involved parties will not eventually occur. If it is somehow avoided in the clinic, it will occur later in the community. The intimacy of rural life does not allow providers, including Dr. Cohen or his staff, to live in a reclusive bubble of isolation. However, while the office staff can appreciate Rev. Andrew's desire to obtain the medical information, they need to understand the circumstances in which the law shields a minor's medical information from parents and when it does not.

As is the case in many states, Rev. Andrews has no right to see his daughter's medical information in this situation. Ethically, Dr. Cohen must protect her privacy. However, Dr. Cohen should strongly reinforce to Tammy Andrews how important it is for her to share her health information, despite her perception that it will create conflict within the family. He needs to inform Ms. Andrews about the disease, its management, and the precautions she will need to take regarding contact with any current or future sexual partners. Dr. Cohen will also need to reinforce to the clinic staff that privacy and confidentiality are both an ethical and legal obligation—essential to a trusting relationship between patients and providers. If Dr. Cohen shares the health information it must be done with Ms. Andrews' concurrence. If she refuses to disclose, or allow Dr. Cohen to disclose, her health information, Dr. Cohen will need to emphasize to Rev. Andrews when they meet that, like clergy, he is ethically required to maintain confidentiality about information shared in a professional relationship.

ANTICIPATING PRIVACY AND CONFIDENTIALITY CONCERNS

Patients trust health care professionals to foster and maintain privacy and confidentiality. When providers breach this professional and legal mandate, they jeopardize not only their personal integrity but also the moral status of their profession within the community.

Because people in rural settings may be relatives, friends or have frequent contact, health care professionals need to be particularly diligent in maintaining confidentiality. It is simplistic to think that breaches in confidentiality would not occur. Similarly, it would be wrong to think of rural health care providers as infallible, or above the law, or to exclude them from taking careful, rigorous steps to protect health information and from monitoring for breaches of confidentiality.

There are several practical ways that rural providers can seek to address and potentially diminish ethics conflicts regarding privacy and confidentiality. Some of these are required by law, as noted in Box 7.1.

BOX 7.1

ADDRESSING CONFIDENTIALITY AND PRIVACY ETHICS CONFLICTS

- Clarify confidentiality and privacy policy with patients
- Conduct informative discussions about confidentiality and privacy with the community in general
- Review medical record management for potential privacy breaches

Health care professionals should ensure that they are following the legal requirements for providing notice of their privacy practices and that the written information available for all patients about their policy regarding confidentiality is clear. Providers should discuss their position regarding confidentiality with all new patients. Health care professionals should proactively participate in discussions and education programs in the community regarding these topics. Community programs can include various providers who have similar professional rules of conduct and confidentiality, as in the case involving Dr. Cohen and Rev. Andrews. Members of the community would have an opportunity to express their concerns, thus fostering an increased community-wide understanding of privacy and confidentiality issues.

Health care professionals should also have regular training and ongoing discussions with staff about their legal obligations and the importance of confidentiality for maintaining trust and professionalism. Hospitals, clinics and provider offices should regularly review patient record maintenance protocols to prevent any breaches in personal health information. As in Dr. Cohen's case, when staff members understand the ethical foundations for such policies and know how to best manage records, they are more equipped to maintain ethics goals.

Despite the ethical mandate to adhere to patient confidentiality that is the foundation for a good provider-patient relationship, there are several morally justified exceptions to preserving confidentiality that may be permitted by law, depending on the particular jurisdiction. Some possible exceptions are noted in Box 7.2.

BOX 7.2

EXAMPLES OF POSSIBLE EXCEPTIONS TO MAINTAINING CONFIDENTIALITY

- Testifying in court
- Reporting communicable disease (and notifying partners)
- Reporting gunshot or other suspicious wounds if criminality is questioned
- Reporting potentially impaired drivers
- Warnings by physicians to persons at risk, when there is a legally recognized duty to warn
- Reporting in workers' compensation cases
- Reporting of child abuse, domestic violence, or elder abuse

These limited exceptions are intended to protect the public and, in some cases, the patients themselves. Unless there is a clear and unambiguous legal exception obligating the clinician to disclose information, health care providers should dedicate themselves to maintaining patient confidentiality and privacy.

CONCLUSION

The discussions of ethics issues that occur in rural settings resonate differently than they would in non-rural settings. Rural culture is embedded in both cases discussed in this chapter. In rural towns, health care professionals and other members of the community frequently encounter one another. Regular contacts within the community may lead people to ask providers for information about patients more often than would occur in non-rural settings. While providers might try to avoid the questions, the very intimacy of rural life does not allow them to live in a reclusive bubble of isolation. Such overlapping relationships can create ethics conflicts. For example, if a doctor were to consistently refuse to answer questions that involve disclosing protected health information about mutual neighbors, this might cause another neighbor, or even the entire community, to question a provider's broader responsibility to the community and its values.

Because many rural patients frequently receive their personal caregiving from family and friends, or people whom they know at some level outside of a health facility, community members sometimes feel they need to know about health issues in order to provide assistance. Sensitivity to these values in rural settings is important for any health care provider, but also fosters ethics challenges. Though it may be difficult at times, providers need to maintain confidentiality. However, awareness of, and sensitivity to, community values and culture should be a part of the patient-provider discussion to make a shared decision regarding how a patient's private, protected health care information may or may not be communicated.

REFERENCES

1. *Opinion 5.05 - Confidentiality. Code of Medical Ethics:* American Medical Association, Council on Ethical and Judicial Affairs. http://www.ama-assn.org/ama/pub/physician-resources/medical-ethics/code-medical-ethics/opinion505.shtml. Accessed July 2, 2009.

2. Edelstein L. *The Hippocratic Oath: Text, Translation and Interpretation.* Baltimore, MD: Johns Hopkins Press; 1943.

3. Siegler M. Sounding Boards. Confidentiality in medicine--a decrepit concept. *N Engl J Med.* Dec 9 1982;307(24):1518-1521.

4. Annas GJ. HIPAA regulations - a new era of medical-record privacy? *N Engl J Med.* Apr 10 2003;348(15):1486-1490.

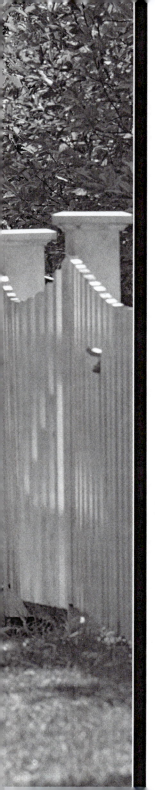
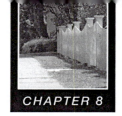

CHAPTER 8

Ethics Conflicts in Rural Communities:
Shared Decision-Making

Denise Niemira

Ethics Conflicts in Rural Communities: Shared Decision-Making

Denise Niemira

ABSTRACT

Shared decision-making is a collaborative interaction between the provider and patient in making treatment decisions in the informed consent process. Shared decision-making is based on trust, truthfulness, and respect for the patient's choice. Good communication is the vehicle that fosters this process within the patient-clinician relationship. A pivotal aspect of the shared decision-making process is a dialogue in which both parties share information, leading to a decision regarding the patient's health care. For the patient the subjects of discussion may include his or her life goals, values, religious and cultural beliefs, and finances. For the clinician, the discussion should include the risks and benefits of possible treatments as well as the likely outcome of no treatment. How information is shared, and what information is shared may influence the patient's choice. Clinicians may find themselves challenged by patient choices that, medically, do not seem in the patient's own best interest. At an ethical level, there is a tension between patient autonomy and beneficence that may not be easily resolved. For rural clinicians, the process may be challenging when the patient is a friend, and boundary issues are intensified; when multiple members of the same family are patients, and wish to participate in decisions of other family members; or when conflicts of loyalty seem to pit the interests of the patient against those of a struggling local medical community. Shared decision-making in the rural setting should be facilitated by open, honest communication between provider and patient, and includes the treatment expectations and boundary issues of each party. Ethics conflicts, especially involving family members, should be anticipated in shared decision-making. When possible, such conflicts should be addressed proactively rather than in a crisis setting.

CASE STUDIES

CASE 8.1 | The extent of information provided
in the consent process

Dr. Jonah Smith, a primary-care provider, is discussing with a patient, Sam Tanaka, the need for a referral for major surgery for a condition that is potentially life-threatening. The surgical procedure could be done at the small, rural hospital; however, the general surgeon has limited experience with the needed procedure. The surgery is one whose outcome is statistically volume-sensitive, i.e., the more procedures the surgeon and institution perform, the better the outcome. Mr. Tanaka does not ask where the best location for performing the procedure is, but says, "Just tell me what to do, doctor." The local community hospital is struggling financially. Contributing to the problem is the number of referrals to large facilities away from the rural community. The surgeon's experience with the particular surgery remains limited because of the frequency of referrals to large, distant hospitals. Dr. Smith is uncertain about how to respond to Mr. Tanaka. How do the economic needs of the rural facility influence Dr. Smith's discussion with the patient about the options and alternatives? Does the discussion change if Mr. Tanaka specifically asks, "Where would you have the surgery done?"

CASE 8.2 | A patient's refusal of needed diagnostic evaluation

Dr. Joan McDougall, a primary-care provider, has recommended additional diagnostic testing for an 80-year-old patient, Ursula Mueller, who may have a malignancy related to a long-standing blood abnormality. Mrs. Mueller has recently been treated for anemia, and she accepted blood transfusions when she becomes symptomatic. Dr. McDougall explicitly states her concerns about cancer with Mrs. Mueller. Though the patient fully understands Dr. McDougall's concerns, she declines further assessment for financial reasons. Ursula Mueller and her husband, who live on the income made from the sale of their farm, are still paying off the hospital bills from her previous testing and treatment. She wishes not to incur further debt at this time. Dr. McDougall treats other members of Mrs. Mueller's family and suspects that they would want their mother evaluated and would help with financial issues. Mrs. Mueller refuses to give Dr. McDougall permission to discuss this matter with her family.

OVERVIEW OF ETHICS ISSUES
Shared decision-making is a collaborative interaction between the provider and patient in making treatment decisions in the informed consent process. Communication is the heart of a good patient-clinician relationship and of shared decision-making. In the shared decision-making model of the doctor-patient relationship, the goal of communication is to enable patients to make informed, autonomous choices regarding their medical care. These choices are made within a dialogue in which the health care professional's clinical experience and fiduciary responsibility are used to inform and guide the patient's choice among the various options for treatment according to the patient's personal preferences and goals. The importance of this process is captured in the American College of Physicians Ethics Manual.[1]

The shared decision-making process attempts to balance the often-conflicting demands of patient autonomy (self-determination) and beneficence (promoting patient well-being and preventing harm), as discussed in Chapter 3 of this *Handbook*. A patient who voluntarily agrees to the treatment recommended by the clinician in the course of this dialogue has given informed consent. A patient who refuses the recommended treatment has given informed refusal.

Elements of Informed Consent[2]
There are several criteria for informed consent. These include:

- *Full Disclosure of Adequate Information:* Communicating all information necessary to understand the medical condition, treatment options, and the risks and benefits of reasonable treatment(s) and non-treatment
- *Voluntariness*: The ability to make treatment decisions free of coercion or undue influence
- *Decision-Making Capacity:* The ability to understand and process information and arrive at a preference-for-treatment decision

Full Disclosure of Adequate Information: Informed choice entails a dialogue in which clinicians provide patients with relevant, understandable information about their medical condition, the types of treatments available for the condition, and the risks and benefits of the treatment(s) or non-treatment for the condition. While there may be an ethics debate about the extent of specific information that must be provided, there are a few generally accepted norms guiding disclosure. The disclosure may be tailored to the patient's desire for information, but the information provided should be truthful. All relevant information that could significantly impact a patient's choice should be disclosed. The standard for disclosed information is shifting from a professional-centered one (what a reasonable practitioner would reveal), to a patient-centered one (what a reasonable person would want to know).[3] Patients may choose to forgo discussions regarding risks and benefits of treatment, or may defer the discussion and/or decision to family members (a process that is common in certain cultural and ethnic traditions). In these settings, clinicians should clarify the patient's desires regarding disclosure and how voluntary is the patient's decision to forgo or defer discussion.

Clinicians exercising beneficence may guide, but not coerce patients in their choices. They can help patients translate personal needs, values, and lifestyle goals into concrete medical choices that will best support these needs and goals. Clinicians may make recommendations in favor of a treatment option based on their clinical judgment of what is best for the patient.

Voluntariness: Patients have the right to accept or refuse any procedure or treatment offered to them. The patient should make a decision based on his or her goals and disease, without having to experience undue force or pressure from clinicians that would erode their voluntary decision. Patients may not always agree with the recommendations of their health care providers. They might reject the recommended treatment. Clinicians faced with this situation often question the patient's choice. Did the patient hear the information that was presented? Did the patient understand the information? Is the patient capable of processing the information to make an informed, voluntary choice? When it is clear that patients understand their disease and the consequences of their choice(s), their decisions should be respected. It is appropriate for clinicians to challenge a patient's ability to make informed decisions when it is unclear whether the patient has a capacity to understand and process information about his or her medical condition. This challenge should be based not on the decision the patient has made, but on how they have come to make it—did the patient have reasonable reasons for their decisions?[4]

Decision-Making Capacity and Competency: When patients lack the ability to understand their disease state and appreciate the consequences of the decision they are being asked to make, they are said to lack decision-making capacity.[5] While decision-making capacity is sometimes equated with competency, competency is a legal determination that a person lacks the cognitive capacity to make reasoned decisions. When a court determines that a person is incompetent to make medical decisions, that person is unable to consent for treatment, even if he may understand his medical condition and the options and outcomes of treatment. The status of incompetent adults is similar to that of minors, particularly older minors who, regardless of understanding and decision-making capacity, are legally unable to consent to treatment. Clinicians in these situations often try to reconcile legal and ethical responsibilities to their patients by fostering their participation in the treatment discussion as much as possible and by obtaining their assent to the treatment.

Lack of decision-making capacity is a clinical determination.[6] It may be obvious, as in patients who are unconscious, floridly delirious or severely demented. In other cases, lack of decision-making capacity may be considerably less obvious—even questionable. There is no single test or standard for determining decision-making capacity. Clinicians must rely on clinical interviews and findings, responses to neurological and psychological testing, and reports from family and significant others. In difficult cases, professionals may need to consult with colleagues, specialists such as psychologists or psychiatrists, hospital counsel, or a risk-management or ethics committee. Since the lack of decision-making capacity may be a temporary condition, clinicians should treat any reversible causes.

When a provider determines that a patient lacks decision-making capacity, an alternative decision-maker, or surrogate, must make treatment decisions. Depending upon the medical circumstances, geographic location, hospital policies, local customs and relevant legal statutes, family members or appointed surrogates may become involved.

Surrogate Decision-Makers
Surrogate decision-makers are individuals who are duly authorized to make decisions for patients who lack decision-making capacity. There are three basic types of recognized surrogates which are defined in Box 8.1.

These three types of surrogates are appointed or selected in several ways. The court, through a guardianship procedure, can appoint the surrogate.

BOX 8.1

BASIC TYPES OF RECOGNIZED SURROGATES

- Court-appointed guardian for health care decisions
- Advance-directive documented surrogate or Durable Power of Attorney agent (proxy)
- Next of kin

Surrogates can be named in a legal document or advance-directive document to assume decision-making when the person naming them is no longer able to make decisions. A frequently used document is the Durable Power of Attorney to make such a designation. Surrogates may also be based on the next-of-kin status. The order of kinship with responsibility to make decisions is generally spouse, adult child and parent. Most states have statutes regarding how to designate surrogate decision-makers, including the order of kinship. The Department of Veterans Affairs has a specific order of surrogates in their national Informed Consent Policy. Surrogates may also be determined by local custom in the absence of specific legislation or regulation to make decisions for relatives or significant others who have lost decision-making capacity. Clinicians should consult with legal counsel to be familiar with the laws and appropriate forms and customs in their state.

The authority of surrogate decision-makers varies with the circumstances of their appointment and relevant legislation. Surrogates are to provide "substituted judgments" based on clear and specific directives from the patient who once had the capacity to decide for himself or herself, or to provide what the surrogate believes is in the "best interest" of the patient lacking capacity, if the patient never specifically clarified his or her desires. More about the surrogate's role, including advance directives, can be found in Chapter 11.

Clinicians as Moral Agents and Informed Consent

In the informed-consent process, clinicians have a moral as well as a professional responsibility to act for the benefit of their patients. Their disclosure and advice should be based on what will best serve their patients' needs, and should not be compromised by self-interest, employers, colleagues or community institutions.[7] When these conflicts are present and cannot be avoided, clinicians must ensure that they do not influence the extent of disclosure to patients, or manipulate the presentation of treatment choices. In general, disclosure of non-patient loyalty conflicts is ethically required.

Clinicians must respect the autonomy and right to privacy of their patients who have decisional capacity. When clinicians question a patient's decision-making capacity, they may query family members about the patient's mental status without specific consent, but should not pursue such an option solely due to disagreement with the patient's choice.

When patients request or even demand a treatment that will cause harm, or have no promise of benefit based on empirical assessments, clinicians may refuse to order or provide such treatment. Clinicians should consider the request, but are not morally required to provide any treatment that they believe lacks scientific validity. Clinicians may also refuse to participate in any treatment(s) to which they are morally opposed. Clinicians have an obligation to inform patients of their moral opposition and to make referrals to other providers when possible.

CASE DISCUSSION

The discussion of the following cases is based on the analysis method presented in Chapter 4.

CASE 8.1 | The extent of information provided in the consent process

Dr. Smith must discuss a surgical referral with a patient, Mr. Tanaka, who needs major surgery for a condition that is potentially life-threatening but not an emergency. This is an illustration of the informed-consent discussion, focusing on the elements of full disclosure and voluntariness. At issue in the informed-consent process is not only the decision to seek surgical treatment but also the location of that treatment. Specialist surgeons who practice at larger community hospitals and medical centers usually do the surgery in question. The outcome of this procedure is statistically better when the hospital and surgeon perform greater numbers of the surgery. This volume might not be achieved in a small rural hospital, even if most patients from the community chose to have it performed there. While the issue is framed in the context of a surgical referral, it applies to other complex care provided in the rural setting, including diagnostic modalities and intensive care.

Dr. Smith realizes that his surgeon colleague and their community hospital are caught in a challenging situation regarding this surgery and other volume-sensitive procedures. If patients like Mr. Tanaka are routinely sent out of the community to larger referral centers with more experience, the community hospital will not improve its outcomes.[8] Dr. Smith realizes that when the medical community loses the experience to manage such cases, fewer talented surgeons and other specialists will choose to practice in the community, and will instead go where their skills can be utilized in a more challenging way. The loss of revenue is detrimental to the small facility, and may threaten its long-term viability. There is an issue of divided loyalties, the extent of which may vary depending upon the practitioner's relationship to the local surgical colleague and hospital, as well as the institution's response to referrals outside the area. Is the practitioner in partnership with the surgeon, or employed by the hospital? Is there an overt pressure to refer within the institution?

The patient in this case, Mr. Tanaka, appears to be short-circuiting the disclosure process by deferring the decision to the clinician's recommendation. This might be a measure of respect for, and trust in, the physician, or of deference to the role of the practitioner in a rural community. It could suggest a paternalistic model of the patient-clinician relationship. It may be an expected social convention. While patients have the right to waive informed consent, health care professionals should accept the role only with the utmost caution; they should ensure that it is truly what the patient wants and is a voluntary request. If the clinician accepts this role, he or she should openly and clearly review his or her thinking with the patient. This is especially important in circumstances where there are conflicts of loyalty.

The primary care practitioner has an ethical duty to be truthful in his or her disclosures and to offer recommendations that will benefit the patient. The clinician also bears a responsibility to the community to maintain and foster the availability of health care treatment. Regardless of the community need, however, the primary-care provider must first act for the benefit of the patient.

CASE 8.2 | A patient's refusal of needed diagnostic evaluation

Dr. McDougall faces an elderly patient, Ursula Mueller, who is refusing recommended diagnostic evaluation for a potentially serious illness. The focus of the ethics issues is on the validity of an informed refusal, including the elements of decision-making capacity and voluntariness of the patient. The clinician's recommendation is based on Mrs. Mueller's abnormal blood test and the knowledge that the patient's condition could transform into a cancer. Mrs. Mueller's refusal to undergo further evaluation at this point will impact future treatment decisions and outcomes. She is able to articulate an understanding of her condition and the clinician's concerns about cancer, but is unwilling to proceed with the recommended testing. Mrs. Mueller appears to have decision-making capacity, but the reasons for her decision—her current financial indebtedness to the hospital and a desire not to incur further debt—seem short-sighted. The clinician wonders if this choice is truly voluntary. Does the patient feel pressured by demands to make payments for past care? Are there social services agencies that can assist or guide the family in addressing the financial issues? Does Mrs. Mueller feel the need to sacrifice for other family members? Are the risks of forgoing evaluation enough to challenge the decision? And how much challenge constitutes coercion on the part of the clinician?

Dr. McDougall faces additional ethics challenges in accepting Mrs. Mueller's refusal of further evaluation. She also treats two of the patient's children, who are mindful of the doctor's confidentiality policy and respectful of their mother's independence, but have expressed concern about their parents' aging and unwillingness to seek health services for financial reasons. The children have stated their willingness to become involved and to help financially when needed. Dr. McDougall has responded to these conversations with a suggestion that a family discussion be held to discuss these issues. However, the patient refuses to participate in such a discussion with other family members. The prior conversations raised by the patient's children led Dr. McDougall to believe that they would want their mother to have the diagnostic work-up and that they would address their mother's financial concerns. She also feels that they would most likely exert pressure on their mother to have the testing done, but would likely accept her refusal if cancer were diagnosed and she did not want treatment. Dr. McDougall believes that the children expect Mrs. Mueller to involve them in this situation. Should the doctor override her patient's refusal to discuss the matter with them?

RESPONDING TO THE SHARED DECISION-MAKING CONFLICTS

CASE 8.1 | The extent of information provided in the consent process

In Dr. Smith's case, Mr. Tanaka's casual remark, "tell me what to do, doctor," should not be taken as an invitation to make a recommendation about the risks and benefits of the surgery, as well as where it should be done, without further discussion. Dr. Smith should explore what the patient knows about the planned surgery, and review any concerns Mr. Tanaka might have, what his support network would be after surgery, and what his preference is regarding the location of the surgery. Mr. Tanaka may have reasons for choosing a location for surgery independent of any statistics, such as having family members in that area. Dr. Smith should ask about Mr. Tanaka's preferences because the patient may need specific information that will shape the discussion. Dr. Smith should be aware of what Mr. Tanaka considers important in arriving at his decision, and of the influence that he, as the doctor, may have exerted on that decision.

The issues involving the community hospital and local surgeon in this case are not without moral relevance, but they do not supersede the need for the provider to disclose to the patient any information that is important when making medical decisions. Practitioners can shape and frame their disclosure of information with patients, including how they present the statistical data or offer recommendations, in ways that will impact the patient's ultimate choice. For example, if the patient is inclined to have the procedure done locally, the primary care practitioner should acknowledge that the medical center hospital has more experience with the procedure, and that statistically this means that results are potentially better. The practitioner may then discuss the local surgeon's experience and offer the patient a choice between the local setting, with its perceived benefits to the patient, and the tertiary setting, with its greater expertise, without favoring one place of surgery or the other.[9]

If the patient asks the clinician whether the procedure should be done elsewhere, the clinician should answer honestly. If the clinician suspects that the patient should not have the procedure in the community, for any reason, this must be disclosed. If the clinician lies, fails to disclose information a patient considers important, or persuades a patient who was inclined to go to the tertiary center to instead remain in the community for a high-risk procedure, the harm of a poor outcome is far worse for the community and the clinician than the loss of the local procedure. And naturally the outcome is far worse for the patient – resulting in a lose-lose situation all around. It is the betrayal of a patient-clinician relationship grounded in trust.

CASE 8.2 | A patient's refusal of needed diagnostic evaluation

The purpose of informed consent is to enhance the patient's autonomy. This means that the professional must respect choices with which he or she disagrees. It does not mean that the provider must accept such choices without question, nor does it preclude him or her from attempting to persuade the patient otherwise, as long as such attempts are not coercive or manipulative. Respect for autonomy also includes the provider's respecting the confidentiality of patients who are competent to make decisions, in spite of pressure from concerned third parties, such as family members. In cases when family members are likely to be involved as future caretakers and/or surrogate decision-makers, it is important that patients be encouraged to involve them earlier in the decision process, so that such conflicts may be discussed and hopefully avoided.

Dr. McDougall should enhance Mrs. Mueller's autonomy in shared decision-making. The doctor's concerns about the voluntariness of Mrs. Mueller's refusing a diagnostic work-up should be discussed—independently of the doctor's knowledge of and relationship to other family members.[10] Dr. McDougall should not override Mrs. Mueller's objections by involving the family, unless she believes that Mrs. Mueller's choice is not autonomous, and the situation warrants that the doctor involve family members regardless of her relationship with them. Mrs. Mueller is not in imminent danger from a life-threatening condition, and has accepted symptomatic treatment. Her refusal to undergo further testing may be a form of denial or an unwillingness to confront a diagnosis of cancer. Her concern about finances might not only involve the proposed diagnostic work-up, but the treatment that could ensue. Mrs. Mueller may simply need more time to process the news. Giving the patient the time and opportunity to revisit the issue, either alone or with her family, allows her to process the information and then have the choice to either change her mind, or to further articulate her goals. It also allows her to remain autonomous and independent, and involve to her family as she chooses.

Since Mrs. Mueller's illness is unlikely to be hidden from her family, Dr. McDougall should encourage her to discuss her plans with them, particularly if Mrs. Mueller continues to deny evaluation and/or treatment. Dr. McDougall should remind Mrs. Mueller that if she becomes incapable of making decisions in the future, her family might need to become involved as surrogate decision-makers. If Mrs. Mueller does not discuss her goals with her family now, they may try to intervene in her future treatment in a way that is inconsistent with Mrs. Mueller's wishes. Suggesting a group meeting to include the doctor, patient and patient's family to review and discuss the issues would serve several purposes: it would involve the family, it would allow Mrs. Mueller to clarify her values in a comfortable setting, and it would allow Dr. McDougall to articulate all the potential risks and benefits of further evaluation to all family members. Dr. McDougall should avoid the temptation to use the family meeting as a forum to coerce or manipulate Mrs. Mueller or her family.

Clinicians faced with patients refusing care should ask themselves what values are at stake from the patient's perspective: how great is the therapeutic benefit and what is the projected loss? Knowledge of the therapeutic benefit may be of little comfort to a patient who has limited savings; and if she were to pursue treatment, she might not be able to afford a final vacation, or might leave a surviving spouse destitute. Death or significant morbidity from an illness that is easily, though perhaps not inexpensively, treated is difficult to explain to family members and patients. The degree to which a clinician persuades or considers coercion should parallel the overall therapeutic benefit to the patient, as well as the immediacy of the situation. Often this is a matter of clinician judgment, based on best guesses or population-based benefits.

When a patient with decision-making capacity persists in refusing a treatment or evaluation, despite multiple attempts at persuasion, the clinician should generally respect the decision. In such situations, the clinician might consider consulting with a colleague or an ethics committee to review alternatives. The clinician should not use the threat of termination of care as a method of coercion to force an unwanted treatment. Even after accepting the patient's refusal of further evaluation, the clinician should continue to see the patient for follow-up visits regarding symptomatic support, and to be a resource in the event that the patient later changes his or her mind and does decide to pursue treatment.

ANTICIPATING SHARED DECISION-MAKING ETHICS CONFLICTS

The patient-clinician relationship does not exist in isolation from its rural context. The social contexts of the community in which both the physician and patient reside exert an influence on their interaction in shared decision-making. This can create conflicts and potentially disrupt the bonds of trust and respect on which the patient-clinician relationship is based. It is important that such conflicts be anticipated and recognized, so that the integrity of shared decision-making is maintained.

Conflicts Arising Within the Health Care Institution

Rural primary-care practitioners and their local hospital(s) share a mutual commitment to the health of the community served. Rural hospitals and clinicians are dependent upon each other to provide quality care to meet their community health needs and expectations. They are also dependent on factors that ultimately affect the direction and shape of their activities, including financial pressures, population base, provider expertise, hospital technology, and geographical location. These factors often determine limits to the possible services offered, and force painful choices about what kind of care the local hospital should provide. For example, as a result of community demands, financial need, or efforts to recruit talented clinicians, rural hospitals may attempt to expand services in areas for which they do not have the population base or clinical services to adequately sustain. The rural hospital might then expect local providers to support such new services through referrals without reservation, and without adequate disclosure to patients, as noted in the first case.

Rural clinicians should work with their medical colleagues, professional associations, hospital boards, administrators, and ethics committees to ensure that local hospitals provide quality care, emphasize shared decision-making, and conduct ongoing efforts to upgrade and maintain clinical competency. Hospitals should solicit and address concerns from practitioners regarding the quality of services provided. Hospitals and physicians should work toward an understanding that supports and encourages local care without limiting or manipulating a patient's right to know or choose.

Both clinicians and institutions should develop policies and procedures that address issues involving potential informed consent, conflicts of interest, confidentiality and privacy. The basic components of policies regarding informed consent and conflicts of interest may be found in Box 8.2 and Box 8.3 respectively.

BOX 8.2

COMPONENTS OF AN INFORMED-CONSENT POLICY

- Define informed consent and the need for shared decision-making
- List and describe the elements of valid consent and refusal
- Delineate what procedures and treatments require a signed informed consent
- Clarify the requirements for documenting informed consent
- Identify the resources for clarifying the informed-consent policy, such as an ethics committee

BOX 8.3

COMPONENTS OF A CONFLICT-OF-INTEREST POLICY[2]

- Define conflict of interest
- Affirm that the patient's interests are primary for the organization
- Delineate how, when, and to whom conflicts of interest (or potential conflicts) are to be disclosed
- Indicate the implications of violating the conflict-of-interest policy
- Identify a facility resource to clarify questions regarding the policy

When Conflicts Arise with Family Members

Primary care providers practicing in rural areas should anticipate conflicts around shared decision-making because of overlapping relationships with multiple members of the same family. The provider's establishment of ethics-grounded practice guidelines is essential in order for him or her to define the boundaries for what patient information is shared with whom. The provider's articulating and sharing a policy with patients, as part of the office routine, will emphasize that the guidelines are an expectation. Such information-sharing can be easily and efficiently implemented as part of a patient handout or handbook that the provider gives to all patients. The language does not have to be complicated; however, the guidelines and their reasons should be clear. Such a document is often better when it is short and somewhat lighthearted—something that can be referred to when ethical challenges occur. A sample is provided in Example 8.1

EXAMPLE 8.1

AUTHOR'S CLINIC CONFIDENTIALITY STATEMENT

Confidentiality: The information in your records is confidential. It will not be shared without your permission unless there is a legal requirement to do so. You sign a release when you join the practice to release information for billing purposes and for government review. If you wish to share information about your visit with your family, it is your prerogative to do so. Doctors, nurses or other medical staff cannot share your medical information without your permission. If you wish that your provider may speak to your family members, please let him or her know. (This applies to hospitalizations as well.) Please respect your family members' and friends' right to confidentiality and do not ask medical providers about their health or whether and when they have been to the clinic.

Having articulated the ground rules for shared decision-making, it is important for the clinician to follow through in action, and for him or her to deflect requests that would be contrary to the stated practice guidelines. Patients and family members will learn quickly how serious a practitioner is about protecting information.

Use of Advance Directives

Staff of rural health facilities and clinics should actively encourage the use of advance directives to decrease the potential for ethics conflicts, and to improve the quality of end-of-life decision-making. Clinicians should routinely raise the topic of advance directives, especially with any patient in a potentially life-threatening or terminal situation. Clinicians can encourage patients to discuss the issue with their family members, and can offer to include family members in discussing future health care decisions. Clinics and hospitals should also obtain, and make available to patients, written material that describes the purpose and process for making advance-directive decisions. The elements of advance health care planning are listed in Box 8.4.

BOX 8.4

ELEMENTS OF ADVANCE HEALTH CARE PLANNING

- Anticipate potential conflicts in shared decision-making involving family members
- Initiate conversations about advance health care planning
- Make use of state-based advance care planning material
- Involve the patient's family when this would be acceptable to the patient
- Share the clinic and/or hospital's policy regarding sharing advance health care planning information
- Document advance health care planning in the patient's chart
- Adhere to the policy described to protect patient confidentiality
- Advocate for patient autonomy through the implementation of the advance care planning

Family involvement in discussions about advance health care planning should be encouraged without endangering patient autonomy. Such discussions would also allow patients to share fundamental personal values that influence health care decisions, and to identify a family member or members who can speak for these values when patients are unable to speak for themselves.

CONCLUSION

Shared decision-making is a joint effort between the clinician and patient to promote the patient's goals and preferences in health care decisions. It is more than a recitation of risks and benefits followed by a recommendation. Shared decision-making is a conversation that explores the patient's desires and values. It recognizes and respects the rights of patients with decision-making capacity to pursue their particular visions of health care. Shared decision-making reflects the professional's duty to inform and clarify the choices, and to ensure as much as possible that decisions are voluntary, and reflect the patient's stated health goals. Shared decision-making occurs in a larger social matrix and is subject to influences from that sphere. Shared decision-making may be enhanced through several practical approaches as noted in Box 8.5.

BOX 8.5

PRACTICAL WAYS TO ENHANCE SHARED DECISION-MAKING

- Develop policies and procedures about informed consent, conflict of interest, confidentiality and privacy
- Share with patients the expectations and boundaries regarding these issues
- Recognize and protect patients' interests if conflicts of interest occur
- Maintain good communications skills, especially listening
- Identify and develop methods to anticipate and possibly avoid complex problems before they develop
- Promote the use of advance care discussions and decision-making through an open discussion of potential future health issues
- Practice truthfulness and embrace choice

Shared decision-making can be flawed when patients do not fully understand the future implications of their choices, or when professionals are too quick to accept patients' abrogation of choice. "Do whatever you think is best, doc" is the beginning and not the end of a conversation. It should evoke a response, such as, "Tell me what is important to you with this particular health issue and I will help you figure out what is best."

Shared decision-making can be compromised when patients do not have the ability to understand and make choices. It can also be compromised when outside parties attempt to coerce patients in their decisions, or to influence clinicians in their disclosure or recommendations.

Issues and problems arising with shared decision-making vary in the ease with which they can be recognized and rectified. Sometimes clarity can be achieved through salient questions: Would I question decision-making capacity if this patient were agreeing with my recommendation? Would I let my spouse have this procedure done here? Would I be thinking about talking to this patient's family without her consent if they were not also my patients? If I were 80 years old might, I feel differently about pursuing aggressive therapy than if I were 40? Questions regarding how competent a patient is, i.e., what their decision-making capacity is, can be thorny, and may require a psychiatric or neurological consult to help resolve. At times, the issues have legal implications. Identifying experts who can provide help in these types of situations is important, particularly if such expertise is not available locally.

To enhance the shared decision-making process in practice settings, clinicians should develop policies and procedures around informed consent, confidentiality and privacy. Clinicians should communicate with patients about their ethical thinking regarding boundary issues, recognizing and protecting patients' interests, and maintaining communication. Clinicians should identify and develop clinical, ethical, and legal resources to address problems when they arise. And, most importantly, providers must practice truthfulness and embrace choice.

REFERENCES

1. Ethics manual. Fourth edition. American College of Physicians. *Ann Intern Med.* Apr 1 1998;128(7):576-594.

2. Lo B. *Resolving Ethical Dilemmas: A Guide for Clinicians.* 2nd ed. Philadelphia, PA: Lippincott Williams & Wilkins; 2000.

3. *Canterbury v Spence,* 464 F. 2nd 772, 797 (D.C. Circuit 1972).

4. Culver CM, Gert B. *Philosophy in Medicine: Conceptual and Ethical Issues in Medicine and Psychiatry.* New York, NY: Oxford University Press; 1982.

5. President's Commission for the Study of Ethical Problems in Medicine and Biomedical and Behavioral Research. Making health care decisions: the ethical and legal implications of informed consent in the patient-practioner relationship. 1982;Volume 1: Report. http://www.bioethics.gov/reports/past_commissions/making_health_care_decisions.pdf. Accessed March 19, 2009.

6. Ganzini L, Volicer L, Nelson WA, Fox E, Derse AR. Ten myths about decision-making capacity. *J Am Med Dir Assoc.* Jul-Aug 2004;5(4):263-267.

7. Beauchamp TL, Childress JF. *Principles of Biomedical Ethics.* 5th ed. New York, NY: Oxford University Press; 2001.

8. Ward MM, Jaana M, Wakefield DS, et al. What would be the effect of referral to high-volume hospitals in a largely rural state? *J Rural Health.* 2004;20(4):344-354.

9. Engelhardt HT. *The Foundations of Bioethics.* New York, NY: Oxford University Press; 1986.

10. Roberts LW. Informed consent and the capacity for voluntarism. *Am J Psychiatry.* May 2002;159(5):705-712.

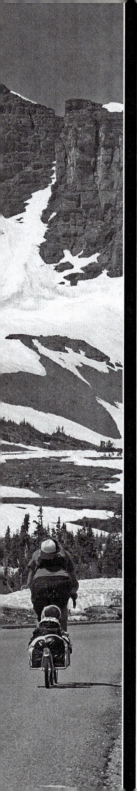

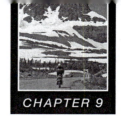

Ethics Conflicts in Rural Communities:
Allocation of Scarce Resources

Paul B. Gardent, Susan A. Reeves

Ethics Conflicts in Rural Communities: Allocation of Scarce Resources

Paul B. Gardent, Susan A. Reeves

ABSTRACT

Allocation of scarce resources is a reality for health care professionals and organizations. Resource allocation issues can be particularly challenging for rural communities, where resources are not enough to meet all needs and fewer alternatives exist to resolve conflicts between competing needs. In addition, the ramifications of decisions may be more visible in the rural setting. Decisions regarding allocation of resources can be troubling for clinicians and administrators to make, at both the personal and professional levels. Such decisions can be at odds with providers' deeply held beliefs about benefiting others without harm. Resource allocation decisions can create conflicts for personal, professional, organizational, and community priorities and commitments. Though resource allocation issues are economic in nature, they inherently raise issues relating to organizational mission and ethics. The philosophical method chosen to resolve resource allocation conflicts can influence both the way in which decisions are framed, and how the decisions are made. When responding to resource allocation conflicts, it is difficult to prioritize and identify a primary fiduciary duty or responsibility. Resource allocation conflicts are characterized by multiple constituencies, complex relationships, and myriad benefits and harms—which may or may not be apparent. All of these factors make resolving ethics conflicts related to scarce resources in rural settings both difficult and emotionally troubling.

CASE STUDIES

CASE 9.1 | Granite Hospital budget restrictions

Granite Hospital owns and operates a small, two-provider primary care practice in a community 25 miles from its main campus. Within the remote practice, two highly regarded family medicine practitioners provide practically all of the primary care to the small town. The hospital has received numerous comments over the years, attesting to the quality of the physicians and the secure feeling that is provided by their presence. The hospital originally established the primary care practice at the edge of its service area in response to anticipated capitation contracts that never materialized. Granite Hospital serves a large geographical area that has a low population, and the facility has received accolades and awards for its efforts to meet community health needs and offer preventive services to residents. The hospital is not strong financially, but has been able to subsidize its primary care businesses with extra income from its acute care services. Recently, deep Medicaid reimbursement cuts have negatively impacted the financial condition of the hospital and, in response, the Board of Trustees and administration have had to consider cutting operating costs. Questions have been raised about the hospital's ability to continue to subsidize the distant primary care practice. Board members are distressed by the devastating impact such a decision could have on the small town. Of course, if the community were to find out, they too would be devastated, and their anger might create a PR nightmare for the hospital.

CASE 9.2 | Moving procedures from hospital to office

Dr. Patel is a general surgeon in a rural community. He has seen his financial situation slowly deteriorate over the last several years, due to reduced reimbursement. He currently does many procedures in the small hospital's operating rooms, despite the fact that they could be done adequately in an office-based procedure area. Dr. Patel is thinking of moving the procedures to his office where he would receive greater reimbursement. The hospital administrator is very upset because the hospital relies on this revenue to support charity care and primary care services for the community. Dr. Patel understands this, but feels a financial obligation to his family. He also feels that the hospital has other opportunities to regain lost revenue. Finally, he believes he could charge less than the hospital, and thereby more directly benefit his patients.

OVERVIEW OF ETHICS ISSUES

Despite the fact that we live in one of the wealthiest nations in the world, the access to adequate health care continues to challenge many communities. These challenges are often magnified in economically disadvantaged geographic locales. For example, rural communities, in particular, struggle to recruit and retain qualified health professionals who are capable of providing basic health services to residents.

Rare is the rural health care professional who believes that there are adequate resources available to meet the demands for patient care. Decisions regarding the allocation of scarce resources are part of the everyday work life of rural health care professionals. Such decisions are often troubling, as they often result in the creation of "haves and have nots." The majority of health care professionals, who by definition have chosen to devote their careers to meeting the health care needs of others, are driven by a strong sense of beneficence. These are individuals who possess strongly ingrained personal and professional values. Such values are often enhanced during professional education, which dictates that harming or wronging others is to be avoided at any cost. This philosophy can include a belief in the right of all individuals to needed health services. The professional's inability to provide adequate health care services to all residents of the community may cause him or her to suffer moral distress. Therefore, the provider's need to consider allocating scarce resources can create conflict between deeply ingrained values and the realities of modern hospital financing in an era of managed care.[1]

Resource Allocation Decision-Making

The first step in ethical decision-making involves identifying the nature of the conflict that surrounds the allocation of scarce resources. The nature of such conflicts can be described in a conflict typology along two dimensions, the focus of moral conflict and locus of values, shown in Figure 9.1. Such value conflicts are often expressed by citing principles of obligation, loyalty, and duty to others.

The "locus of values" may manifest among any combination of personal, professional, organizational, and community values. Deeply held beliefs

FIGURE 9.1

ALLOCATION OF SCARCE RESOURCES CONFLICT MATRIX				
Focus of Conflict	**Locus of Values (Perceived Obligation, Loyalty or Duty)**			
	Personal	Professional	Organizational	Community
Stakeholder 1				
Stakeholder 2				
Stakeholder 3				

typically express themselves as personal values, which often are a result of faith, culture, upbringing, and life experiences. Professional values are expressed as professional Codes of Ethics in medicine, nursing and other health professions, and become ingrained during the individual's professional development and formation (e.g., American Medical Association Ethics Manual; Code of Ethics for Nurses; American College of Healthcare Executives' Code of Ethics). Organizational values are expressed through the sense of obligation felt to an organization. These values often relate to an individual's sense of responsibility for supporting the organization's mission, value statements, and policies. Finally, and particularly for people living or working in rural communities, there can be a deep cultural sense of dedication and obligation to the community.

The focus of the ethics conflict is on the competing values of the various stakeholders. The stakeholder conflict can be an internal personal conflict; a conflict among professionals; a conflict between professionals and the organization; a conflict between the organization and the community, or some combination of these. A personal conflict may be experienced when an individual is confronted with trying to adhere to competing values. Inter-professional conflicts occur among and between professionals due to conflicting personal moral principles or while trying to adhere to values held within a different locus. Often conflicts are heightened when the priorities between these dimensions vary among the professionals involved in decisions regarding allocation of scarce resources.

Frequently, trying to allocate limited resources becomes a problem of deciding how to rank the various competing values within the context of the organization's priorities. A suggested ranking is outlined in Box 9.1.

BOX 9.1

PRIORITY RANKING OF COMPETING ORGANIZATIONAL VALUES

- Patient's quality of care
- Professional excellence
- Organization's financial stability

Professor Werhane has noted that the stakeholder theory of decision-making should drive the reflection process for ethical decision-making done by health care organizations, in cases when there are competing values within the context of organizational decisions. The stakeholder theory, she writes, "…argues that the goal of any firm and its management is, or should be, the flourishing of the firm and all (of) its primary stakeholders,"[2] as compared to a goal of maximizing the welfare of the shareholders. This line of priority setting would require that the primary mission of the health care facility be to provide quality patient care. Therefore, excellence in patient care is the first priority. Because the integrity, and possibly the survival of the organization, is dependent on the professional's ability to offer competent, quality care, the staff would be the second priority. The third priority would be the long-term organizational viability, including its financial stability.[2]

The process of applying Werhane's proposed priorities is complicated by the fact that specific situations vary. For example, an acute financial crisis may require heightened attention to the organization's financial priorities. The proposed ranking is not an absolute algorithm. But it can provide a starting point for providers and administrators to reflect and discuss the concept of setting priorities, such as in situations when the "locus of values" matrix highlights stakeholder differences, e.g. in conflicts between personal and organizational values.

General Ethics Approaches for Consideration

Despite the proposed priority ranking of competing values, there is no quick answer to the problem of inadequate health care resources. Conflicts surrounding allocating resources will continue to be a reality for those charged with the distribution of available resources. Therefore, the questions become: What approach should be the basis for allocation decisions? What type of process would be best used to mitigate the negative impact of such decisions? And are there strategies to reduce the inevitable moral distress perceived by those with decision-making responsibilities?

The philosophical approach chosen by providers and administrators to resolve resource allocation conflicts can impact both the way decisions are resolved and how decision-making is approached. For example, the health professional may use a utilitarian approach (based on the theory that if an action or practice is right, when compared to an alternative action, it leads to the greatest possible balance of good consequences), which would call for the delineation of derived benefits by the recipients, with a choice to favor the decision that ultimately benefited the most people.[3] Such philosophical approaches tend to leave out disadvantaged groups with small numbers (e.g., a small town or an individual practitioner).

A "communitarian" approach is used to derive decisions which benefit the community as a whole over decisions that benefit individuals.[4] Each of the cases introduces the complexity of defining "community." For example, the community of interest for the Granite Hospital is the patient population it serves, comprising several towns around the hospital, whereas the remote small town that would be impacted by the primary care center closure is defined much more narrowly. For the practicing clinician, the community of interest may be even more restricted. Again, it is important to be clear around the definition of "community."

Deontological approaches, unlike utilitarianism, are used to decide what is right according to a duty to basic beliefs. These types of approaches are expedient, but often ill-suited for providers to apply to resource allocation issues, because of the focus on an action's intent rather than its result.[5] Deontological approaches by nature are contextual, and they often fail to resolve conflicts among competing values. As such, the application of this type of ethics approach is difficult.

Health Care Ethical Principles
In addition to the general ethics theories just discussed (philosophical, communitarian, utilitarian and deontological approaches) there are widely accepted and applied health care ethical principles, which include beneficence, nonmaleficence, autonomy, justice, veracity, and fidelity[4, 6]—all discussed in Chapter 3. These principles are frequently captured in a hospital's mission, vision and values statements, as well as in the staff practice standards.

The principles of veracity (honesty), fidelity (loyalty), and justice are also embedded into many resource allocation cases, including those presented here. The various providers and the hospital have many loyalties. The plight of the individual physician who attempts to juggle personal, professional, community and organizational loyalties is particularly difficult. Hospitals are torn between serving the community and surviving in a business market, and thus may not always be completely honest with the community. When designating programs or funds, honesty is typically the best policy, particularly when financial situations change. An "honesty" policy will reduce the amount of public relations backpedaling that the hospital will need to do if programs must be cut. For example, Granite Hospital may have entered the remote community market as a business strategy, with the intent to make a profit, but likely did not communicate the establishment of the practice as such to the local townspeople. It is more likely that the strategy was described as one that fulfilled the hospital's care mission. While both strategies are likely true, the marketing of the clinic establishment may have been less than forthcoming.

When confronting decisions regarding the allocation of necessary yet scarce resources, a number of moral issues are raised that challenge these core principles. Such decisions often challenge a provider's values and beliefs about what is morally right and wrong, particularly in situations where there are no good alternatives. The resulting moral distress can be debilitating to the decision-maker. And, such distress can be divisive and destructive within organizations and communities. So what happens when there are both good and harmful effects of such decisions? How does one decide what is the right thing to do?

Decision-Making Methodologies for Situations That Involve Scarce Resource Allocation

Making decisions in situations where scarce resources must be allocated is inherently difficult, and often challenges the clinician's desire to do what is right. The methods that providers use to make such decisions, including cost/benefit calculations, can be helpful in resolving allocation issues, although they do not entirely resolve providers' feelings of moral distress. In cost/benefit calculations, the clinician or administrator must first identify all the parties who may be involved and impacted by a decision. Ideally, representatives of the various parties would contribute to the cost-benefit discussion process to gain the best and most comprehensive inventory of costs and benefits. A listing of the costs and benefits that accrue to each of the parties should be clearly identified, taking care to include costs and benefits that are non-financial in nature. Relative measures of risk/harm and benefit/good should be made as objective and quantifiable as possible. Often, the use of a skilled facilitator to work with the various parties is a useful adjunct to this type of process.

The decision-making team should always conduct a further evaluation after an open and inclusive cost/benefit analysis. Their evaluation should examine whether a severely disadvantaged or marginalized group has borne a disproportionate burden of harm or cost as the result of the decision. Members of such groups, and their needs, are often poorly represented in medical decision-making processes. For example, Granite Hospital might argue that it is preferable to require the citizens of the remote community to drive the 25 miles to the hospital for services, as opposed to having the hospital go out of business all together. But for members of a disadvantaged group (e.g., those without any transportation), there is little difference between losing their primary care practice and being able to access the hospital, as the hospital would effectively be inaccessible to them.

When confronted with allocation decisions, the concept of distributive justice can be employed in a manner that allows the allocation methodology to promote equity and fairness.[5] While there are various methodologies that health care management can apply in decision-making, transparency is essential when choosing the type of methodology, and the consistent application of that methodology. Potential justice distribution methodologies include those listed in Box 9.2.

BOX 9.2

POTENTIAL JUSTICE DISTRIBUTION METHODOLOGIES[3]

- To each person an equal share
- To each person according to need
- To each person according to effort
- To each person according to contribution
- To each person according to merit
- To each person according to free-market exchanges

A related justice concept, procedural justice, is defined as, "The belief is that if the process is fair, the outcome will likely be fair as well."[7] Procedural justice, akin to stakeholder analysis, attempts to describe and understand the impact of a decision, including the costs and benefits to all who may be affected by it.[2] Important characteristics of procedural justice include consistency, objectivity, representation and transparency. For instance, a hospital's diminishing reimbursement may require budget reductions in various programs and services. However, prior to any decision, the executive leadership and clinicians need to explore and understand the ramifications of such a decision on all the related stakeholders. For the long-term health of the organization, it is important for the process to be conducted fairly and for decisions to be perceived as just by those affected by such decisions. Specifically the process for budget reductions should include the criteria provided in Box 9.3.

BOX 9.3

BUDGET REDUCTIONS DECISION-MAKING PROCESS

- Clear criteria, which are consistently applied
- An objective process for determining the facts related to the impacts upon the targeted programs and services
- Opportunities for affected parties to have their voices heard and for all parties to consider alternative ideas and proposals
- Complete transparency of all processes and decision-making elements

Health care leaders should seize the opportunity to structure a process so that it is fair, inclusive, and transparent.[8] Again, the use of a qualified facilitator, skilled in drawing out difficult issues, would enhance the process and outcome.

At the beginning of any decision process, the organization's leadership should make clear to all the involved parties how the decision will ultimately be derived and what criteria will be used, since a path forward does not always emerge from a discussion that entails ranking competing priorities among multiple constituencies. This is an important step to ensure that all parties know the ground rules and how power is distributed. A procedural-justice approach should never be considered if, in essence, a decision has already been made, and the process of involving stakeholders is simply being used to co-opt the participants. Inevitably, such processes backfire, creating an even bigger backlash against the decision-makers than what might have occurred initially, had they been honest and forthcoming at the outset.

CASE DISCUSSION

The discussion for the following cases is based on the analysis method discussed in Chapter 4 in this *Handbook*.

CASE 9.1 | Granite Hospital budget restrictions

Due to limited resources, Granite Hospital is faced with closing a primary care practice in a distant community in order to protect the viability of the rural hospital. This raises concerns about ethical responsibility among communities, to individual communities, and to an organization.

The hospital had initially established the primary care practice during a different Medicare reimbursement environment, intending to earn a profit from the practice, and perhaps, having a secondary motive to demonstrate commitment to the medical needs of a distant community. The community need is still apparent, and the hospital's focus on community service has become an important hallmark and expectation. It is not clear how acute the financial situation is for the hospital, or what alternatives exist to address these problems. Whatever the original reason was for establishing the primary care practice, the hospital has a responsibility to its board, staff, and its local and remote community to make decisions based on current circumstances.

The case also suggests that there may be differing feelings by clinicians, administrators, and the board about whether the distant community is really as important as the local community in which Granite Hospital is located. This raises questions about the boundaries of professional and organizational duty. Do we have a higher responsibility to our local community than to a more distant community? Also, there may be different perspectives among the administrative, trustee, and clinician leadership regarding whether to close the remote practice.

While the resource allocation conflict is framed from the perspective of the hospital organization and its members, there is also the perspective of the distant community and its two primary care physicians to consider. In a rural environment, resource allocation conflicts are intensified by the visibility of the benefit and harm to the individuals involved. These decisions can impact friends, neighbors, and colleagues. A characteristic of rural communities is that residents tend not to be transient and, as a result, the long-term memories of rural community members remain remarkably vivid—often spanning generations. Accordingly, resource allocation decisions have not only an immediate impact on the community, but may have long-term impacts on future relationships, with and within the community, that may last decades. These impacts can include the way the hospital is perceived, future contributions to fund-raising, staff recruitment and retention, and patient and physician loyalty to the hospital.

Granite Hospital leaders are unsure about how to proceed. They are deeply distressed by the idea of closing the distant clinic, but know that the hospital does not have the funding to continue the clinic's operation. Can they close the clinic without causing undue risk to patients, without undermining the hospital's mission, and without damaging the hospital's image?

CASE 9.2 | Moving procedures from hospital to office

In the case of Dr. Patel, the surgeon considering the relocation of some procedures to his office, personal and inter-professional conflicts are raised, as well as conflicts of loyalty and duty. Dr. Patel is confronted with personal conflict when he has to weigh the benefits for his family and patients versus the potential harm to the hospital and possibly his community. He is also confronted with an inter-professional conflict with the hospital administrator.

For Dr. Patel, it will be beneficial to his practice (and thus, to him and his family) to move the location of his procedures to his clinic. However, for the hospital, the loss of procedural revenue will cause a significant financial strain. This conflict arises from the difference in the locus of the perceived duty that each party has to their constituencies. The surgeon may feel a deep responsibility to his family and patients, while the administrator feels a duty to the community hospital for which he has a fiduciary responsibility, and to its trustees and financial stakeholders.

Dr. Patel knows that moving some of his procedures to his office will hurt the hospital, but this would be beneficial to him and his patients. Dr. Patel's ultimate allegiance is to his patients, but he knows that the hospital is important to them as well, and to him since it would likely provide many of his referrals. Can the surgeon move his procedures to his own clinic, and still maintain support for the hospital and a good relationship with the hospital staff?

RESPONDING TO RESOURCE ALLOCATION ETHICS CONFLICTS

CASE 9.1 | Granite Hospital budget restrictions

Granite Hospital leaders are considering the closure of the distant ambulatory practice. Is the closure of the primary care practice one of several options available to control Granite Hospital's operating losses? Are there other options for expense reductions that might respond to the financial crisis, or is the financial situation dire enough so that any source of operating loss is intolerable, thereby placing the viability of the hospital at risk? The answers to such questions are highly relevant and will serve to better inform the decision-making process.

The governing board of the hospital can play an important and helpful role in larger decisions affecting the broader community. An active and broadly representative board of trustees is able to simultaneously embrace two critical roles. First, a representative board can reflect the values and articulate the interests of the community. Also, a board member from the local community is able to communicate more easily with that community, and to explain the challenges and trade-offs facing the hospital. In situations such as the one facing Granite Hospital, it is important to involve the trustees in the decision regarding the ambulatory practice. It conveys to the community that the hospital understands the significance of the decision, and will use a process that is fair and thoughtful.

Neither the utilitarian nor the communitarian approach adequately addresses the degree of harm or benefit to the various parties in this case. While there may be small benefits to each individual of a large group, there may be extraordinary harm to a small group. In addition, neither approach adequately deals with differences in the perceived degree of loyalty or duty that the decision-makers feel. Such differences can exacerbate inter-professional conflicts, and make it difficult to reach a resolution that is morally justified in the eyes of the participants.

The establishment of the primary care clinic in the remote town has been very positive for the Granite Hospital organization, as it has not only been profitable until recently, but also affirmed the hospital's value of acting beneficently. Clearly, closing the primary care practice and the resulting lack of access to care has significant potential to cause harm to the residents of the community. However, as discussed, it may be preferable to lose a remote primary care practice than to risk losing the entire hospital to the region.

While Granite Hospital may have entered the remote community market as a business strategy, it likely did not communicate the establishment of the practice as such. It is probable that the strategy was described as one of fulfilling the organization's care mission. While both strategies may be true, the marketing of the care facility establishment might have been less than forthcoming.

Given that the decision to potentially close the ambulatory practice raises not only economic but also organizational mission and ethics issues,

Granite Hospital leaders decide to involve the board in the decision-making process. Fortunately this includes a board member from the community where the practice is potentially to be closed. The hospital forms a small ad-hoc board committee to develop a process, collect facts, and make a recommendation to the full board. The process is widely communicated to all participants. It includes an opportunity for a public meeting to explain to the community the financial difficulties the hospital is facing. Throughout the process, several potential savings are identified that might be implemented via significant changes in the ambulatory clinic's operations. Although such changes would be disruptive and not particularly provider-friendly, the local physicians decide they are willing to try them.

In addition, the hospital sets specific milestones and timelines that need to be met in order to keep the practice open. This particular process step insures that everyone knows what financial performance levels must be achieved for the practice to remain open. Interestingly, the hospital includes a member of their clinical ethics committee on the *ad hoc* board committee. The *ad hoc* committee finds that many of the concepts used in clinical ethics decisions turn out to be helpful in crafting this organizational resource allocation decision.

CASE 9.2 | Moving procedures from hospital to office

Resolving the conflict of the surgeon who is considering moving his procedures from the hospital is more difficult if it is viewed simply as the result of financial motivation. It would be easy to see Dr. Patel as just wanting to enhance his finances. Similarly, the administrator may be viewed as concerned only with the bottom line of the hospital. Framing the differences in this limited manner, though, minimizes the important moral reasoning that supports each of the player's views. If the conflicting positions are instead examined and addressed in a positive manner, the sense of isolation and unhappiness that professionals in rural settings frequently feel could be reduced. This might then lead to more stability in professional turnover and, thus, to improved health care.

In this case, Dr. Patel is troubled by the thought that the hospital administrator and the board might not understand his situation or motives. While he knows that he might make the decision to move his procedures to his clinic without the permission of the hospital, he doesn't like the idea of disrupting what has been a positive relationship of several years' duration. Thus, he decides to meet with the hospital's chief executive and chairman of the board to discuss his situation. He approaches the meeting with a clear understanding of his own needs, but also with a willingness to discuss alternative approaches.

During the discussion it becomes apparent to Dr. Patel that the chief executive and chairman have not appreciated the challenges of the present situation. Dr. Patel is also surprised that the hospital executive acknowledges the long-term benefit of moving services to an office-based setting, including lower costs and ease of access for patients. The executive notes that the hospital can focus on procedures that require an acute-care setting. They discuss a cooperative physician-hospital relationship which provides the opportunity for more coordinated planning for the community's needs and the possibility of some type of shared joint arrangement where both parties benefit. Dr. Patel and the chief executive agree to work together to move some procedures to Dr. Patel's office, while keeping some in the hospital. They also agree to meet on an annual basis to discuss planning for other services that should be moved out of the hospital. A year later, these discussions ultimately will evolve into an ambulatory facility joint venture between the hospital and some other physicians, including Dr. Patel.

In both of these cases, it is difficult for the clinician or administrator who is faced with resource allocation conflicts to identify a primary fiduciary duty or responsibility. When determining responsibility, it is important for such individuals to explicitly define what ethics and economic questions are being raised. Multiple constituencies, complex relationships, and myriad benefits and harms often characterize resource allocation conflicts. For example, these conflicts can impact hospital staff, physicians, payors, departments and services, providers in the community, and the community itself. There are a number of steps that individuals and groups can take that help them arrive at more ethical decisions. It is particularly important to make the process transparent to all of the individuals involved, as openness and honesty build trust among the participants. For a helpful overall process for resolving conflicts, see Chapter 4.

ANTICIPATING ALLOCATION OF SCARCE RESOURCE CONFLICTS

As with most situations, prevention of conflict is always preferable to having to solve conflict once it occurs. When establishing business strategies, organizations and individuals can work to both anticipate future conflicts and challenges, and to proactively eliminate or mitigate them—these steps are noted in Box 9.4.

BOX 9.4

MECHANISMS FOR HOSPITAL ADMINISTRATORS AND CLINICIANS TO PREVENT AND MITIGATE RESOURCE ALLOCATION ETHICS CONFLICTS

- Consider the long-term implications of decisions
- Maintain ongoing communication and dialogue
- Be deliberate when establishing service-area boundaries
- Identify the extent to which community service is owed or expected for service area(s)
- Promptly address imbalances in benefits and harms
- Consider the addition of an ethicist to the strategy/leadership team

Consider Long-Range Implications of Decisions

Rural health care providers, hospitals, and clinics should always consider the long-range implications of organizational decisions, particularly when such decisions are financially based. When Granite Hospital initially elected to establish the remote primary care practice, the decision was based on market and financial factors, with anticipated reimbursement conditions. The improvement of health care in the remote community was congruent with the hospital's mission; however, it was not the main reason behind the clinic's opening. Ironically, the decision to discontinue the practice is now one of mission and community service, because closing the clinic is expected to help keep the main hospital open. However, for patients in the remote area, the decision to discontinue the practice will be perceived as inconsistent with Granite Hospital's mission and values. Thus, this case should serve as a good warning for non-profit, service-based groups who also have businesses to run. In the future, financial strategy should always first be tied to mission, then second to market conditions, due to the volatility of such markets. People will remember that an organization is committed to improving care in their community. They won't recall that it was only there for as long as the venture was remunerative.

Maintaining Ongoing Communications and Dialogue

Health care providers and institutions should also publicly communicate specific quality and financial performance reports to the communities they serve, so that there can be broad understanding and engagement in support of the organization in an ongoing way—not just during a crisis. Such communication can take the form of town meetings or other special events that mesh with the culture of the community. In addition, the organization's trustee configuration should continue to broadly represent the service area.

Once established, service areas should not fluctuate according to short-term strategic imperatives. They should be entered for the right reasons, with the proper investments, and service continued until there is a mutual decision to make different arrangements.

Promptly Address Imbalances in Benefits and Harms

The legal structure among hospitals and providers may take many forms, but mutual interdependence is common, and this provides the foundation for successful, long-term, sustainable relationships. There should be routine, transparent reporting of financial and quality measures between related health organizations and providers, so that as market and reimbursement conditions fluctuate, each partner can support the other(s). Similarly, regular communication that centers on building relationships is critical to weathering those times when conflicts occur. Routine communication and meetings are essential for establishing trust, respect, and rapport among providers, patients, and administrators during non-crisis situations. Creating such positive relationship elements is essential during conflict situations to balance the benefits and harms to the parties involved, particularly regarding patients. These elements are also helpful to clarify the motivations and commitments of all parties.

It is much easier to resolve ongoing conflicts when it is clear that the parties share trust, respect, and common interests. For example, Dr. Patel ultimately decides to openly discuss his concerns for his patients, himself, and even the hospital with the hospital administrator. As he transitions some procedures from the hospital with the chief executive's blessing, Dr. Patel should communicate with his patients and the administrator to ease any tensions surrounding this change, while maintaining his own (Dr. Patel's) support for the hospital and its goals.

Consider the Addition of an Ethicist to the Leadership Team

Since resource allocation issues in health care inevitably raise ethics questions, it may be a good preventative measure to routinely include an ethicist as a member of the organization's operating or strategy team. For instance, it may be helpful for an ethicist to join the hospital's governing board. Also, ongoing training for administrators and providers on the ethical dimensions of governing and decision-making will enhance the effectiveness of health care organizations' governing boards and senior management teams.[9] The role of the ethicist in such forums is to make more explicit the ethics questions that emerge from various allocation methodologies. If used proactively during strategy-formation sessions, a more thoughtful strategy may be the result, and a more informed decision may be the ultimate benefit.[10]

Of course, it may prove challenging for a rural health organization to access a qualified ethicist. Often, local clergy or college-employed philosophy professors with the requisite expertise are available. While these professionals may not understand the nuances of health care per se, their command of ethics knowledge is what they bring to the table. And, as is often the case, those who are not involved with the intricacies and emotion of resource allocation decisions may be better able to introduce insightful and unbiased thoughts and questions.

Increased ethics help is also available via technology. This might include teleconferencing with ethics professionals based at an academic medical center, or conducting web seminars with ethicists associated with professional organizations or with philosophy professors based at large universities. Finally, if there is an operating ethics committee at the local hospital or health agency, often the baseline expertise exists within the group, and can easily be expanded and modified to apply to more administrative-based ethics conflicts or challenges.

CONCLUSION

Decisions on how to allocate limited resources are always difficult, particularly in rural areas where community relationships, as well as geographic and economic limitations, can create unique challenges for health care providers. Choosing a philosophical and methodological approach that is appropriate to the resource situation is a key part of the decision-making process.[11]

Identifying the nature of the conflict when resource allocation decisions are involved is an important first step for clinicians and administrators. The "conflict matrix" can be helpful in clarifying both the locus of values and the involved stakeholders in these conflicts. Having a basic understanding of the concepts and processes for dealing with ethics conflicts is a good start, but it can be particularly helpful to involve an expert in organizational ethics to facilitate significant or intractable conflicts.

Finally, anticipating allocation of scarce resources conflicts through preventive strategies may be the most important way to prevent and mitigate ethics conflicts for clinicians and administrators. Open and honest communication within the health care organization, as well as with the communities served, will ultimately prove the most important preventive strategy to reduce the ethics challenges associated with allocating limited resources that inevitably face all rural health care providers and administrators.

REFERENCES

1. Gilbert JA. *Strengthening Ethical Wisdom: Tools for Transforming Your Health Care Organization.* Chicago, IL: Health Forum, Inc.; 2007.

2. Werhane PH. Business ethics, stakeholder theory, and the ethics of healthcare organizations. *Camb Q Healthc Ethics.* Spring 2000;9(2):169-181.

3. Hinderer DE, Hinderer SR. *A Multidisciplinary Approach to Health Care Ethics.* Mountain View, CA: Mayfield; 2001.

4. Purtilo R. *Ethical Dimensions in the Health Professions.* 4th ed. Philadelphia, PA: Saunders; 2005:15-16.

5. Pence GE. *Classic Cases in Medical Ethics: Accounts of Cases That Have Shaped Medical Ethics, With Philosophical, Legal, and Historical Backgrounds.* Boston, MA: McGraw-Hill; 2004.

6. Beauchamp TL, Childress JF. *Principles of Biomedical Ethics.* 5th ed. New York, NY: Oxford University Press; 2001.

7. Nelson WA. An organizational ethics decision-making process. *Healthc Exec.* Jul-Aug 2005;20(4):8-14.

8. Ozar D, Berg J, Werhane PH, Emanuel L. Organizational ethics in healthcare: toward a model of ethical decision-making by provider organizations. American Medical Association, Institute of Ethics; 2000. http://www.ama-assn.org/ama/upload/mm/369/organizationalethics.pdf. Accessed April 11, 2009.

9. Ritvo RA, Ohlsen JD, Holland TP. *Ethical Governance in Health Care: A Board Leadership Guide for Building an Ethical Culture.* Chicago, IL: Health Forum; 2004.

10. Perry F. *The Tracks We Leave: Ethics in Healthcare Management.* Chicago, IL: Health Administration Press; 2002.

11. Danis M. The ethics of allocating resources toward rural health and health care. In: Klugman CM, Dalinis PM, eds. *Ethical Issues in Rural Health Care.* Baltimore, MD: Johns Hopkins University Press; 2008:71-96.

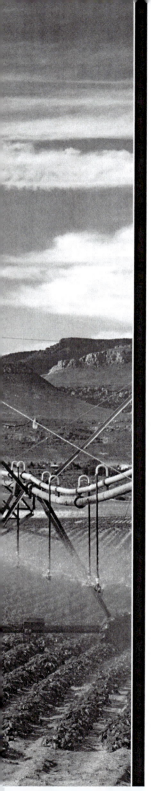

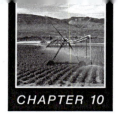

Ethics Conflicts in Rural Communities:
Stigma and Illness

Aruna Tummala, Laura Weiss Roberts

Ethics Conflicts in Rural Communities: Stigma and Illness

Aruna Tummala, Laura Weiss Roberts

ABSTRACT

Stigma is defined as a negative perception that is assigned to an individual because of an attribute that, in the eyes of others, deeply discredits and diminishes him or her from a whole and usual person to one who is tainted and discounted. Stigma always occurs in a context. In rural health care settings, stigma takes on special importance because of the interdependent and overlapping relationships that exist in small communities. To be viewed negatively by others, to be avoided, and to be seen as less than a full member of the community is an extraordinary burden for a person in a rural community. Stigma comes with implications for the rural person's life and family, at the current time and in the future. This chapter discusses the implications and effects of stigma and stigmatizing illnesses in rural communities, and the related ethics conflicts. Such conflicts include ethics dilemmas pertaining to the rights to privacy and confidentiality, or to the allocation of scarce health care resources, and are exacerbated by the unique stressors in the rural health care provider's experience. These ethics conflicts can be minimized, or even avoided, by following certain practical guidelines. When dealing with patients who have stigmatizing illnesses, confidentiality and establishing trust are of paramount importance. Rural health care providers should also be their patients' advocates and be proactive in mitigating stigma by educating the general public about common stigmatizing illnesses.

CASE STUDIES

CASE 10.1 | Confidentiality, overlapping relationships, and unwillingness to seek care

Nancy Smith is a 25-year-old woman living in a small town. She works at the local grocery store that her family owns. Several months into the relationship with a man from a neighboring community, she found out that her partner was HIV-positive. Following testing at a distant family planning center, her fear is confirmed that she is HIV-positive. She realizes that she needs treatment, and talks to her primary care physician, Dr. Russell, about the situation. Ms. Smith is hesitant about seeking care at the only primary health care clinic in her town, because the main nurse of the clinic and the lab technician are both regular customers at her store, and are also friends of her family. She fears the possible stigma and discrimination that her illness may cause, and isn't sure that her diagnosis can be kept a secret from her family or the community.

CASE 10.2 | Limited access to health care resources in rural communities

Greg Becker, a Vietnam War veteran, is a prominent leader in his rural community. He is now running as an elected official in his local town. For some months, privately, he has been experiencing difficult memories from his war experiences, including intrusive thoughts, nightmares, irritability and an inability to relax. He feels depressed and has occasional thoughts of suicide. His wife has "nagged" him about drinking until he reluctantly has agreed to see Dr. Chen, the family practice physician in his town. Mr. Becker is uncomfortable discussing his wife's fears about his drinking with Dr. Chen, and he fears his disclosure may hurt his campaign. Dr. Chen recommends Prozac for depression, but Mr. Becker later develops side effects, and chooses to be non-compliant. Dr. Chen suspects alcohol issues, but does not know how to broach that topic. Dr. Chen soon feels overwhelmed by the situation and recommends referral to a psychiatrist located 100 miles away. Mr. Becker agrees, and stops seeing Dr. Chen. However, due to his fear of being labeled a "psych patient," Mr. Becker does not see the psychiatrist.

OVERVIEW OF THE ETHICS ISSUES

Coined by the Greeks, the word 'stigma' originally referred to a mark or sign on the physical body of a person that identified the bearer as being morally flawed and thus inferior to his fellowmen—someone to be avoided, especially in public places. In an important 1963 article, sociologist Erving Goffman defined stigma as "an attribute that is deeply discrediting," where a person is diminished "from a whole and usual person to a tainted, discounted one."[1] Stigma is essentially the devaluing of an individual's social identity.

Stigmatization is best understood as a 'situational threat' where one's stigma could influence how one is treated or judged. Link and Phelan state that stigma exists "when elements of labeling, stereotyping, separation, status loss, and discrimination co-occur in a power situation that allows the components of stigma to unfold."[2] Thus, for stigma to occur, the stigmatized individual must have a labeled attribute that is different and distinguishable from the stigmatizer. Next, dominant cultural beliefs link such labeled persons to negative stereotypes. Thirdly, labeled persons are placed in distinct categories to accomplish separation of "us" from "them." Finally, labeled persons experience status loss and discrimination that lead to unequal outcomes. And, all of this is dependent on social, economic, and political power. It takes power to stigmatize, and being empowered (i.e., having control over the outcomes of self/others) reduces one's vulnerability to being stigmatized.[3] Stigma research[4] provides insight into an individual's experience of stigmatization. These experiences are portrayed in Box 10.1.

BOX 10.1

THE "STIGMA EXPERIENCE"

- Prejudice and discrimination, wherein the stigmatized person encounters barriers to employment, housing, accessibility to health care, and acceptance in social groups and/or communities
- Awareness of the devalued quality of one's social identity, such as when teenage African-Americans are aware of the prejudice against their group[5]
- Threat from a stereotype, such as the negative attitudes experienced by any person wearing a turban, who may have been assumed to be a Muslim terrorist, following the 9/11/01 attacks

Stigma associated with illness, disability, and physical and mental limitations in particular, can create tremendous difficulties for rural residents as well as for the clinicians who provide their care. Certain illnesses are more stigmatizing in some communities. For instance, in some Alaskan villages, alcohol use and dependence are commonplace, and do not appear to have socially adverse consequences, whereas in other villages, stigma and alcohol are tightly linked. Link and colleagues[6] have studied how stigma may be more closely associated with other perceptions, such as how "biologically based" an illness is, as opposed to being more of a "psychological problem" or a "lack of will power." Other factors identified in the same study that increase the stigma of an illness are shown in the Box 10.2.

BOX 10.2

PERCEPTION ISSUES THAT INCREASE THE STIGMA OF AN ILLNESS

- Responsibility or blame for the illness' cause, for example, acquiring HIV by IV drug use or multiple unprotected sexual contacts, versus by blood transfusion for needed surgery
- Negative, stigmatizing labels associated with certain conditions, for example, the labels "lazy" or "stupid" associated with ADHD/ADD/Mental Retardation/Autism
- Potential for danger, most highly associated with mental illness and substance use
- Perception of "contagiousness," and, hence, a desire for distance; for example, AIDS/HIV, substance abuse, mental illnesses, other STDs are more stigmatizing than diabetes or heart disease[7]

There are certain core ethical principles and concepts that should guide every patient-provider encounter; definitions are shown in Box 10.3.

These principles are also discussed in detail in Chapter 3 of this *Handbook*.

The ethical principles are severely tested while dealing with stigmatizing illnesses, be it in an urban or rural setting. However, treating stigmatizing illnesses in rural areas becomes even more complicated, due to specific characteristics of the rural health care system. Some of these rural patient-provider characteristics, as enumerated in the Hastings Center report,[8] and the resultant ethics conflicts are listed in Box 10.4.

BOX 10.3

GUIDING PRINCIPLES FOR HEALTH CARE PROVIDERS

Autonomy
The right to self-rule or self-determination, closely linked to concepts of privacy and voluntarism

Respect for Persons
All persons are worthy of respect due to inherent personal worth and dignity, irrespective of race, ethnicity, socio-cultural background, sexuality, etc.

Beneficence
The obligation to "do good," "do right by patients," and to "use one's expertise to treat the ill"

Justice
Equitable distribution of power and resources

Ethical Use of Power
The use of power by a provider in an ethically directed manner, as determined by intent (i.e., to do good and to minimize harm) and by the outcome of the provider's actions

Confidentiality
A promise to not disclose personal information, linked to the concept of respect for a person's privacy

Do Your Duty
The adherence to profession and organization established standards of ethical behavior including professional codes of ethics

Nonmalefience
Seek to avoid risks and ensure that potential benefits of care outweigh burdens and harms

Veracity
Telling the truth in a clear and open manner

Overlapping Relationships and Conflicting Roles

In rural health care settings, stigma takes on special importance because of the interdependent and overlapping relationships that exist in small, closed communities.[8-10] In rural and frontier communities, health care providers routinely interact with patients in non-medical roles. Among

BOX 10.4

ETHICS CONFLICTS INHERENT IN THE RURAL
PATIENT-PROVIDER RELATIONSHIP

- Overlapping relationships and conflicting roles
- Challenges in preserving confidentiality
- Respect for cultural values in relation to professional standards
- Limited access to health care resources in rural communities
- Issues of clinical competence
- Exceptional stresses on caregivers in rural settings

physicians practicing in communities with fewer than 5,000 inhabitants, Paul Ullom-Minnich and Ken Kallail[11] found that two-thirds of physicians or their staff interacted on a non-medical basis with more than 5% of their patients. Nearly half of the physicians reported that more than 5% of their patients were friends or family. In such situations, ethics conflicts pertaining to principles of autonomy, ethical use of power, confidentiality, and right to treatment may arise. Consider an example in which the physician is the patient's uncle. The patient's (niece's) sense of autonomy may be undermined by the physician's role in her personal life. The physician-uncle wields significant power that should be used to be of beneficence to the patient-niece. Constructive approaches to this dilemma include, but are not limited to, separating personal and professional roles to the extent possible; making it feasible for members of the clinical team to excuse themselves gracefully from especially sensitive cases; discussing the awkwardness of overlapping relationships with patients; seeking collaboration, supervision, and/or consultation when a provider's personal feelings predominate in a clinical case; and referring patients to neighboring communities when overlapping roles create conflicts of interest.

The conflicts related to overlapping relationships are also shown in the example of a physician who has diagnosed alcoholism in his friend/patient. The stigma of alcoholism may prevent the friend from seeking care, or being compliant with his physician/friend's treatment. A physician's anonymity is sometimes helpful in treating people with stigmatizing conditions. The physician in this type of situation has the option of referring his friend to a neighboring health care provider; referring the friend to local mental health professionals or clergy for counseling; or continuing to treat his friend, by separating personal and professional roles to the extent possible. Separating personal and professional roles can be accomplished by maintaining a professional demeanor while in the clinic, including addressing patients more formally, openly discussing the awkwardness of the dual relationship, and assuring patients that you and your staff follow confidentiality procedures as a matter of routine. Ensuring that both staff and patients understand confidentiality policies will help the provider to mitigate the effects of stigmatizing illnesses.

Challenges in Preserving Confidentiality

Respect for a patient's privacy is central to quality health care, and is especially important in the care of patients with stigmatizing illnesses. Maintaining confidentiality helps in establishing trust in the patient-provider relationship, but is very difficult in a small community where many people know each other, and many people talk or gossip about others' business. Also, for providers, being the town's "carriers of secrets" exacts a heavy toll. If confidentiality were breached by anyone on the health care team, this could result in a lack of patient trust in the provider and the team, and might form a barrier to needed, ongoing care. For example, a patient diagnosed with HIV might forego necessary labs and medication to avoid being "found out," as in the case of Nancy Smith.

Heightened Cultural Dimensions of Health Care

Cultural values and beliefs can influence patients' illness perception, care seeking, and acceptance of caregivers. For example, an urban-trained physician in a rural setting has to understand cultural differences, because lack of awareness may lead to patient mistrust. Some conditions may be especially stigmatizing in a particular ethno-cultural group while not viewed that way in other groups, and such acceptance or lack thereof may be entirely different from the physician's own cultural beliefs and understanding of that particular illness' stigma. For the rural provider, enhancing his or her knowledge of a community's culture, history, and current concerns, and becoming attuned to individual patient's cultural experiences, will be helpful in mitigating any potential cultural ethics conflicts.

Limited Access to Health Care Resources in Rural Communities

The case of Greg Becker, the troubled Vietnam Vet who is trying to hide his problems because he is running for town office, highlights the problem of limited resources and access to needed health care, which has become a major source of health care disparity in rural communities.[12, 13] In *Health Status and Access to Care*, Braden and Beauregard[14] reported that one out of every seventeen rural counties in the United States had no physician providing patient care. Although health care needs of rural patients do not differ significantly from their urban counterparts, rural patients have to contend with limited resources and, sometimes, inadequate care. Rural health care providers are called upon to work long hours and are sometimes at risk of exhaustion and burnout. They are asked to make difficult ethics decisions regarding the allocation of scarce resources, and to provide services clearly beyond their levels of expertise, which bring forth ethics dilemmas pertaining to competence of care. A system-level solution needs to be implemented to resolve these myriad issues. Health care providers need to become advocates for rural health care funding. Local and nationwide involvement of consumer groups; professional organizations, such as the National Rural Health Association; and community leaders may help with bringing funds to address rural health care needs. Finally, when faced with difficult ethics questions, consultation with colleagues or community leaders may provide helpful support.

Issues of Clinical Competence
The case of Greg Becker (Case 2) also illustrates the ethics issue of clinical competence, and of clinicians being called upon to provide services beyond their training and expertise. This ethics problem appears to arise directly from issues of scarce resources. Rural providers (physicians, nurses, nursing assistants, social workers, and "deputized" local citizens) are called upon to make health care decisions clearly beyond their scope of training or practice. This often happens as rural patients are faced with a lack of family support, lack of transportation, or financial limitations that do not allow them to pursue needed care in far-off urban centers. As mentioned previously, a system-based solution needs to be implemented to increase funds to rural clinics.

Exceptional Stresses on Caregivers in Rural Settings
Based upon the special characteristics of rural practice, it is clear that rural clinicians face unique clinical and ethical challenges. The stressors specific to rural caregivers are listed in Box 10.5.

These factors place exceptional stress on rural caregivers. How does the rural clinician balance the patient's need for confidential care with the need for public health concerns in the community? How does the clinician, who is also a family member, friend, and/or neighbor, navigate the challenges of caring for the patient? How does the clinician protect the patient's dignity and privacy when "everyone knows everyone and everything?" How does the clinician deal with the absence of adequate health care resources, or (perhaps an even more difficult task) allocate a

BOX 10.5

STRESSORS SPECIFIC TO RURAL CAREGIVERS

- Personal and professional isolation, especially in their role as the town's "carrier of secrets"
- Cynicism associated with exhaustion and burnout
- Increased patient risk when rural clinicians are called to work extreme overtime to the point of fatigue, to make decisions beyond their level of expertise, and/or to cope with limited resources

fraction of already scarce resources to an individual who may be disliked or devalued by others in the community (who may include some of the clinician's patients, family, friends, and neighbors)?

CASE DISCUSSION

The following cases were explored using the analysis method presented in Chapter 4 of this *Handbook*.

CASE 10.1 | Confidentiality, overlapping relationships, and unwillingness to seek care

Stigma and the related fear of potential discrimination interfere with individuals' willingness to seek needed care.[15, 16] Nancy Smith's case exemplifies the general problem of disease stigma in small rural communities. Her reluctance to seek treatment stems from fear of the stigma and discrimination of having a sexually transmitted disease. This fear has clearly undermined her autonomy, making her choose to forgo treatment even though she knows it is needed. If Ms. Smith were living in an urban setting, she might be able to go to a different clinic where she could maintain anonymity. However, in rural settings, overlapping relationships and limited resources in the community create health care disparities rarely seen in urban settings.[12, 13] Ms. Smith is also lacking in trust that her diagnosis will be kept confidential by the nurse or the technician, especially since both know her family well.

There are several ethics issues that Ms. Smith's primary care provider, Dr. Russell, will need to address to foster quality health care for her, including Ms. Smith's diminished autonomy due to the disease stigma, the patient's expectation of a respectful encounter without prejudice or chastising, and the patient's concerns about maintaining confidentiality.

CASE 10.2 | Limited access to health care
resources in rural communities

In the case involving Mr. Becker, the ethical principles of justice and ethical use of power are sorely tested. Justice in this case relates to the lack of mental health resources in Mr. Becker's community. The ethical use of power and professional responsibility relate to Dr. Chen's maintaining the confidentiality of sensitive information within the context of the provider-patient relationship. Mr. Becker is reluctant to discuss his mental health issues and substance abuse, because he fears the information could sabotage his campaign. Dr. Chen also faces ethics challenges, because he is under pressure to provide mental health care services to Mr. Becker that are beyond his training and expertise.

In both vignettes, the principles of confidentiality, professional responsibility, and respect for people are also put into question. Physicians are people as well, whose inherent values, morals, and judgment systems may clash with those of certain patients depending on what the problems and diagnosis may be. For instance, Dr. Chen may have an inherent sense of disgust toward alcoholics and drug abusers, possibly from his own experiences with an alcoholic father. This may undermine Dr. Chen's ability to respect and be compassionate toward Mr. Becker. In addition, clinicians dealing with patient problems are also faced with the dilemma of beneficence toward an individual versus toward society. For instance, should a doctor disclose a school bus driver's struggle with alcoholism to the school authorities?

RESPONDING TO STIGMATIZING ILLNESS ETHICS CONFLICTS
In general, the clinician's decision-making in resolving ethics conflicts should be guided by clinical-illness factors, ethical principles, legal mandates governing the situation, collateral and corroborative information, and conscientiousness to pursue the least restrictive/intrusive intervention, and thorough documentation of the decision-making process. The provider should approach ethics conflict situations on a case-by-case basis. Ethical principles are not mandates, but can provide fundamental guidelines to help approach and solve ethics dilemmas. Box 10.6 lists basic ethics skills that are useful to clinicians. Rural health care providers should be trained in these ethics skills, or be able to access research material, such as this *Handbook*, that will help them identify ethics issues and inform their practice.[17-19]

BOX 10.6

FUNDAMENTAL ETHICS SKILLS[20]

- The ability to identify the ethical features of a patient's care
- The ability of a provider to see how his or her own life experiences, attitudes, personal values, and knowledge may influence his or her patient care.

    For example: In the treatment of stigmatizing illnesses, recognizing one's attitudes to such illnesses is paramount. Research has shown that there is sometimes a marked discrepancy between expressed attitudes and behavior towards stigmatized persons. Awareness of a person's stigmatized status may activate unconscious negative stereotypes, which will in turn influence subsequent behavior with the stigmatized person.

- The ability to identify one's areas of clinical expertise (i.e., scope of clinical competence) and to work within those boundaries
- The ability to anticipate situations that are ethically risky or problematic
- The ability to gather additional information, and to seek consultation and additional expertise in order to clarify and, ideally, resolve the conflict
- The ability to build additional ethical safeguards into the patient-care situation

CASE 10.1 | Confidentiality, overlapping relationships, and unwillingness to seek care

In this case, there are a number of ways in which the rural physician, Dr. Russell, and his staff can respectfully support Ms. Smith and her autonomy, and also ensure confidentiality of her records. The physician and his staff may conduct public discussion forums to educate the public about common diseases, including stigmatizing illnesses. One hopes that knowledge and awareness might at least partly mitigate stigma. Dr. Russell and his staff should also practice respectful encounters as a "routine" with all their patients. They should be aware of diseases that are stigmatizing; be mindful of their personal values and feelings towards patients; take steps to prevent these values/feelings from affecting patient interactions; and be mindful of the potential for stigma to affect or cause certain illness behaviors, including reluctance to seek care.

The staff should practice confidentiality in all patient scenarios. They should constantly evaluate confidentiality leaks, and take steps to prevent them. There could be collaborative teamwork among the clinic staff to evaluate and provide constructive criticism and feedback regarding each other's patient interactions, confidentiality practices, and the effect of personal moral/value judgment systems on patient interactions. The clinic may spread its message of confidentiality and respect for all people through its actions, thus supporting patients with stigmatizing illnesses, like Ms. Smith, to seek services at the clinic. The clinic should be open to feedback; should have a formal system of receiving feedback from patients, such as comment cards placed in a box in the office; and should implement changes in response to this feedback. Additionally, the patient should be made an equal collaborator in her care, thus enhancing her autonomy.

If Ms. Smith refuses treatment of her HIV, should the physician respect her right for autonomy or, in view of beneficence to society, report this illness to health agencies? Such a situation needs to be handled with compassion and respect, with the provider educating the patient about the illness, its treatment, and its prognosis with and without treatment. The provider will thus ensure that the patient is making informed decisions as an engaged collaborator in treatment. If Ms. Smith is adamant about not pursuing ongoing HIV treatment and support from Dr. Russell and others at the clinic, he should strongly encourage her to seek and obtain the needed treatment and care in a location where she would be more comfortable. Additionally, Dr. Russell should reassure Ms. Smith that if she changes her mind about where to receive care, she would be welcome to return to see him and others on the staff.

In situations where the physician is mandated to report an illness to an agency, the physician should first discuss the issue with the patient. The information provided in such a discussion is highlighted in Box 10.7.

Furthermore, when patients are fully informed about their right to confidentiality, and the practices that have been implemented to ensure confidentiality, they are more likely to cooperate fully and, perhaps, will be more likely to seek treatment even in those cases when reporting might be mandated. Maintaining confidentiality in these cases might be enhanced by using the measures listed in Box 10.8.

These steps will help patients to receive appropriate treatment, without giving up their right to confidential care. Such steps also can help to reduce the overall stigma associated with certain illnesses.

BOX 10.7

Informing Patients About Mandatory Reporting — Information the Clinician Should Communicate with the Patient Prior to Making Any Report

- The name of the agency requesting the report
- Who will complete the report
- In what form the reporting will be completed (fax, e-mail, regular mail, etc.)
- What information about the patient will be disclosed (name, age, gender, work details, address, etc.)
- Who will have access to this information
- The purpose for reporting each item of information mentioned above
- What measures are taken to ensure confidentiality, and to make sure that the information reaches only those for whom it is intended

BOX 10.8

Measures to Enhance Confidentiality

- Be mindful of confidentiality's importance to patients
- Discuss with the patient the strategies for maintaining confidentiality
- Direct patients to a mail-order pharmacy where medications can be obtained
- Educate colleagues and staff about confidentiality in effective patient care, making it routine practice with every patient and following up on any "leaks"
- Keep records out of public view and/or keep sensitive records separate from other health care documents
- Have collaborative clinics where all kinds of care, such as treatment of medical, psychiatric, HIV, and substance abuse conditions, are given under one roof, thus making stigmatizing conditions less obvious
- Conduct community forums to educate the public about stigmatizing illnesses and dispelling related myths
- Maintain a collaborative network with neighboring health care clinics and providers where patients can be referred to support anonymity

CASE 10.2 | Limited access to health care
resources in rural communities

Due to a lack of mental health providers in his community, Mr. Becker
turns to Dr. Chen. But Dr. Chen is not trained to deal with Mr. Becker's
psychiatric problems, beyond simple attempts to diagnose or try
antidepressants. Dr. Chen may also be responding to his unconscious
feelings towards alcoholics, and thus not following through with Mr. Becker.
Ideally in such scenarios, clinicians need to be aware of their unconscious
negative feelings toward patients with stigmatizing illnesses and take steps
to understand how these feelings impact patient interactions. There could
be a discrepancy between how clinicians and their patients view illnesses.
For instance, some conditions may not be considered stigmatizing by
a clinician but may be potentially stigmatizing to patients. If unaware of
such discrepancies, patients may perceive a lack of sensitivity. Health care
providers should routinely evaluate their patients' illness experiences and
associated feelings.

Dr. Chen may, with sensitively and compassion, broach the topic of Mr.
Becker's potential war-related PTSD symptoms, including the excessive
use of alcohol. He may educate Mr. Becker that alcohol dependence is
a medical condition that requires specialized treatment with therapy and
medications, and acknowledge that he (Dr. Chen) lacks such training. Since
their community has no mental health providers, Dr. Chen and his team
may establish a collaborative and complementary network of services with
neighboring health care clinics and providers, as some services may be
better provided in Dr. Chen's clinic while others may be best provided in
other neighboring clinics. Dr. Chen should be aware of the services and
location of Veterans Hospitals, and the many Community Based Outpatient
Clinics to which Mr. Becker can be referred. In such an endeavor, a system
of transportation may be established which can be used by patients to
travel between clinics. This requires funding for which the support of local
politicians may be enlisted, as well as the cooperation among local health
care agencies. The rural health care provider thus has to wear the mantle
of activist for the welfare of his patients—a skill that is, unfortunately, not
taught in medical school.

ANTICIPATING STIGMATIZING ILLNESS ETHICS CONFLICTS
Following the old adage, "prevention is better than cure," rural clinicians
may take steps early on to recognize ethics conflicts that stem from
stigmatizing illness, and prevent them from occurring. Rural clinicians

have the advantage of being aware of their community's pulse; however, an individual patient's perception of his or her illness may still vary from the norm. Hence, clinicians should approach each situation on a case-by-case basis, and be aware of the patient's feelings, perceptions and understanding of his or her own illness as well as community-wide myths and beliefs. Such awareness could positively change the interaction between patient and clinician in both of the cases presented. Asking patients like Nancy Smith and Greg Becker about their feelings and ideas would educate their clinicians about what they can expect in a given situation. All patient interactions must be conducted in a sensitive, compassionate, and respectful manner, and these interactions, including clinical practice, must be ethics-directed. Having all interactions be ethics-directed will mitigate ethical mistakes, including those in cases where patients have stigmatizing illnesses. Because confidentiality is of paramount importance with regard to potentially stigmatizing illnesses, clinicians need to ensure that confidentiality is maintained. By preserving confidentiality as a routine practice, providers can encourage other people with stigmatizing illnesses to seek necessary care.

In addition, community-wide education programs can be useful in decreasing the negative impact of stigmatizing diseases. For example, community forums can be facilitated in collaboration with neighboring clinics and/or small rural hospitals, to improve the community's understanding and diminish misperceptions regarding diseases that all too often carry stigma. The development and implementation of community-wide programs can be further enhanced if such programs are planned in collaboration with respected community officials or leaders, such as police officers or clergy.

CONCLUSION
Disease stigma combines with the special characteristics of the rural provider-patient relationship to cause further dilemmas in the ethical practice of health care. Rural clinicians are faced with such challenges on a continual basis. Rural health care practice, despite its limitations, must be guided by ethical principles to the greatest extent possible. Education and training in ethics skills, and training in handling sensitive or stigma-related conditions, are essential for rural providers to undergo so as to enhance their ethical practices. Education of the general public, through community "forums" about various stigmatizing illnesses, may help to dispel associated myths. Such education may mitigate stigma, mobilize financial resources, invite public participation, and help in providing care for

the stigmatized group. Policy-makers at the local, state, and federal levels must be made aware of this problem in rural communities, so that more funding and research is made available to help individuals with stigmatized illnesses. Providers should work as advocates for their patients, and be active participants in local policy-making and resource allocation. Such involvement can be enhanced through establishing collaborative networks of health care with neighboring providers. Collaborative relationships can be effective for fostering patient referrals and working with the county, state, or national agencies to advocate for financial resources to enhance rural health care delivery systems. Finally, compassion and respect for individuals must be essential features of all provider-patient interactions.

REFERENCES

1. Goffman E. *Stigma: Notes on the Management of Spoiled Identity.* Englewod Cliffs, NJ: Prentice-Hall; 1963.

2. Link BG, Phelan JC. Conceptualizing stigma. *Annu Rev Sociol.* 2001;27:363-385. Accessed Dec. 13, 2008.

3. Fiske ST. Controlling other people. The impact of power on stereotyping. *Am Psychol.* Jun 1993;48(6):621-628.

4. Crocker J, Major B, Steele C. Social stigma. In: Gilbert DT, Fiske ST, Lindzey G, eds. *The Handbook of Social Psychology.* Vol 2. Boston: McGraw-Hill; 1998:504-553.

5. Rosenberg M. *Conceiving the Self.* New York, NY: Basic Books; 1979.

6. Link BG, Phelan JC, Bresnahan M, Stueve A, Pescosolido BA. Public conceptions of mental illness: labels, causes, dangerousness, and social distance. *Am J Public Health.* Sep 1999;89(9):1328-1333.

7. Phelan JC, Bromet EJ, Link BG. Psychiatric illness and family stigma. *Schizophr Bull.* 1998;24(1):115-126.

8. Roberts LW, Battaglia J, Smithpeter M, Epstein RS. An office on Main Street. Health care dilemmas in small communities. *Hastings Cent Rep.* Jul-Aug 1999;29(4):28-37.

9. Simon RI, Williams IC. Maintaining treatment boundaries in small communities and rural areas. *Psychiatr Serv.* Nov 1999;50(11):1440-1446.

10. Stockman AF. Dual relationships in rural mental health practice: An ethical dilemma. *J Rural Comm Psych.* 1990;11(2):31-45.

11. Ullom-Minnich PD, Kallail KJ. Physicians' strategies for safeguarding confidentiality: the influence of community and practice characteristics. *J Fam Pract.* Nov 1993;37(5):445-448.

12. Merwin E, Snyder A, Katz E. Differential access to quality rural healthcare: professional and policy challenges. *Fam Community Health.* Jul-Sep 2006;29(3):186-194.

13. Johnson ME, Brems C, Warner TD, Roberts LW. Rural-urban health care provider disparities in Alaska and New Mexico. *Adm Policy Ment Health.* Jul 2006;33(4):504-507.

14. Braden J, Beauregard K. Health status and access to care of rural and urban populations. National Medical Expenditure Survey Research Findings 18.Rockville, MD: AHCPR; 1994.

15. Roberts LW, Battaglia J, Epstein RS. Frontier ethics: mental health care needs and ethical dilemmas in rural communities. *Psychiatr Serv.* Apr 1999;50(4):497-503.

16. Purtilo R, Sorrell J. The ethical dilemmas of a rural physician. *Hastings Cent Rep.* Aug 1986;16(4):24-28.

17. Niemira DA. Grassroots grappling: ethics committees at rural hospitals. *Ann Intern Med.* Dec 15 1988;109(12):981-983.

18. Perkins DV, Hudson BL, Gray DM, Stewart M. Decisions and justifications by community mental health providers about hypothetical ethical dilemmas. *Psychiatr Serv.* Oct 1998;49(10):1317-1322.

19. Roberts LW, Johnson ME, Brems C, Warner TD. Preferences of Alaska and New Mexico psychiatrists regarding professionalism and ethics training. *Acad Psychiatry.* May-Jun 2006;30(3):200-204.

20. Roberts LW, Dyer AR. *Concise Guide to Ethics in Mental Health Care.* Washington, DC: American Psychiatric Publishing; 2004.

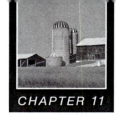

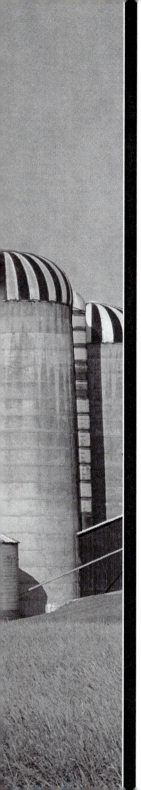

Ethics Conflicts in Rural Communities:
End-of-Life Decision-Making

Denise Niemira, Tom Townsend

Ethics Conflicts in Rural Communities: End-of-Life Decision-Making

Denise Niemira, Tom Townsend

ABSTRACT

Caring for people at the end of their lives can be one of the most challenging and personally rewarding aspects of primary care. The proximity to death intensifies and transforms the medical encounter calling upon both the emotional and the clinical competence of the medical provider. As people live longer with chronic illnesses, and as life-prolonging interventions become routine, death frequently involves a decision to forgo or limit care. Such decisions can generate moral conflict, even when the ethical and legal principles governing decisions are well defined and widely accepted. Family members, may feel that withdrawing life support is morally different than withholding such therapy in the first place. Surrogates named in advance directives may want to keep their loved ones alive rather than follow directives, even when the patient's wishes are clearly articulated. The clinician's responsibility is to support the autonomy of the dying person, while recognizing the emotional needs of the family. This has become more challenging in cases where there is no ethical consensus about either the decision to be made, and/or the legal requirements for its enactment, such as the withdrawal of artificial nutrition or terminal weaning from a ventilator. Ethical challenges in end-of-life care are heightened for rural providers who often have multifaceted relationships with patients and their families. Rural providers are sometimes the sole recipients of oral directives, and may have less experience than urban providers with complex end-of-life care. Rural clinicians should enact procedures to help their patients and patient's families prepare for the end-of-life process to reduce both ethics conflicts and undue stress for all parties involved.

CASE STUDIES

CASE 11.1 | Surrogate wishes run counter
to advance directives

Dr. Mark Townes, a family practitioner, returns from a vacation to find
Frank Foote, a 72-year-old patient with multiple illnesses, including
heart failure and end-stage COPD, on a ventilator in intensive care.
Brenda Foote, Frank's wife of 48 years, greets Dr. Townes, saying, "I'm
so glad you're back. His breathing got so bad I had to call 911. Your
partner put in a breathing tube, and now he's been on the ventilator
for six days. The antibiotics for the pneumonia aren't working so well.
Your partner told me he should go to the University Hospital, because
his breathing isn't getting better and he may need a tracheotomy.
I'm so scared I might lose him. They say he's not responsive, but
he seems to calm down when I speak to him and act up when they
poke him to draw blood." A reading of the medical record confirms
Mrs. Foote's story. Dr. Townes' partner, following Mrs. Foote's lead,
has pursued aggressive care and Mr. Foote is in full code. The chart
indicates that Mr. Foote had no advance directive, although Dr. Townes
and Mr. Foote had discussed it at his last visit, and Mr. Foote assured
Dr. Townes that an advance directive had been completed, but had
not yet been witnessed. Two unsuccessful attempts have been made
to wean Mr. Foote off of the ventilator. Based on previous discussions
with the patient, Dr. Townes knows that continued care including
intubation is not what Mr. Foote would want. However, Mrs. Foote
is also Dr. Townes' patient, and he knows that she has a hard time
confronting death — both her own and her husband's. Dr. Townes
also knows that withdrawing Mr. Foote's ventilator will not be a typical
procedure at his small hospital, and that there exists no policy for
terminal weaning. The doctor is uncertain as to how to proceed.

CASE 11.2 | Colleagues disagree with end-of-life decisions

Dr. Rachel Dennis, a general internist, has recently discharged Mr.
Coulter to a nursing home for permanent placement, following a
hospitalization for complications related to a fall. Mr. Coulter, 80
years old, has end-stage Alzheimer's disease, with a swallowing
disorder that has been worsened by his recent illness. Prior to

discharge, Dr. Dennis had conducted a lengthy discussion with the Coulter family about Mr. Coulter's condition, specifically regarding his swallowing problems. At that point, the doctor had discussed the option of a feeding tube with Mr. Coulter's wife of 50 years, but Mrs. Coulter, the Durable Power of Attorney for Health Care, had rejected this option. Dr. Dennis believed that she had been clear in her description of the benefits and risks of the feeding tube, and she had felt that the family was clearly committed to a palliative care course, without supplemental nutrition, by the time that she had discharged Mr. Coulter to the local nursing home. The nursing home is generally known for its commitment to end-of-life care, and his staff understood the proposed plan of care. The administrator did tell Dr. Dennis that a new medical director had just been employed, and that he would need to review the proposed plan of care.

Several days after the hospital admission, Dr. Dennis receives a frantic call from Mrs. Coulter, who has just authorized the transfer of her husband to the hospital emergency room for evaluation. This has followed a discussion with the nursing home medical director, who thinks Mr. Coulter is dehydrated and probably has elevated sodium. Mrs. Coulter is upset following this conversation, and by remarks she has overheard from other staff members about her husband starving to death. She wants to reconsider her decision to withhold a feeding tube. Her family is confused by this abrupt change in plans, especially since it seems that their father might not be allowed to return to the nursing facility without a feeding tube.

OVERVIEW OF ETHICS ISSUES

Providing care for those at the end of life can be one of the most challenging yet rewarding tasks in medicine. It requires health care providers to competently address and manage the broad array of clinical, emotional, social, and spiritual issues that frequently arise in the dying process. It also requires providers to address many potential ethics issues in the end-of-life decision-making process. Despite the intensity of such challenges, providing competent, quality care at the end of life can be professionally fulfilling and reflects the health care professional's respect for their patient's life and values.[1]

Modern medicine is highly specialized, and technological interventions are commonplace, allowing people with chronic illnesses to live longer lives.

As illnesses progress and the burdens of life-maintaining interventions increase, patients often exercise their autonomy by refusing continued treatment or requesting that current therapy be withdrawn. Clinicians who are aware of illness trajectories should initiate these discussions as part of the informed-consent process, when new treatments are proposed, or when reviewing the patient's current status in end-stage disease.[2-6] In either case, clinicians should respect and maximize the patient's present autonomy, and anticipate and arrange for a future in which the patient may lack decision-making capacity. Such discussions form the heart of advance-care planning, and the preferences that patients express about future care constitute advance directives.[7, 8]

Advance Directives

Advance Directives are oral or written instructions regarding an individual's choices for what medical care is to be given during a future illness when the person articulating such choices is no longer able to express his or her desires.[7] The three general categories of advance directives are noted in Box 11.1.

BOX 11.1

ADVANCE DIRECTIVES

- Oral statements made to family, friends, or providers
- Written statements or documents
- Naming a proxy or surrogate to make health care decisions

Both the fields of health care ethics and the law generally recognize these various forms of advance directives as an extension of a competent person's autonomy, to be used in those situations when a person lacks competence or decision-making capacity. Advance directives seek to respect patients' values and preferences to direct their care when they no longer may be capable of making health care decisions. Written directives are preferable, since they are less easily challenged and, if executed properly, have legal standing. Written advance directives may take several forms, as noted in Box 11.2.

Patients may supplement these typical forms with more extensive expressions of values or desired treatment in specific clinical situations.[3] Almost all states have laws that specifically address the right of a competent adult to make known his or her wishes about medical

BOX 11.2

TYPES OF WRITTEN ADVANCE DIRECTIVES

Living Will
An expression of a person's desires regarding their own future treatment when death is imminent

Durable Power of Attorney for Health Care
Naming a specific person as a surrogate decision-maker

Terminal Care Document
A document which names a decision-maker and expresses choices about specific treatments, often including choices of mechanical ventilation, nutrition, and hydration

treatment through some form of legal document. While states vary in their laws, preferences expressed in living wills are most often upheld and referred to in court decisions regarding end-of-life care, even in states that do not recognize this specific document. Withholding certain therapies, such as hydration and artificial nutrition, however, may be subject to specific requirements in some legal jurisdictions. States may also define the necessary conditions, such as witnessing requirements, for a legally binding advance directive document. The state-specific law may define or limit the scope of the surrogate decision-maker, including who cannot be a surrogate, and which decisions a surrogate may not make without specific written instructions. In most states, the patient's health care providers are excluded from being appointed as surrogate decision-makers. Rural health care professionals are urged to be aware of their state's statute.[9]

Providers are expected to assist surrogates in making the most appropriate decisions based on their medical knowledge and understanding of the patient's desires and health care values.[6] As extensions of their patients' autonomy in decision-making, clinicians are expected to treat advance directives with the same respect as they would with other patient choices. If the provider disagrees with the patient's choices, he or she has an ethical obligation to inform the patient when the document is executed, and to either resolve the conflict, or arrange for transfer of care. The same is true if the surrogate decision-maker presents the document at a later stage.

Surrogate Decision-Makers

Chronically ill or dying patients often lose their decision-making capacity prior to death, when care is ongoing and decisions still need to be made. For those who have executed a Durable Power of Attorney for Health Care (DPOAHC) according to the statutes of their state, the agent named is their legal surrogate decision-maker. Other potential surrogate decision-makers are listed in Box 11.3.

BOX 11.3

SURROGATE DECISION-MAKERS

- Agent named in Durable Power of Attorney for Health Care (DPOAHC)
- Guardian
- Spouse (may include domestic partners, depending on legal status or custom)
- Adult children
- Parents
- Siblings
- Other relatives or friends

Unfortunately, the option to formally identify a surrogate decision-maker in a DPOAHC is not often exercised. Therefore, other mechanisms for establishing surrogate decision-makers have evolved.[3] In most states, statutes list the individuals who can consent in the absence of an appointed agent or guardian with health powers, and in what order of priority. In some states, legal statues define the need, the role and the process for establishing guardianship in certain end-of-life decision-making situations. In other states, the law is silent or defers to kinship. Barring a legal requirement, most health care providers rely on those people who are most intimately knowledgeable with their patient's wishes, usually spouses and family members. When state law does not define a kinship hierarchy, many institutions will have a policy defining such a hierarchy for surrogates that usually lists, in the following order: spouse, adult children, parent, sibling, other relative or friend. The role of non-spousal domestic partners is often ambiguous in states where such relationships have no legal standing, and providers should strongly encourage people in such relationships to execute a proxy document if they wish to have their partner, rather than their family, be their decision-maker.

However surrogates are chosen, their role in decision-making is to represent the values and wishes of the person for whom they are deciding.

The surrogate's decisions must be guided by standards that have a basis in law as well as in ethics.[2, 3, 9] Rural health care professionals should be aware of their state's related statutes.

There are generally two recognized standards for surrogate decision-making, as indicated in Box 11.4.

BOX 11.4

STANDARDS FOR SURROGATE DECISION-MAKING

Substituted Judgment
Based on the patient's clear and specific previous expressed values, desires, actions, or beliefs

Best Interest
Based on a comparative assessment of the burdens and benefits of the current treatment options in relationship to the patient's condition

The first standard for surrogate decision-making is an autonomy-based standard, which includes clear, specific, previously expressed oral and written directives that reflect the decision the patient would chose. The decision-maker's role is to make decisions based on the patient's expressed desires. These desires form the basis for what is known as "substituted judgment."

The second level of surrogate-decision-making standard is the best-interest standard. This standard attempts to maximize the net benefit of treatment by weighing the burdens versus the benefits of treatment options, given the patient's current condition. Surrogates are directed to make decisions on the basis of the first standard, unless there are no reliable expressed wishes or actions from which to make a substituted judgment.

Unless specifically stated in the DPOAHC or guardianship document that legally authorizes them, surrogates do not have the authority to make treatment decisions based on their own personal values or desires. Physicians caring for the dying have an ethical obligation to their patients to gently but firmly challenge the decisions of surrogates who ignore advance directives and instead base decisions on their own values or emotional reactions to impending loss. Providers should review treatment options with dying patients who retain decision-making capacity, or with surrogates.

Clinicians must honor their ethical commitments to truthfulness, fidelity and respect for all people. Many of these commitments have been reviewed in Chapter 8 of this *Handbook*.

End-of-Life Decision-Making

End-of-life care decisions are challenging, because emotions and ethics are attached to actions that can lead to the hastening or perceived hastening of death.[7, 10] There are fairly universal legal and ethical prohibitions for certain actions, such as active euthanasia, which is the direct killing of a person. However, other actions, such as physician-assisted suicide, are now legal in Oregon and Washington. In addition, there are other actions that are legally and ethically permissible, but are considered morally objectionable by certain individuals or groups, often centered in faith and/or geographic communities. These actions include withdrawal of nutrition and hydration,[11] withdrawal of ventilator support, and use of sedation for extreme pain and other symptom control (known as palliative sedation, previously called terminal sedation).[12]

What makes end-of-life decision-making even more challenging for the provider, especially during discussions with patients and surrogates, is that the end-of-life terminology that is often used, (such as allowing to die, euthanasia, assisted suicide, physician-assisted death, etc.) can have different meanings to different people. Providers need to be clear in their use of terminology, ensuring that the patient or surrogate is using the term in a manner similar to the provider.[13]

Health care providers must be sensitive to, and respectful of, the diversity of moral beliefs surrounding end-of-life care, and must clearly understand the moral justifications for actions that may be perceived as hastening death. For example, the "principle of double effect" is often invoked to justify the use of high doses of narcotics to effectively treat pain in terminal illness (although hospice advocates would argue that it is irrelevant here) and the use of sedation to treat intractable symptoms.[4] Most doctors and nurses who work in end-of-life care know that, although the narcotic is given to treat increasingly unbearable pain, drugs like morphine given in increasingly high amounts that produce unconsciousness can also hasten death.

The principle of double effect (see Box 11.5) allows one to perform such actions if the action has two effects—one that is good and desired and one that is bad and foreseen but not desired. Additional requirements are that the bad effect is not the means to the good effect and that the good effect outweighs the bad.[5]

BOX 11.5

Principle of Double Effect

- Planned action must have good as well as bad effect
- Only the good effect is desired
- The bad effect cannot be the means to the good effect
- The good effect must outweigh the bad effect

Health care providers must also be aware that while legally and ethically, there is no difference between withholding therapy in the first place and withdrawing therapy once it has been started, family members may feel differently. While a clinician's moral obligation is to his or her patient during end-of-life care, the patient-family unit is more often the object of care, even when other family members are not actually patients. Clinicians may have moral duties to the family unit as well as to the patient, especially when end-of-life-care choices run counter to prevailing community sentiments.

Do Not Resuscitate/Do Not Attempt Resuscitation Orders (DNR/DNAR)

Choosing to forgo resuscitation is the most common end-of-life care decision. This decision, based on patient or surrogate consent, is enacted when a clinician issues a Do Not Attempt Resuscitation (DNAR) order, which instructs medical personnel not to begin cardiopulmonary resuscitation (CPR) when a patient suffers a cardiac or respiratory arrest.[14] At one time CPR was seen as a medical obligation, rather than a therapy that could be withheld at a patient or surrogate's request. As statistics of survival to hospital discharge after CPR have accrued, it has become apparent that survival rates after CPR are dismal for most people with end-stage diseases, and that resuscitation offers little or no benefit to the terminally ill; in many cases it simply prolongs their suffering. This dilemma has sparked discussions among ethicists about futility and CPR;[15] specifically about whether there is a need for informed consent before initiating a DNAR order in certain terminally ill patients.[5, 6]

Currently, patient or surrogate consent is generally required before a DNAR is issued. The issue of how to handle a situation in which the patient or surrogate insists on CPR despite the fact that it would be medically futile is an area of intense debate.[13] At least two states have enacted statues that address this situation.[15]

While withholding resuscitation for the dying makes clinical sense to those in the medical profession, patients and family members may see these decisions as an attempt to limit other therapies or restrict care. DNAR discussions between provider and patient are, in fact, often the logical starting point for broader discussions about therapy limitation(s); since a DNAR order, by itself, only limits one specific therapy, cardiopulmonary resuscitation. It is important that patients, their surrogates and hospital staff all understand the limited nature of a DNAR order and appreciate that it is consistent with both aggressive disease-fighting care as well as comfort measures only. By emphasizing the limited nature of DNAR and sensitively exploring patient goals for care, clinicians can help their patients understand and navigate other potential treatment decisions that might arise. Providers can also uncover and address any inconsistencies in choices; for example, patients who request resuscitation, but simultaneously refuse treatment for the underlying condition that will likely result in cardiopulmonary arrest.[13, 15-18] Even after a decision is made, the clinician and patient can discuss the issue of resuscitation again when a related therapy decision needs to be made.[7]

DNAR discussions with patients and families should always involve honest and sympathetic dialogue, with the health care provider trying to determine as clearly as possible what are the patient's or surrogate's wishes. To further emphasize the value of such discussions, one study noted that in almost one in three cases, the patient's preferences not to use CPR were different than the physician's perception of what the patient wanted.[19] The study reinforces the importance of DNAR discussions and other end-of-life issues with patients or surrogates.

End-of-Life Care and the Rural Setting
The ethical principles underlying end-of-life care are the same, regardless of whether that care is given in rural or urban settings.[20] Certain characteristics of rural life and society, however, may pose unique ethics conflicts to rural-based clinicians doing end-of-life or palliative care. The close-knit relationships among people in small and rural communities, while a source of support in times of crisis, are often a threat to medical privacy and confidentiality. When patients and surrogates make end-of-life choices that stray from the moral values of the community majority, it is important to safeguard their privacy in ways that may not be necessary in larger, more anonymous settings. These same close-knit relationships often make it likely that the same physician will care for multiple family members. Balancing the desires of the dying with the needs of the living

and the available choices of care can be difficult. Compromises and accommodations are often necessary, but the clinician should never permit pain and suffering for the dying.[17, 18]

Rural practitioners also need to honestly evaluate the type of palliative care they can provide in their community. Ideally, a patient's death will occur in a local setting, surrounded by family and friends, and attended by the patient's trusted family physician. There are circumstances, however, where the burden of disease and suffering requires expertise in pain and symptom management, as well as supportive staff who are comfortable administering large doses of opiates and sedatives for refractory symptoms. Such circumstances require clinicians to have not only a commitment to symptom relief, but also an understanding that such activity is not intended to be euthanasia, but is a morally acceptable treatment for intractable symptoms.[21] Without both medical and ethical competence, rural providers must question whether they should provide end-of-life care for some highly complex patient situations.

CASE DISCUSSION
Each of the cases in this chapter involves ethics conflicts centered on advance directives. Each also attempts to illustrate the emotional turmoil that families experience when they are faced with the impending death of a loved one, and are asked to make decisions that will impact that outcome. Even when such situations have been discussed in advance and family values are congruent, grief and loss can cause families to question their previous choices. Clinicians who are sensitive to the needs of family members will realize that what the medical team sees as ethically and medically appropriate is not necessarily seen the same way by the family.

The interpretation for the following cases is based on the analysis method discussed in Chapter 4.

CASE 11.1 | Surrogate wishes run counter to advance directives

Dr. Townes is obligated to both Frank and Brenda Foote as their primary care provider. He has obligations to respect Mr. Foote's autonomy by carrying out his wishes for end-of-life care, and to help Mrs. Foote by minimizing the psychological and emotional trauma of her impending loss. Dr. Townes wonders to what extent the need to avoid or minimize harm to Mrs. Foote trumps Mr. Foote's autonomy?

Dr. Townes' discussions with Mr. Foote constitute an oral advance
directive, but there is no existing written document, other than chart notes,
which substantiates Mr. Foote's wishes. A problem may arise if Mrs. Foote
insists, in the future, that her discussions with Mr. Foote on end-of-life care
differ from Dr. Townes' recollection of the oral discussions. A copy of the
document Mr. Foote wrote, though not witnessed, might further clarify
his wishes and form the basis for a discussion with Mrs. Foote about
substituted judgment.

A further and independent dilemma exists for Dr. Townes, regarding the
appropriate location for terminal weaning, since this is an anticipated
outcome of the decision-making process. He should evaluate whether he,
or someone in the hospital or clinic, is competent in providing pain and
symptom relief as the ventilator is withdrawn. How does the nursing and
respiratory therapy staff feel about removing a ventilator from someone
who is not ready to be extubated, not permanently unconscious, and who
will need pain and anxiety medications during the process? If potential
participants say, "This is euthanasia, but I am willing to participate because
it is the right thing to do," is it the right thing to do?

Dr. Townes knows that his first duty is to his patient, Mr. Foote, and he
must discuss options with Mrs. Foote. But he is unsure how exactly to
proceed, given his relationship with Mrs. Foote and the capabilities of the
rural hospital.

CASE 11.2 | Colleagues disagree with end-of-life decisions

Dr. Dennis is faced with a dilemma: a colleague has a disagreement with
her about whether to withhold artificial nutrition and hydration (ANH) from
a patient with advancing Alzheimer's disease who is unable to maintain
adequate hydration through oral intake. The colleague's disagreement has
challenged the decision of the patient's family. The family members are now
confused and question the decision they previously made. The patient's
advance directive was executed years before, and does not contain
specific mention of ANH, further complicating the situation. Fortunately, the
state the Coulters live in does not require a specific directive regarding ANH
before nutrition and hydration can be withheld.

Dr. Dennis is unsure about the extent of her colleague's ethics
disagreement—or its implication for Mr. Coulter's future care, if he
should return to the facility. Does the facility require a feeding tube in all

circumstances similar to Mr. Coulter's? If not, under what conditions do they allow withholding or withdrawing? Does her colleague believe that nutrition and hydration must never be withheld, in any circumstance or by any means? If so, will that become an institutional policy?

While Dr. Dennis feels that she had come to a clear understanding with the family before transfer to the nursing home, she is now unsure whether they fully understood Mr. Coulter's condition, and what could happen if the feeding tube were withheld. Why are they changing their decision? Were they unprepared for such rapid deterioration? Are they ethically challenged by the consequences of their decision, reframed as starvation? How can Dr. Dennis rectify the situation to Mr. Coulter's greatest benefit?

RESPONDING TO RURAL END-OF-LIFE ETHICS CONFLICTS
End-of-life conflicts are fueled by the emotional intensity of the dying experience. Family members want to believe that they are doing the right thing, and that medical providers are treating their loved ones with professional competence, compassion, and respect.

CASE 11.1 | Surrogate wishes run counter to advance directives

First, Dr. Townes must examine the implications and implementation of various options, including where withdrawal of ventilator support in a terminal weaning situation should occur. If Mrs. Foote decides to support Mr. Foote's wishes, and if she allows ventilator withdrawal, it is important that it be done in a clinically and ethically competent way. If withdrawal cannot be done locally, Dr. Townes should consult the palliative care service at the referral center about arrangements to transfer Mr. Foote.

Family members sometimes need time before they can abandon their own wishes and accept the clinical reality and the previously expressed wishes of a loved one. If Dr. Townes begins slowly, addressing the seriousness of Mr. Foote's condition and the generally poor outcome of resuscitation, he may negotiate a DNAR order, opening further discussions of limiting therapy with the patient's wife. Given time and support, Mrs. Foote may accept Mr. Foote's impending death, and honor his wishes for how his death with dignity should occur. Mrs. Foote has a right to expect that Dr. Townes will be honest with her, and will not knowingly deceive or coerce her into conforming to Mr. Foote's wishes. If a transfer is arranged to the tertiary center, Mrs. Foote should be aware of the intent, whether that is aggressive or palliative therapy.

If Mr. Foote will be transferred regardless of the type of care he will receive, Dr. Townes should not leave the discussions of end-of-life care to the clinicians at the tertiary center. He has had long-standing relationships with Mr. and Mrs. Foote. He should advocate for Mr. Foote's choices, both in discussions with Mrs. Foote about the transfer, and in talks with the tertiary center about Mr. Foote's wishes. He should also prepare Mrs. Foote for the possible discussions and decisions she may face at the tertiary center, and inform her of the helpful services available there, such as social workers and ethics committees. Mr. Foote may not return as Dr. Townes' patient after the transfer to the tertiary center, but Mrs. Foote will still be his patient. Dr. Townes' future relationship with her will be shaped by the compassion, honesty, and integrity of their conversations now.

Dr. Townes has an overriding obligation to treat Mr. Foote's pain and dyspnea before he attempts to honor his commitments to both Mr. Foote and Mrs. Foote. When Dr. Townes is assured that Mr. Foote is comfortable, he can begin to negotiate goals of therapy and a plan of care with Mrs. Foote. Dr. Townes may find it helpful to address Mrs. Foote's difficulty by reframing her reluctance as love rather than denial. He also must read the written document from Mr. Foote, even if it's not witnessed. If this document echoes the wishes Mr. Foote expressed to him, it can help him to gently lead Mrs. Foote in the direction of substituted judgment. If it is vague, or allows for decisions at Mrs. Foote's discretion, Dr. Townes may need to modify his own thoughts of what should be done.

CASE 11.2 | Colleagues disagree with end-of-life decisions

For Dr. Dennis, whose patient and family have been caught in the crossfire of a disagreement between health care providers, it is important to understand the nature of that disagreement before renegotiating the plan of care. If the nursing home's new medical director has no problems with the ethics of withholding the therapy, but is concerned about legal issues or safeguards, returning Mr. Coulter to the nursing home without a feeding tube can resolve the situation. If there are ethics issues related to feeding tubes, Dr. Dennis should determine if these are universal, regarding allowing a patient to die; or specific to her patient, who is not yet in the very end stages of Alzheimer's. Depending upon her colleague's responses, Dr. Dennis can ascertain the circumstances under which Mr. Coulter may return to the facility without a feeding tube, or the circumstances under which the tube may be removed once he is a patient in that facility. Such discussion may warrant the assistance of a health care ethicist and/or legal counsel. Such a discussion will help shape her discussions with the Coulter family.

For the Coulter family, it is important to know that their initial decision was "right," loving, and consistent with Mr. Coulter's wishes as they interpreted them. Dr. Dennis should explain to the family the disagreement about morality regarding the withholding of intravenous or tube feeding. The remarks about starvation should be explained, though not excused, as the interpretation of those who are morally opposed to withholding artificial nutrition and hydration (ANH) under any circumstances.

Dr. Dennis should offer the Coulters an opportunity to review all options, including hospice referral. She may consider starting the discussion with a review of Mr. Coulter's life—his attitudes, the things he enjoyed, and his beliefs. What he said about his future at the time of his diagnosis and at the time he executed his advance directive may also help the family understand what he would want them to do now. Whatever decision the Coulters make should be supported. Decisions about withholding artificial nutrition and hydration are difficult, even when there is a clear written directive. Support for a decision to initiate tube feeding should not imply that the original decision was wrong or uncaring.

ANTICIPATING RURAL END-OF-LIFE CARE CONFLICTS

Death brings an end to relationships and, in turn, brings loss and grief to those left behind. The moral diversity inherent in these relationships can play out in end-of-life decision-making in ways that may or may not present true ethics conflicts. Families who participate as surrogates are sometimes unable or unwilling to participate as agents of substituted judgment. Rural hospital and nursing facilities may lack policies on important and sometimes controversial end-of-life decision-making, as well as aspects of palliative care. Rural clinicians might be unaware of regulations governing aspects of withdrawal of therapy, especially when these regulations change. These factors combine to create difficult conditions under which patients, health care providers, and families must make choices.

Advance directives are a useful tool, but are only as good as the communication and clarity that goes into their execution. Individuals who know that their spouses will not make the decisions they request, in the event of their becoming incapacitated in the future, should be strongly advised to name another surrogate. Patients should not rely on other family members or the family's PCP to push reluctant agents to agree to the patient's point of view.[22, 23]

Because of the importance of advance directives, some individuals should be encouraged to complete advanced directives more urgently than others. These categories are noted in Box 11.6.

BOX 11.6

PATIENTS WHO SHOULD BE STRONGLY ENCOURAGED TO HAVE ADVANCE DIRECTIVES

- Patients with a life-limiting illness
- Patients who are estranged from their families
- Patients who belong to faith communities with specific limitations of therapy
- Patients who are involved in committed same-sex relationships that are neither sanctioned nor protected by their state's laws
- Patients who are involved in dangerous occupations or recreational activities
- Patients whose values or desires regarding end-of-life care are not shared by family or community members
- Patients who have no family
- Patients of advanced age, even if they do not yet have a life-limiting illness

People who are estranged from their families, or the values of the community, or who are members of faith communities with limitations on health services (such as Jehovah's Witnesses), or who are involved in committed same-sex relationships, in states which don't recognize these, should be strongly encouraged to execute advance directives so that their values and surrogate choice will be respected in end-of-life care. Young people who engage in dangerous occupations (law enforcement, firefighting, the military) or enjoy dangerous recreational activities (extreme sports, rock climbing, professional mountaineers) should likewise be encouraged to initiate discussion and document their desires regarding treatment of a catastrophic injury that results in permanent impairment of decision-making capacity. In states where there are specific requirements regarding withholding of artificial nutrition and hydration, providers should encourage patients to complete specific documentation related to this decision. Providers should also prompt patients to make these documents available to clinicians, the named surrogate, and local health care institution. Patients should also update their documents regularly, particularly with changes in their health and marital status, as well as changes in the law related to end-of-life decision-making.

Rural institutions that provide care for patients at the end of life should develop adequate resources to address potential ethics conflicts that may arise in the provision of this care. Some important resources are listed in Box 11.7.

BOX 11.7

INSTITUTIONAL RESOURCES NEEDED TO ADDRESS END-OF-LIFE CARE ETHICS CONFLICTS

- Clear-cut policies and procedures related to DNAR, palliative care and symptom control, and limitation of therapy including artificial nutrition and hydration
- Relevant education for employees regarding end-of-life issues
- Readily available information about legal aspects of end-of-life care
- Mechanism for conflict resolution

Rural hospitals should have policies and procedures related to end-of-life care, especially in the areas of surrogate decision-making, DNR orders, limitation of treatment and palliative care, and withdrawal and withholding of certain therapies, especially artificial hydration and nutrition. Such policies should reflect current state law(s) and should be periodically reviewed and updated. These institutions should also have an easily accessible source for information related to the legal aspects of end-of-life care that is available to all practitioners. When legal counsel is not readily available through a hospital or medical society to discuss specific situations, health care professionals can review up-to-date and accurate Web sites. Rural institutions should also identify and meet the educational needs of their staff regarding end-of-life practices, particularly those that have some degree of moral ambiguity. Staff members must understand institutional policies. Institutions and staff must commit to privacy and confidentiality regarding end-of-life decisions for individual patients. A family's decision to withhold artificial nutrition and hydration is not a matter for discussion by hospital members outside of the treatment setting. The institution should also have a mechanism for arbitrating conflict about end-of-life care, especially if this involves disagreement between members of the treatment team. Such a mechanism might include an ethics committee, a mediation group, or a referral to an outside ethics resource.[24-26]

Because of the close ties between rural hospitals and the communities they serve, hospitals should consider extending their educational efforts around end-of-life care into the community. This can be done by developing educational materials, such as pamphlets and brochures about end-of-life care choices; by sponsoring community forums about advance care planning; and by promoting advance directive use through partnering with local faith communities. Such activities foster an understanding of end-of-life decision-making and treatment options that patients and families might need to consider. These activities encourage communication within families, and between patients and their health care providers, and may lessen the difficulty for surrogate decision-makers as they grapple with hard choices.[25, 27]

CONCLUSION

Caring for patients and guiding families through the dying process are a natural conclusion of the patient-clinician relationship for rural physicians. Once, unfettered by technology and the choices it engenders, this was a simpler, if not necessarily gentler, scenario. Pain and dyspnea were still there, and families still grieved and wrestled with unresolved guilt and conflict, but treatment options were fewer, and family values were more congruent. As life and technology have changed, the experience of death has undergone the same medicalization in rural and urban settings. People are living longer, and families are more fragmented than they were in the past. The additional burden of making decisions about modern medical advances including resuscitation, food and fluid administered through tubes rather than being swallowed, and breathing machines are add to the stress of end-of-life decision-making.

As patients and families have struggled with the new options available to them, questions and conflicts have arisen about the limits of intervention and choice. "Can life-sustaining care, once started, be stopped?" "If I say it is okay to turn off his respirator, am I killing him?" Patients and family members see these issues from one perspective, while practicing clinicians may view them from another. The challenge for rural clinicians in guiding their patients and families through the dying process is to anticipate conflict and reframe options and choices in ways that resonate. To be done well, end-of-life care calls for both clinical and ethical competence. With foresight and planning, rural physicians can meet the challenge.

REFERENCES

1. Field MJ, Cassel CK, eds. *Approaching Death: Improving Care at the End of Life.* Washington, DC: National Academy Press; 1997.

2. Lynn J. Why I don't have a living will. *Law Med Health Care.* Spring-Summer 1991;19(1-2):101-104.

3. Doukas DJ, McCullough LB. The values history. The evaluation of the patient's values and advance directives. *J Fam Pract.* Feb 1991;32(2):145-153.

4. Quill TE. Perspectives on care at the close of life. Initiating end-of-life discussions with seriously ill patients: addressing the "elephant in the room". *JAMA.* Nov 15 2000;284(19):2502-2507.

5. Lynn J. Perspectives on care at the close of life. Serving patients who may die soon and their families: the role of hospice and other services. *JAMA.* Feb 21 2001;285(7):925-932.

6. Singer PA, Martin DK, Kelner M. Quality end-of-life care: patients' perspectives. *JAMA.* Jan 13 1999;281(2):163-168.

7. Ethics manual. Fourth edition. American College of Physicians. *Ann Intern Med.* Apr 1 1998;128(7):576-594.

8. Patrick DL, Curtis JR, Engelberg RA, Nielsen E, McCown E. Measuring and improving the quality of dying and death. *Ann Intern Med.* Sep 2 2003;139(5 Pt 2):410-415.

9. Meisel A, Snyder L, Quill T, American College of Physicians--American Society of Internal Medicine End-of-Life Care Consensus P. Seven legal barriers to end-of-life care: myths, realities, and grains of truth. *JAMA.* Nov 15 2000;284(19):2495-2501.

10. Lo B. *Resolving Ethical Dilemmas: A Guide for Clinicians.* 2nd ed. Philadelphia, PA: Lippincott Williams & Wilkins; 2000.

11. Lo B. The persistent vegetative state. In: *Resolving Ethical Dilemmas: A Guide for Clinicians.* 2 ed. Philadelphia, PA: Lippincott Williams & Wilkins; 2000:162-165.

12. Lorenz KA, Lynn J, Dy SM, et al. Evidence for improving palliative care at the end of life: a systematic review. *Ann Intern Med.* Jan 15 2008;148(2):147-159.

13. Lo B. Confusing ethical distinctions. In: *Resolving Ethical Dilemmas: A Guide for Clinicians.* Philadelphia, PA: Lippincott Williams & Wilkins; 2000:119-128.

14. Lo B. Tube and intravenous feedings. In: *Resolving Ethical Dilemmas: A Guide for Clinicians.* Philadelphia, PA: Lippincott Williams & Wilkins; 2000:145-150.

15. Cantor MD, Braddock CH, 3rd, Derse AR, et al. Do-not-resuscitate orders and medical futility. *Arch Intern Med.* Dec 8-22 2003;163(22):2689-2694.

16. Gazelle G. The slow code--should anyone rush to its defense? *N Engl J Med.* Feb 12 1998;338(7):467-469.

17. Covinsky KE, Goldman L, Cook EF, et al. The impact of serious illness on patients' families. SUPPORT Investigators. Study to Understand Prognoses and Preferences for Outcomes and Risks of Treatment. *JAMA.* Dec 21 1994;272(23):1839-1844.

18. Halevy A, Brody BA. A multi-institution collaborative policy on medical futility. *JAMA.* Aug 21 1996;276(7):571-574.

19. Teno JM, Hakim RB, Knaus WA, et al. Preferences for cardiopulmonary resuscitation: physician-patient agreement and hospital resource use. The SUPPORT Investigators. *J Gen Intern Med.* Apr 1995;10(4):179-186.

20. Summaries for patients. Treatment of seriously ill patients who are near the end of life: recommendations from the American College of Physicians. *Ann Intern Med.* Jan 15 2008;148(2):I42.

21. Van Vorst RF, Crane LA, Barton PL, Kutner JS, Kallail KJ, Westfall JM. Barriers to quality care for dying patients in rural communities. *J Rural Health.* Summer 2006;22(3):248-253.

22. Planning ahead. National Hospice and Palliative Care Organization. http://www.caringinfo. org/PlanningAhead. Accessed May 10, 2008.

23. National Rural Health Association. *Providing Hospice and Palliative Care in Rural and Frontier Areas.* Kansas City: National Rural Health Association; 2005. Available from: http://www.capc.org/palliative-care-across-the-continuum/hospital-hospice/Rural-Toolkit-READER.pdf/view?searchterm=Providing%20hospice%20and%20palliative%20care%20 in%20rural%20and%20frontier%20areas. Accessed Dec. 13, 2008.

24. Jennings B, Kaebnick GE, Murray TH. *Improving end of life care: why has it been so difficult?.* . Garrison, NY: Hastings Center; 2005. http://www.thehastingscenter.org/pdf/ improving_eol_care_why_has_it_been_so_difficult.pdf. Accessed Dec. 13, 2008.

25. Tulsky JA. Beyond advance directives: importance of communication skills at the end of life. *JAMA.* Jul 20 2005;294(3):359-365.

26. Steinhauser KE, Christakis NA, Clipp EC, McNeilly M, McIntyre L, Tulsky JA. Factors considered important at the end of life by patients, family, physicians, and other care providers. *JAMA.* Nov 15 2000;284(19):2476-2482.

27. Perkins HS. Controlling death: the false promise of advance directives. *Ann Intern Med.* Jul 3 2007;147(1):51-57.

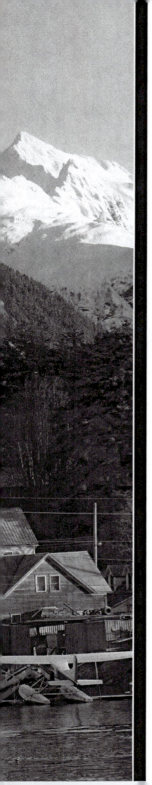

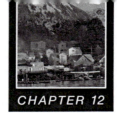

Ethics Conflicts in Rural Communities:
Recognizing and Disclosing Medical Errors

Ann Freeman Cook, Helena Hoas

Ethics Conflicts in Rural Communities: Recognizing and Disclosing Medical Errors

Ann Freeman Cook, Helena Hoas

ABSTRACT

This chapter explores the ethical responsibility of health care providers to administer safe clinical care. It further explores the challenges that such providers can experience in recognizing, reporting, and disclosing medical errors. Medical errors can cause serious harm (to the patient, provider and institution or clinic) and can prove to be expensive, stressful, time-consuming, and personally devastating. While rural health care providers frequently underscore their desire to provide safe care, they also report that it is very difficult to develop and implement strategies that reduce the risk of making errors. Studies show that there is limited agreement among health care providers when defining, reporting, disclosing, or resolving error. Providers who wish to actively pursue strategies that heighten safety may become inhibited by this lack of agreement. This chapter presents findings from empirical ethics studies involving rural participants from 14 states. These studies shed light on the ethics issues surrounding medical errors that occur in physicians' offices and hospitals. The two case examples that this chapter presents reflect both the experiences of rural health care providers, and the complexities that can accompany the search for ethically-attuned processes for error disclosure and resolution.

CASE STUDIES

CASE 12.1 | Addressing questionable quality of care

Dr. Bristol practices in a rural hospital where he and other physicians perform colonoscopies to detect or biopsy lesions that may indicate colorectal cancer—a common cancer in the United States, and one that has a high cure rate if found and treated at an early stage. In rural settings, family physicians sometimes conduct this procedure. Colonoscopy has provided an important source of revenue for Dr. Bristol, compared to the reimbursement rates for many other health care services, which are often inadequate in rural settings. Unfortunately, Dr. Bristol has been less thorough than other physicians when conducting the examination, and has frequently failed to reach the cecum to complete the procedure. The nurses who assist the physicians have been aware of the discrepancy and, believing that Dr. Bristol has not performed the test correctly, repeatedly have sought the intervention of the hospital administrator. The nurses have also spoken to other members of the medical staff and asked for an intervention. The administrator and the medical staff were hesitant to intervene. After two years of repeatedly lodging complaints with the hospital administration and struggling with their moral obligations to provide safe care, the nurses announced that they would no longer assist Dr. Bristol when he was performing the procedure. Faced with pressure from the nurses, the hospital administration agreed to study and respond to this clinical and ethical problem.

CASE 12.2 | The use of a wrong clinical management care plan

Dr. Simpson diagnosed his 83-year-old patient, Mr. Desrosiers, with atrial fibrillation (AF). During atrial fibrillation, the heart's two small upper chambers (the atria) quiver instead of beating effectively. Blood may not be pumped completely out of the upper chambers, and may pool and clot. If a blood clot in the atria leaves the heart and becomes lodged in an artery in the brain, a serious stroke will result. To reduce stroke risk in people with AF, physicians may prescribe anticoagulant and antiplatelet medications, which thin the blood and reduce clotting. Long-term use of appropriate medications in patients with AF can greatly reduce the chances of stroke, but such therapy requires careful monitoring in order to avoid unanticipated events, like hematomas. Mr. Desrosiers was admitted to the hospital for evaluation, his heart rate was controlled, and he was started on two medications, Heparin and Coumadin. When Mr. Desrosiers' blood test showed that his INR (International Normalized Ratio, used to determine the clotting tendency of blood) had reached an acceptable value of 2.5, Dr. Simpson discharged him. Mr. Desrosiers was given a prescription of 5 mg/day of Coumadin, and told to return to the clinic for a scheduled visit and follow-up laboratory tests in three weeks. No tests were ordered prior to that visit. The patient arrived at the Emergency Room one day before his scheduled appointment with a dangerous INR value of 14.7, and pain from an expanding spontaneous hematoma on his thigh. The ER staff notified hospital leadership that the patient had been given an inappropriate clinical management plan.

OVERVIEW OF ETHICS ISSUES

Since publication of the 1999 Institute of Medicine (IOM) report *To Err is Human*,[1] intensive national efforts have focused on how providers and management can identify and implement error-reduction strategies in hospitals. According to that report, an error is defined either as the failure of a planned action to be completed as intended (i.e., an error of execution), or the use of a wrong plan to achieve an aim (i.e., error of planning). As noted in the report, medical errors are one of the leading causes of death in the U.S. Medical errors may rank as high as the fifth leading cause of overall death in the U.S., exceeding the number of deaths that occur from motor vehicle accidents, breast cancer, and AIDS combined. In the years since the IOM report was published, research has revealed that errors are a growing problem in the family practice setting, and upon discharge from the hospital.[2] Errors can affect anyone, but often strike the weak and helpless.[3]

While errors do not always create ethics problems, the manner in which health care providers in clinics and small rural hospitals respond to errors may pose ethics concerns. Errors may not be recognized. Many hospitals and clinics lack mandatory reporting policies, so errors are not reported or charted. Even when policies are in place and errors are recognized, health care providers might feel such guilt and blame, or fear of retribution, that they choose not to acknowledge or document errors. In other cases, errors are discussed only behind closed doors between providers and administrators; patients and families aren't told when errors have occurred, or that corrective actions are needed. Thus, certain kinds of errors re-occur, and the risk for patient harm increases.

When health care providers do not recognize, report, or disclose errors, they fail to act in the best interest of the patient. This failure compromises patient autonomy and informed decision-making. The failure to report and disclose errors also compromises the principles of beneficence, fidelity, and justice, discussed in detail in Chapter 3 of this *Handbook*.

Seeking Safer Care: Goodness and Truth
In order to provide safe, ethically attuned care, a growing number of public, governmental and private entities have encouraged health care providers to adopt a systems approach to patient safety. Advocates suggest that a systems approach helps good caregivers give good care. Such an approach defines error, fosters the recognition of error, and promotes open discussion of errors and prevention strategies. A systems approach also promotes policies for honest reporting and disclosing of errors, offers apologies to patients and families, and seeks fair compensation for treatment needed as a result of the error(s). Since 2001, The Joint Commission has required disclosure of adverse outcomes to patients.[4] This standard reflects the national trend towards greater transparency. Indeed, initiatives like the *Sorry Works* Coalition and the Institute for Healthcare Improvement (IHI) have demonstrated the compelling need to disclose errors, and the benefits of such disclosure.[5] Patients, health care providers and the systems in which they work all benefit from such disclosure. Studies show that disclosure may help patients get treatment to offset the results of an error, may award them fair compensation, and may help restore trust in the health care provider.[6, 7] Thus, the honest, forthright disclosure of an error, including an apology, is an important component of an ethically-attuned patient-safety agenda.

While a systems approach to disclosing medical errors sounds reasonable, logistical problems can complicate such a systems implementation. The process of reporting and disclosing medical errors requires agreement among health care professionals about what constitutes an error; how errors should be reported; and when, how, and by whom they should be disclosed. A systems approach presumes that all parties involved can handle the consequences of reporting and disclosing errors. A systems approach is based on the assumption that the hospital has an ongoing willingness to keep patient safety a high priority, in spite of financial and other organizational pressures.

Lessons from Rural Empirical Ethics Studies

The empirical ethics studies that the authors have conducted over the past 12 years have shed light on conditions that can hinder the recognition and resolution of ethics-related problems that occur in rural health care settings. Rural nurses in our ethics studies reported that they lacked the vocabulary to talk about ethics issues with either peers or patients, and were, therefore, hesitant to initiate conversations about or bring attention to incidents that had ethics implications. Unclear lines of communication within the hospital further hindered the providers' identification or discussion of ethics issues. Our studies have also shown that there is little agreement among health care providers regarding how ethically challenging situations should be resolved. When rural health care providers were asked if the honest disclosure of error to patients would increase or decrease levels of trust in their institution, responses were evenly split.

Related findings emerged from the four-year Advancing Patient Safety study that the authors conducted in 30 rural health care settings in a multi-state area. This study showed that doctors' recognition and reporting of errors was selective, and tended to depend upon the type of error that had occurred, and to whom it would be disclosed. When doctors assessed cases that involved medication errors that could be attributed to nursing (e.g., overdosing of medication), most agreed that an error had occurred (97%) and should be reported on a system level (96%). But levels of agreement diminished when doctors considered disclosure of the error to the patient. Agreement among doctors was also drastically reduced when participants considered the recognition, reporting, and disclosing of errors associated with diagnosis and treatment—and so attributable to physicians.[8]

Our research showed that even when hospitals have policies for mandatory reporting and disclosure of errors, and even if health care providers believe that there is a "no shame, no blame" approach to error in their setting, professional disagreements about what constitutes an error hinders the provider from recognizing, reporting, and disclosing any problematic events. When participating in a case-based intervention on patient safety, health care providers almost uniformly acknowledged that the case problems being analyzed had occurred, or could occur in their setting. But even when cases met the Institute of Medicine definitions of error, health care providers were still hesitant to identify problematic events as errors. Physicians, for example, often used words like "sub-optimal outcomes" or "practice variance" or "clinical judgment" when discussing the errors depicted in the case studies. Nurses used terms such as "not right" or "unfortunate" or "poor care." Administrators explained that they "lack(ed) the clinical skills to make the call as to whether an error had occurred." At times, health care providers alluded to a general sense of a bad outcome or unfortunate care, but were unwilling to tag the event as an error. If the event was not clearly recognized as an error, the provider's need to report on the system level or to disclose to the patient was thus deemed unnecessary.

When quality improvement staff from rural health care settings analyzed 13 case studies, they uniformly agreed that the issues depicted could and did occur in their settings. They also noted that these issues would probably not be recognized, reported, or disclosed. In their hospitals, these kinds of issues would also not be referred to the ethics committees, if such committees existed, nor referred to medical staff committees or to quality improvement officers. Many of the problems depicted become normalized over time; they become part of what "just happens" when delivering health care.

This "institutional hesitancy" can be reflected in policy documents developed by hospitals and clinics for reporting and disclosing errors. Policies may use words such as "incidents" or "events" when describing issues of medical errors that compromise care. The word "error" may not be used, and the need for an apology may not be stated. So, it is not surprising that health care providers have a difficult time determining the appropriate language and disclosure practices to use when facing errors, given the fact that their own management is not clearly communicating about this topic, and the fact that specific training for providers may not be available.

CASE DISCUSSION

It is important to consider the background information given in the cases presented when trying to develop interdisciplinary strategies for providing safe, ethical care. The two cases in this chapter each depict a different kind of error. The first case depicts an error of execution, and the second case describes an error of planning. Although the cases are different in nature, both show the organizational, professional, and personal features that are in play when providers try to respond in an ethical manner.

CASE 12.1 | Addressing questionable quality of care

In the case of Dr. Bristol and his colonoscopies, the nurses lodged their complaints because they believed that Dr. Bristol was not meeting the standard of care when performing these procedures. To respond to the concerns of the nurses, the administration needed to determine whether patients undergoing this procedure had received the standard of care, and to clarify the hospital's ethical obligation to address the situation if errors had occurred.

Those struggling with the colonoscopy case quickly realized that they faced a complicated situation involving hospital staff, other local physicians, individual patients, and community members. Administrators assembled a team and sought advice and assistance from the hospital's legal counsel, insurers, outside risk managers, and other medical experts, including a group of board-certified gastroenterologists. The team first needed to determine whether a problem truly existed with Dr. Bristol's procedure. Did he fail to meet practice standards, and if so, did that failure compromise the provision of safe care? The team explored a number of questions in order to better understand the scope of the problem, including those listed in Box 12.1.

As the administrative team and their legal counsel began to respond to the questions listed above, the ethical dimensions of the case became apparent. These included the professional and organizational responsibilities associated with maximizing benefits, preventing harm, truth-telling, autonomy, and informed consent.

Maximizing Benefits and Preventing Harm

The investigation's findings suggested that Dr. Bristol's procedures had not met the clinical performance standards. That failure appeared to be linked to Dr. Bristol's skill level. The team then attempted to determine the ethical implications of that failure. Had Dr. Bristol failed to maximize benefits for his patients by failing to meet the standard of care? Had the technique used by Dr. Bristol placed patients at risk by under-diagnosing cancer or pre-cancerous conditions? Did patients have sufficient information about the skills required for this procedure and their own screening results to make informed decisions? If corrective efforts are not taken, will the levels of risk or potential harm for current and future patients escalate?

Related issues surfaced as the administrative team grappled with the implications of these questions. Since the procedure was performed in the hospital, what ethical obligations did the hospital face? If, for example, the hospital recognized an ethical obligation to require remedial training in order to prevent harm, would Dr. Bristol respond by accepting such a mandate, or would he choose to leave the community? Many rural hospitals fear losing physicians, and indeed that fear contributed to the administration's hesitation to address this problem when it was first reported. Medically

BOX 12.1

QUESTIONS TO ASK WHEN GATHERING INFORMATION REGARDING QUALITY OF CARE

- What performance standards should be met when conducting this test?
- Is there any way to determine Dr. Bristol's overall success rate?
- If complaints are accurate, why did Dr. Bristol fail to reach the cecum?
- Does the failure to perform the test correctly place patients at risk or cause harm?
- If complaints are accurate, what are the hospital's ethical responsibilities?
- If there is a need for additional training, how should such training be implemented?
- If concerns are validated, does the hospital have an ethical obligation to tell Dr. Bristol's patients?
- What are the implications of disclosure for the hospital and the community?
- Who should be involved in the disclosure process and how should it be accomplished?
- If repeat examinations are recommended, who is responsible for the cost?
- What impact would disclosure have on Dr. Bristol's reputation within the hospital and the community?
- If, after additional training, Dr. Bristol continues to perform this procedure, how should his competency be assessed and monitored?
- What new policies, procedures, or guidelines are needed to ensure clinician competence?
- What policies, procedures, and guidelines are needed to create a more open and ethically attuned environment within the hospital?

underserved communities report that it can easily take two years and many thousands of dollars to recruit a new physician. The team members grappled with the notion that some care may be better than no care.

Professional Responsibility, Truth-Telling, and Informed Consent

While the administrative investigative team acknowledged that truth-telling is an important ethical principle, they did not want to unduly alarm patients or community residents. They were also very conscious of the potential financial implications, for both the physician and the hospital, of telling the truth in this case. If community members were to learn of the problems with Dr. Bristol's colonoscopy skill level, they might lose trust in him, and might seek an alternative health care provider. Dr. Bristol might not be able to maintain a financially viable practice and the hospital could lose a source of reimbursement. However, if the hospital chose not to inform patients that their cancer screening might have been inadequate, would the hospital then be violating its ethical obligation to be truthful? When would the failure to disclose important information adversely impact a patient's autonomy? When might the lack of information about benefits, risks, and skill level compromise the informed consent process? The administrative team recognized that patients might already have been harmed, but questioned the extent to which the moral obligation for honesty and truth-telling would entail an obligation to compensate for or mitigate past failings.

As this case unfolded, the obligations that physicians have to their profession became a topic of discussion. The American College of Physicians' Charter on Medical Professionalism states that, "Professionalism is the basis of medicine's contract with society. It demands placing the interests of patients above those of the physician, setting and maintaining standards of competence and integrity, and providing expert advice to society on matters of health."[9]

Dr. Bristol's physician colleagues were aware of his performance-related problems, but were hesitant to question his procedures. They pointed out that they were "call partners" and depended upon one another in a resource-strapped environment. Losing a call partner would have major implications for the working conditions and quality of life of the remaining physicians and staff. Dr. Bristol's physician co-workers acknowledged that they operated under an unspoken code. They "did not look over one another's shoulders," and "did not look in one another's charts." Physicians explained that they "live in glass houses." They also pointed out that Dr. Bristol had provided appropriate care, and even extraordinary care, in many circumstances. Dr. Bristol was a trusted member of the community, and they did not want to jeopardize his standing. The nurses countered by referencing their professional and moral obligations to protect their patients' well-being. Thus they expressed a moral obligation to seek corrective action.

The hospital also faced the challenge of addressing organizational ethics issues, including the relationships among staff members. Ross *et al.*

noted that relationships among staff are a key indicator of an ethical environment.[10] In the authors' studies on ethics and patient safety, health care providers have often reported a lack of dialogue and respect among and between members of the various health professions, and noted that these conditions hindered recognition, reporting, and resolution of ethics problems. In the colonoscopy case, nurses expressed concern for more than a year before they were able to get attention focused on what they believed was sub-standard and improper care. As they promoted the need for corrective action, many nurses also noted that they worried about the consequences of their activities. Nurses stated that they are "not supposed to question doctors," and that they are not supposed to move beyond their scope of practice. Some feared they would lose their positions or be re-assigned. Given this backdrop, does the hospital have a moral obligation to have policies that deal with issues such as communication, reporting, and adherence to practice standards?

CASE 12.2 | The use of a wrong clinical management care plan

We have presented this case because the health care providers who participated in our studies explained that problems associated with atrial fibrillation (AF) management occur with some frequency in rural health care settings, but often go unrecognized or undetected. To support recognition, disclosure, and prevention of this type of error, the authors have proposed an information-gathering process that mirrors the one used in the colonoscopy case. Administrators may need to assemble a team, and seek advice and assistance from many departments, including the emergency room staff, quality improvement officers, and admittance and discharge personnel. The team would need to determine if practice standards have been met, benefits of treatment maximized, and harm prevented. The team would need to explore how the physicians' professional obligations and the hospital's organizational obligations might influence their recognition and resolution of this issue. They might ask: Are there procedures in place to help identify this kind of problem? If standards have not been met, can obligations for truth-telling and informed consent be honored?

The ethics issues in this case are similar to those presented in the previous, colonoscopy case, and such ethics issues are present in most cases involving medical errors. These include issues associated with maximizing benefits, preventing harm, truth-telling and disclosure, autonomy, and informed consent. Since both cases emerged through the authors' empirical research project, we have decided to show the process by which the participating health care providers arrived at workable solutions. This "real life" approach shows how difficult it is for well-meaning people to resolve ethics dilemmas.

RESPONDING TO MEDICAL ERROR DISCLOSURE CONFLICTS

CASE 12.1 | Addressing questionable quality of care

The administrative team determined that their priority was to demonstrate a commitment to uphold the integrity of the hospital's mission—"to provide safe, quality, ethical care to patients". In addition to requiring that Dr. Bristol obtain additional training prior to performing any new colonoscopies, they initiated a monitoring process that required a photograph of the cecum to be taken during each procedure to demonstrate that the colonoscopy had been performed correctly.

The hospital recognized that this case was complicated by issues associated with staff relationships and communication, and realized that corrective actions were necessary. The concerns of the nurses should have been heeded when first lodged. The hospital also recognized the need to increase consensus among the involved health care providers, with respect to recognizing, reporting, and responding to errors so that problems of this type could be avoided in the future. Admittedly, it can be very difficult to gain consensus when trying to meet ethical obligations. This difficulty certainly emerged when health care providers analyzed this case. They noted that ongoing training is a reality of medical life, and that the hospital could announce that Dr. Bristol is seeking additional training to make sure that patients receive the best care possible. The health care providers could also envision activities like a "colonoscopy month" during which patients could schedule colonoscopies at a reduced charge.

While some health care providers felt that the gold standard of ethical conduct would have entailed contacting former patients, disclosing that the test may not have been done correctly, and offering options for re-screening at no cost, the administrative team decided that this approach was not feasible or wise. Both the administrative team that faced this issue and the other health care providers within the hospital were reluctant to advocate such a policy, and believed that it could result in unnecessary harm or worry for patients.

CASE 12.2 | The use of a wrong clinical management care plan

While health care providers who discussed the atrial fibrillation (AF) case were hesitant to use the word "error," they acknowledged that the problem was one that occurred with some frequency in clinics and in hospitals. They had many suggestions for preventing the problem in the future. These recommendations included assigning responsibility to pharmacists for management of blood thinners, designing new hospital discharge policies, and enhancing patient education. Even though harm had occurred, most agreed that the patient probably would not be told that the complications he suffered were related to the failure to prescribe an appropriate treatment plan. This failure to disclose could be linked to a number of issues already discussed in this chapter, including lack of agreement of definitions of error, lack of policies for reporting and disclosing errors, concerns about consequences of disclosure, and lack of agreed-upon discharge standards.

Thus the real ethical stumbling block for those addressing this case was the issue of disclosure: what exactly would the patient be told, by whom, and how? In order to uphold the ethical principles and concepts associated with maximizing benefit, preventing harm, truth telling, protection of autonomy, and informed consent, a disclosure plan should be carefully planned and implemented.

**ANTICIPATING RECOGNITION AND DISCLOSURE
OF MEDICAL ERRORS ETHICS CONFLICTS**
An ethically attuned disclosure process requires that health care professionals and institutions implement a change in orientation and culture. The emphasis moves from placing blame on individual providers and health care organizations to developing systems that improve the quality of care. In order to accommodate such a cultural change, health care settings have to promote recognition of error in a manner that engages all stakeholders, including patients. Hospitals can no longer perceive themselves as powerless when errors occur, unable to direct the behavior of physicians, or unable to control the economic impact of errors. Both hospitals and clinicians fear lawsuits, which may tarnish their reputations and lead to lost revenue. These fears have discouraged the use of words such as "error" and "I'm sorry," but practices are gradually changing.

In the AHRQ patient safety study,[8] participants were presented with case examples and a standard set of companion questions that were structured to reinforce recognition of error, foster the use of a common language in discussing error, and provide common experiences when trying to resolve problems. When developing this intervention, the authors considered the use of other error analysis models such as the Root Cause Analysis Model (RCA) and the Failure Mode Effects Analysis (FMEA) model. Many of these models, however, required substantial training, time, and resources, and were less appealing to project participants as a result. Some who had used the RCA process, for example, described it as difficult and unsatisfactory. Participants expressed the need for a model that was accessible, and that provided practical guidance for safer care. We developed the patient safety model illustrated in Table 12.1 as a result of these requests.

TABLE 12.1

PATIENT SAFETY ERROR ANALYSIS MODEL	
Topic and description of problem	Is the diagnosis correct? Is the prognosis/treatment plan correct?
Issues that need to be addressed	Was the treatment provided properly? Were appropriate procedures used?
Ethics Considerations	Explore issues including: • autonomy • justice • beneficence • nonmaleficence • truth-telling • impartiality • publicity • shared decision-making
Learning Points	What are the learning points?
Guides/Standards	What clinical guides could be suggested to solve this problem and avoid future problems? Is there a system plan for reporting, disclosure, and remediation?
Strategies for Improvement	What steps for improvement should be considered? What issues should be disclosed?

This case study methodology proved to be a cost-effective and time-efficient way to disseminate information throughout clinics and hospitals and to enhance the level of dialogue. Responses to the case studies were shared among all team members, shaped into case summaries, and distributed to staff. Hospitals used the case studies to provide continuing education programs for nurses and physicians. The case examples given in this *Handbook* were discussed at staff meetings, and copies, including summaries, were posted at nurses' stations and in clinical staff lounges. The majority of participants reported that the weekly case studies were relevant (92%), useful (92%), valuable (94%) and resembled situations that happen in their hospital(s) (74%). The majority of the participants also reported that the case studies and their summaries had a positive impact on interdisciplinary collaboration, and contributed to a change in the organizational safety climate.

This case-based intervention and the use of the Patient Safety Error Analysis Model helped health care providers recognize differences in their professional beliefs and practices; showed how these differences influence recognition and resolution of error; and showed that change is necessary, desirable, and possible. Since the case studies helped build staff-wide support for patient safety initiatives, they became the basis for implementing new standards and practices. Over the four-year course of the project, health care providers gained skills in addressing the issues in the case studies, and they became more willing to discuss ethically problematic issues that occurred in their own settings. The study manual, *"From good intentions to good actions: A patient safety manual for rural health care settings,"* is available online.

A Call for Disclosure

In order to honor and respect patients, and to maximize benefits, reduce harm, and reflect honesty and truthfulness in the patient/clinician relationship, health care organizations are morally obligated to develop and implement a disclosure policy that promotes open and honest communication. When even minor errors happen, patients and families want to be informed in a timely manner. Failure of professionals to communicate effectively, and to honestly admit to the error in a timely manner, can potentially undermine the hospital's reputation and heighten the risk of litigation.

The disclosure process should be delineated in the institutional policies, and should include issues that are addressed during and after disclosure, including follow-up and remediation. Follow-up and remediation should include a system for fair compensation. While there is no foolproof way to disclose a bad outcome and error(s) in care, the recommendations from a growing body of literature suggest that the issues listed in Box 12.2 be discussed during a disclosure meeting.

BOX 12.2

ISSUES TO ADDRESS WHEN DISCLOSING A MEDICAL ERROR[11]

- Express regret, and apologize
- Explain the nature of the error, including time, place, and circumstances
- Explain the proximal cause
- Explain the known consequences for the patient, and the potential or anticipated consequences
- Explain any actions taken to treat the medical error
- Identify those who will manage the ongoing care of the patient
- Discuss any planned investigation or review of the error
- Explain who else has been, or will be, informed of the error
- Identify actions taken to identify system issues that may have contributed to the error
- Discuss who will manage ongoing communication with the patient and his or her family
- Provide the names and phone numbers of individuals with whom patients and families can address concerns and questions
- Explain how to obtain support and counseling regarding the error
- Explain that any charges directly related to the error will be removed from the patient's account
- Offer a commitment to assist the patient and his or her family in identifying resources to help obtain compensation if actual damages are warranted

It is noteworthy that patient safety advocates stress the importance of disclosure even in situations where there is no error, but when a bad outcome nonetheless occurred. Under that scenario, the steps include:

Step 1: Set up a meeting with the patient, family and attorney
Step 2: Show empathy, answer questions, open records, and prove innocence

Step 3:   Look for genuine resolution; honesty and disclosure can
mitigate the likelihood of unnecessary tension and litigation

Maintaining the Commitment to Disclose Medical Errors

Health care providers may experience a certain relief when disclosure
policies have been crafted and are in place. The goal of patient safety,
however, can still remain quite tenuous in many health care facilities.
Implementing a disclosure process requires a significant change in
previously accepted attitudes, beliefs, and processes.

It is important to realize that change is a complex process, involving
stages that include pre-contemplation, contemplation, planning,
action, maintenance, and sometimes relapse.[12-15] These stages do not
necessarily occur in a sequential fashion. Certainly the pre-contemplation
stage precedes contemplation, but if one's experience is unpleasant, one
could easily revert from the contemplation stage, or even the planning
stage, back to pre-contemplation. Consider the experiences of the nurses
who spent two years in a pre-contemplation phase and then over a year
in a contemplation phase as they tried to focus attention on Dr. Bristol's
colonoscopy procedures. Such a stressful experience might cause a
provider to reconsider identifying an event as an error, or decide not to file
a report when encountering a subsequent error. Indeed, change theorists
caution that only 10-15% of persons who think they are in a change
phase are actually in the action process.[14] And even when change has
been successfully achieved, the maintenance of new behaviors is an
ongoing challenge. When change is hard to maintain, people can easily
backslide and revert to old behaviors and patterns. Stages of change are
outlined in Box 12.3.

Health care professionals need ongoing support in order to recognize
problems, handle the consequences of recognition, and work for
change.[12-15] As part of the Advancing Patient Safety study, the authors
developed an interdisciplinary curriculum that was rooted in change
theory.[16] The curriculum employed weekly case studies that depicted
unsafe situations that actually occur in rural hospitals and clinics. Every
week the cases were delivered via email to three- or four-member
interdisciplinary teams in each participating setting. Even with this level
of support, health care providers noted that it was still hard to disclose
errors, and easy to backslide. So, hospitals and clinics have to cultivate a
high level of vigilance.

BOX 12.3

STAGES OF CHANGE

Pre-contemplation
Is the stage at which there is no intention to change behavior in the foreseeable future. Many individuals in this stage are unaware or underaware of their problems.

Contemplation
Is the stage in which people are aware that a problem exists and are seriously thinking about overcoming it but have not yet made a commitment to take action.

Preparation
Is a stage that combines intention and behavioral criteria. Individuals in this stage are intending to take action in the next month and have unsuccessfully taken action in the past year.

Action
Is the stage in which individuals modify their behavior, experiences, or environment in order to overcome their problems. Action involves the most overt behavioral changes and requires considerable commitment of time and energy.

Maintenance
Is the stage in which people work to prevent relapse and consolidate the gains attained during action.

CONCLUSION

There are no easy road maps for providers who face a complex problem like medical error disclosure. Errors can trigger feelings of shock and anxiety among all parties involved. Indeed, the health care providers we have interviewed report that they carry the pain of past errors for years. As one physician explained, "The guilt from that event has been on my shoulders for 15 years."

Given the personal and professional pain that may ensue when a serious medical error occurs, a provider might be tempted to look away, and so avoid the moral reflection and actions that are needed to acknowledge, report, and then truthfully disclose the error(s).

Health care providers also noted that, in spite of their best intentions, it was often hard to keep patient safety on the "radar screen." Any number of emergency rooms, dealing with staff attrition and replacement, or the need to rely on temporary employees, can divert attention away from recognition and disclosure and toward what seem like more pressing issues. Thus, it is critical to create an environment in which professionals continually evaluate and reinforce ethically-attuned responses to patient-safety issues.

REFERENCES

1. Kohn LT, Corrigan JM, Donaldson MS, eds. *To Err is Human: Building a Safer Health System.* Washington, DC: National Academy Press; 2000.

2. Clark PA. Medication errors in family practice, in hospitals and after discharge from the hospital: an ethical analysis. *J Law Med Ethics.* Summer 2004;32(2):349-357, 192.

3. Wachter RM, Shojania KG. *Internal Bleeding: The Truth Behind America's Terrifying Epidemic of Medical Mistakes.* New York, NY: Rugged Land; 2005.

4. Devers KJ, Pham HH, Liu G. What is driving hospitals' patient-safety efforts? *Health Aff (Millwood).* Mar-Apr 2004;23(2):103-115.

5. Sorry Works! Coalition. http://www.sorryworks.net/. Accessed Dec. 6, 2008.

6. Wu AW, Cavanaugh TA, McPhee SJ, Lo B, Micco GP. To tell the truth: ethical and practical issues in disclosing medical mistakes to patients. *J Gen Intern Med.* Dec 1997;12(12):770-775.

7. Boyle D, O'Connell D, Platt FW, Albert RK. Disclosing errors and adverse events in the intensive care unit. *Crit Care Med.* May 2006;34(5):1532-1537.

8. Cook AF, Hoas H, Guttmannova K, Joyner JC. An error by any other name. *Am J Nurs.* Jun 2004;104(6):32-43; quiz 44.

9. ABIM Foundation, American Board of Internal Medicine, ACP-ASIM Foundation, American College of Physicians-American Society of Internal Medicine, European Federation of Internal Medicine. Medical professionalism in the new millennium: a physician charter. *Ann Intern Med.* Dec. 6, 2008 2002;136(3):243-246.

10. Ross JW, Glaser JW, Rasinski-Gregory D, Gibson JM, Bayley C. *Health Care Ethics Committees: The Next Generation.* Chicago, IL: American Hospital Publisher; 1993.

11. Morath J, Hart LG. Partnering with families: disclosure and trust. Paper presented at: National Patient Safety Foundation/ JCAHO Patient Safety Initiative 2000: Spotlighting Strategies, Sharing Solutions; October 6, 2000; Chicago, IL. http://www.npsf.org/download/Morath.pdf. Accessed Dec. 13, 2008.

12. Emmons K. Commentary: The transtheoretical model of behavior change: Application to clinical practice. *Adv Mind Body Med.* 2006;1:221-223.

13. DiClemente CC, Prochaska JO, Fairhurst SK, Velicer WF, Velasquez MM, Rossi JS. The process of smoking cessation: an analysis of precontemplation, contemplation, and preparation stages of change. *J Consult Clin Psychol.* Apr 1991;59(2):295-304.

14. Prochaska JO, Norcross JC, DiClemente CC. *Changing for Good: The Revolutionary Program that Explains the Six Stages of Change and Teaches You How to Free Yourself from Bad Habits.* New York, NY: W. Morrow; 1994.

15. Lebow J. Transformation now! (or maybe later): client change is not an all-or-nothing proposition. *Psychotherapy Networker.* 2002(Jan/Feb):31-32.

16. Cook AF, Hoas H, Guttmannova K. From Here to There: Lessons From an Integrative Patient Safety Project in Rural Health Care Settings. *Advances in Patient Safety: From Research to Implementation.* Rockville, MD: Agency for Healthcare Research and Quality; 2005. Available at: http://www.ncbi.nlm.nih.gov/books/bv.fcgi?rid=aps.section.1290. Accessed Dec. 6, 2008.

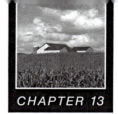

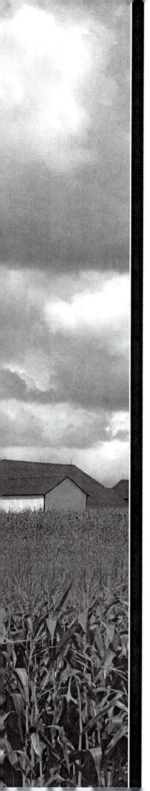

Ethics Conflicts in Rural Communities: Reproductive Health Care

Barbara Elliott, Ruth Westra

Ethics Conflicts in Rural Communities: Reproductive Health Care

Barbara Elliott, Ruth Westra

ABSTRACT

For the rural health care professional, it is essential to create a practice where community members can expect trust, respect, and safety in their patient-clinician relationships. This goal becomes critical when the practice includes reproductive health care, a specialty where providers may experience heightened ethics concerns regarding the management of clinical information. When health care is needed as a consequence of sexual activity that strays from the community's culture or norms, the clinician and clinic can be put into a difficult position. Both medical and social circumstances require appropriate care, confidentiality, truth-telling, and careful boundaries. In order to avoid such conflicts, specific and personal guidelines can be indispensable. When the professional communicates expectations up front, he or she lets patients know that they will receive appropriate care, whatever their circumstances, and that confidentiality of their personal medical information is carefully guarded. Clinician stress is reduced, and patient-clinician relationships are enhanced, when clinicians can establish and maintain clear boundaries in their clinical relationships, and take the time to examine their own views regarding birth control, abortion, and sexual liaisons. These personal efforts on the part of the clinician can assure objectivity and integrity in a practice that includes reproductive care.

CASE STUDIES

CASE 13.1 | Birth control for a minor

Dr. Bennally has been a friend of the Rosenthal family since coming to town 18 years ago as a family physician. The Rosenthal's oldest child, Sally (15 years), has come to the office to have a physical for the school's track team. Her mother has brought her to the office but, as usual, Dr. Bennally sees Sally alone. After taking the history and doing an exam, it is evident that Sally wants to talk. In response to a question about dating, she explains that she has been dating one boy for the last six months. Sally says she really likes him a lot, and although they "haven't done it yet, they have been thinking about it a lot." Sally is wondering if she could start taking birth control pills. Sally also explains that her parents do not know anything about her sexual activity. Sally says that when she tried to talk with her mother about sex, Mrs. Rosenthal just, "got weird—talking about babies having babies, and nobody having morals any more." Sally says that her mother would be very upset if she knew Sally is considering birth control, and asks that Dr. Bennally not share this information with her parents.

CASE 13.2 | Managing and treating sexually
transmitted infections

Dr. Haladay, a family physician, is providing care for Joan Larson, who is 26 weeks pregnant. This is her third pregnancy; her previous two vaginal deliveries went easily and her babies were born at full term. Ms. Larson and her husband attend the same house of worship as Dr. Haladay and her family. When Ms. Larson comes to the clinic for the appointment, she complains of a "sensitive area" that "really hurts" on her perineum. The exam confirms that she has developed herpes simplex infection (HSV). Dr. Haladay explains how this may result in the possible need to plan for a C-section with the upcoming delivery. Joan Larson is horrified, and then somewhat chagrined. She admits to having had an affair with a well-known community member, who is likely the source of the infection. Ms. Larson's husband, Mr. Larson, does not know about the extramarital relationship and she does not want him to know. She is certain that her husband is the father of the child she is carrying. Ms. Larson asks Dr. Haladay to treat the infection—and not to put the information in the chart or tell her husband.

OVERVIEW OF ETHICS ISSUES

Several ethics issues come into play regarding reproductive health issues. These issues are listed in Box 13.1.

BOX 13.1

ETHICAL DIMENSIONS OF REPRODUCTIVE HEALTH CARE

- Confidentiality
- Truth-Telling
- Boundary Issues
- Community and Personal Values
- Paying for Care
- Referrals to Distant, Specialized Providers

Confidentiality

One of the essential concerns in managing ethics tensions in rural settings is the need for confidentiality.[1] This becomes especially important for patients with reproductive health issues in rural settings, given their limited care options, unique community values, and overlapping patient-clinician relationships. Confidentiality can be difficult to maintain in a small community, where the people who work at the clinic are relatives, friends, and neighbors. However, in order to "do no harm," confidentiality is vital. Charts and billing records need to contain information that supports continuity of care. Balancing the ethics burdens associated with confidentiality can also isolate clinicians, adding to clinician stress.[1, 2]

Truth-Telling

Overlapping relationships, community and personal values, and clinician stress all share a common core ethics issue: truth-telling. Questions, such as: how much of the truth is revealed to the patient and when; to what extent should information be placed in the medical record; and so on, are all part of the scope of truth-telling. It is important for the clinician to establish the habit of being honest and objective about medical diagnoses and treatments when talking with patients. This can become socially and emotionally complicated, given the expectations and values of the people involved and the community. Nevertheless, in order to ensure informed consent, provide appropriate medical care, and protect the community's public health, the truth needs to be told.[3, 4]

Boundary Issues

Tensions around boundary issues are brought into patient-clinician encounters by the clinician, the patient, and/or the patient's family.[1, 2, 4] When working with patients regarding sexual or reproductive health diagnoses and treatment decisions, ethics tensions may be increased by differing community and personal values, and by overlapping relationships. Such conflicts can put the clinician in a difficult position regarding how he or she offers recommendations. A clinician's scientific and/or social objectivity may be limited when specific sexual liaisons are revealed, or particular sexual infections are diagnosed. Clinician stress can also be increased in these circumstances.

Community and Personal Values

Ethics tensions are heightened when personal values and the community's culture are part of the clinical decision-making process.[4, 5] Decisions that are impacted by social and/or personal stigma increase the provider's difficulty in decision-making, and complicate patient-clinician relationships. With limited access to alternate care settings,[2, 4] these value conflicts can undermine appropriate medical care, and can add to both the patient's and the clinician's stress.

Smaller communities frequently include less diversity in values.[5] As a consequence, the community's norms are narrower than larger settings and there may be less tolerance for a variety of experiences.[4, 5] For example, if community values include the traditional sexual expectation of "sex only after marriage, and then monogamy," all sexual behavior is assessed in this light. Appropriate and responsible medical care for any sexually active person includes birth control and the prevention and treatment of sexually transmitted infections. These medical interventions should be indicated, and care provided to all patients, even those who are not meeting the community's expectations. Providing this care is made more difficult when the clinician's own values are offended by the patient's sexual activity, and patient-clinician tension is increased.

Paying for Health Care

Clinical settings are fiscally precarious, especially in rural settings where the costs associated with the care of one patient can mean being in the black or in the red.[1, 2] Third-party payers have access to the charted notes regarding care for which they are asked to pay, so billing records need to be consistent with charted care. When confidentiality is necessary because of personal and/or community values, arranging payment for rendered care must also be discrete. The business side of practice can be ethically complex and requires great care, adding to clinician stress.

Referrals to Distant, Specialized Providers
Because rural areas often have limited access to specialized clinicians and resources, referrals to distant hospitals are common.[1, 2, 4] This can result in diminished resources for the local care community, and requires patients to travel far and sometimes spend extended time away from home. This travel issue raises both financial and personal ethics issues for the community, clinician, and patient.[1, 2] The ethics tensions in making these referrals add to the complexity of decisions that need to be made and add to clinician stress.

Rural Characteristics That Intensify Ethics Issues
In rural settings, the ethics concerns that are commonly involved in reproductive health care are heightened by the specific characteristics of rural settings. These characteristics are described in Box 13.2.

BOX 13.2

RURAL CHARACTERISTICS INTENSIFYING ETHICS ISSUES IN REPRODUCTIVE HEALTH CARE

- Availability and/or limited access to care and services
- Overlapping relationships between patients and clinicians
- Community and personal values
- Clinician stress

For example, rural communities offer close support and supervision of family units and sexual behaviors. When health care is needed for sexual activity that strays from the community's culture and norms, the clinician and clinic can be put into a difficult position (re: experiences with HIV and related diseases, etc). Health care that is medically appropriate, but required as a result of socially stigmatized relationships and behaviors, becomes fraught with ethics tensions.[3] The resulting pressures, both from within the patient-physician relationship and without, can actually become barriers to accomplishing the needed care.

Availability and/or Limited Access to Care and Services
One ethics issue that increases providers' concerns in the reproductive health arena is the limited number of clinicians and medical facilities in rural areas.[6] In most settings, few clinicians work in each clinic. Few

options for reproductive health care are available other than the 'local clinic' (e.g., Planned Parenthood, etc). This limitation increases the likelihood that all sexual and reproductive health issues will be treated through one set of clinicians.

Overlapping Relationships Between Patients and Clinicians
The providers who work in the local clinic are also part of the community, and they have relationships beyond their clinical connections.[1, 4] All community residents have opportunities to participate in activities with one another. These overlapping relationships, whether at work, school, a place of worship, ballpark, or neighborhood, can increase the ethics tensions related to needed health care as a consequence of sexual behavior. The expectations of the community and individuals can complicate the clinician's relationships.

Health Care Provider Stress
A clinician needs to manage all circumstances that heighten tensions within the patient-clinician relationship. These circumstances often create additional stress for the clinician, who in turn needs to increase attention to his or her own personal care.[1, 4] Given so many overlapping relationships, the clinician in a smaller community is often in a position where his or her own values need to be set aside when providing care. In many cases, the characteristics of a case can isolate the clinician to the extent that he or she cannot manage the stress by simply talking with colleagues. Instead, the provider needs to develop additional ways to cope with the stress that can arise as a result of these cases.

These characteristics of the rural health care experience especially amplify the ethics challenges related to reproductive health care. The ethics issues that arise in these circumstances are certainly observed in practices everywhere. However, they are especially poignant in rural settings, and become important considerations for rural clinicians who want to create a practice in which community members can expect trust, respect, and safety in the patient-clinician relationship.

CASE DISCUSSION
Neither case presented at the beginning of this chapter involves ethics conflicts that are focused on clinical decisions. However, the clinicians and patients differ somewhat in their view about how best to accomplish the common goal of providing appropriate care. The first patient wants her information kept private from her parents; the second patient wants

information kept private from both her husband and the insurance company. These differences generate ethics conflicts for the clinicians, especially in a rural context. In rural settings, personal, professional, and community issues complicate the clinicians' abilities to deliver state-of-the-art care.

The discussion of the cases is based upon the analysis method presented in Chapter 4 of this *Handbook*.

CASE 13.1 | Birth control for a minor

In this case, the clinician's personal and professional issues are especially poignant. The ethics questions raised by Sally Rosenthal's request are highlighted in Box 13.3.

BOX 13.3

ETHICS QUESTIONS IN THE CASE OF BIRTH CONTROL FOR A MINOR

- Should Dr. Bennally keep Sally's confidence?
- Who, if anyone, should tell Sally's parents about their daughter's sexual activities?
- Should Dr. Bennally prescribe birth control for Sally?

To address these questions, additional information is critical to the clinician in deciding how to proceed. The needed information is related to Sally's maturing identity and relationships, to state laws regarding confidentiality in the treatment of minors, and to the clinician's personal and professional positions on birth control. It is clear that Sally is competent and is speaking for herself when she makes the requests for contraception and for confidentiality. She is at the appropriate developmental level for her age, and does not want to tell or involve her parents in her independent activities. Various states have their own laws regarding the confidentiality of medical information generally and with respect to specific types of information, such as that related to reproductive health care. As is noted in Chapter 7, The Health Insurance Portability and Accountability Act of 1996 (HIPAA) resulted in an overlay of federal privacy regulations. It is important that rural clinicians be aware of what the law requires of them and their staff members with respect to sharing patient information, as well as what it permits.

As is the case in many states, Dr. Bennally has no right to reveal medical information in this situation—the patient can have confidential relationships with clinicians around reproductive health issues.[3] Thus, neither conversations nor medical records about Sally Rosenthal's health care relating to sexual activity are available to anyone else—including her parents—without her permission. State laws on minor consent vary and can apply differently to different types of medical information, so it is important to know the law in one's state. Each clinician has her own personal feelings about prescribing birth control to anyone at any age; each of us needs to know our own heart. The boundary issues and personal values concerns related to this assumption are significant because they can directly impact patient care.

State-of-the-art medical care for Sally indicates that Dr. Bennally should prescribe her requested contraception and should keep this care confidential. To provide this care and protect Sally from the perceived harm of involving her parents, Dr. Bennally faces several ethics challenges. These challenges result from the clinician's overlapping roles in the rural community and the need to maintain confidentiality. The conflicts Dr. Bennally faces are described in Box 13.4.

BOX 13.4

ETHICS CONFLICTS IN THE CASE OF BIRTH CONTROL FOR A MINOR

- Personal and professional conflicts due to overlapping relationships in the community
- Professional conflict, because of concern that confidentiality may be breached in connection with payment or reimbursement for Sally's care and medications
- Anticipated conflicts related to the confidentiality of future care

Dr. Bennally's relationships with Sally, Mr. and Mrs. Rosenthal, and other relevant parties such as clinic staff, make adherence to ethical standards more difficult and add to her stress level. Her friendship with Sally's parents is based on expectations of honesty. How can Dr. Bennally maintain her friendship without sharing the confidential care she is providing for their daughter?

Confidentiality can also be strained when it comes to payment. Sally may need to pay cash for her care, or be billed directly—but not through the insurance company—in order to maintain the privacy she requests. How does Dr. Bennally maintain confidentiality when the billing system works against that process?

Finally, Sally will need to return for more injections or prescriptions in order for Dr. Bennally to provide the best possible care. Reminders about that care will also need to be handled confidentially. If Sally has medical problems as a result of the birth control or her sexual activity, Dr. Bennally may have to explain the circumstances to her parents. What would Sally want Dr. Bennally to say to her parents then? The complexity of maintaining confidentiality becomes a truth-telling issue.

CASE 13.2 | Managing and treating sexually transmitted infections

Professional and community values are especially important in the ethics issues raised by the second case. There are two ethics questions raised by Joan Larson, the wife who'd contracted herpes from an affair, and now wants her medical records not to indicate her STD so as to disguise the affair from her husband (see Box 13.5).

BOX 13.5

> **ETHICS QUESTIONS ABOUT MANAGING AND TREATING SEXUALLY TRANSMITTED INFECTIONS**
>
> - Should Dr. Haladay keep Joan Larson's herpes diagnosis information out of the record?
> - Who should inform Joan's husband, Mr. Larson, and her extramarital partner about the infection, if anyone?

These issues require more information that is critical in order for the provider to move forward. Dr. Haladay needs to obtain more information about Ms. Larson's medical condition and her pregnancy, and to plan for the care of the newborn. The doctor also needs to examine her own personal and professional truth-telling attitudes and skills. Ms. Larson is competent when she requests appropriate treatment for herself, the baby, and her partner, and when she requests confidentiality. She is an adult and does not want to involve her husband in this conversation. Since she is pregnant, Ms. Larson needs to be treated medically for her incident case of HSV, and will need careful monitoring until delivery.[7] If the disease is active when she goes into labor, she will need to protect the baby from acquiring the disease by having a C-section, which will either mean a referral to the obstetrician in a regional center, or else careful planning around a local delivery if there is a local physician who performs C-sections. If a C-section occurs, it will necessitate decisions about how to explain the need for surgery to Ms. Larson's husband.

Though Ms. Larson's condition has implications for her baby, her husband, her partner, and perhaps the community at large, public health guidelines do not require reporting of HSV in most states. However, in order to provide appropriate care, Ms. Larson's partner will need to be informed of these circumstances and be offered treatment to suppress his HSV. Ms. Larson's husband will need to protect himself from the disease by using condoms during intercourse, assuming he has not already contracted the disease.

Each clinician has his or her personal guidelines and habits regarding truth-telling in settings where there is high emotion around a socially sensitive diagnosis. Revealing bad news is a skill all clinicians develop, but certain circumstances involving sexual liaisons and overlapping relationships can be especially sensitive. This case discussion assumes that the clinician, Dr. Haladay, prefers honesty in both conversation and charting.

Given this information, appropriate care for Ms. Larson involves medications, increased monitoring of her pregnancy, and education about protecting others (her fetus and her sexual partners) from HSV. Ms. Larson has requested care and that the information regarding that care be kept confidential. This leads to several specific ethics conflicts for the clinician, as described in Box 13.6.

BOX 13.6

ETHICS CONFLICT ISSUES IN THE MANAGEMENT AND TREATMENT OF SEXUALLY TRANSMITTED INFECTIONS

- Maintaining the challenge of confidentiality is difficult in some cases, including potential the need to make a referral
- Billing for the care and medications will need to document the diagnosis
- Anticipating confidentiality needs for future care
- Boundary issues due to professional and personal contact with patient in the community
- Potential community health issue in the spread of infection

If Ms. Larson's request to keep the medical information confidential is honored, her medical care may be compromised, depending on how the medical and ethical issues are managed. Ms. Larson needs to be treated now for her active HSV infection. Her extramarital partner needs to be evaluated now for suppressive therapy for his HSV infection. Ideally, her husband would also be evaluated for infection and treated as appropriate. However, if Dr. Haladay honors Ms. Larson's request for confidentiality about the infection and does not reveal it to her husband, Ms. Larson and Dr. Haladay will need to decide how to handle the billing for the necessary exams and cultures. If Ms. Larson decides to refuse the indicated tests, there may be an increased risk for harm to the fetus or need for a surgical delivery.[8]

These conflicts result from overlapping roles in the community, truth-telling, the need to maintain confidentiality while making referrals, and paying for care. When Dr. Haladay completes his charting and requests the referral (if a local C-section is unavailable), he will need to explain the reason for the consult, and written information returning from the consultant will include full discussion of the diagnosis. How can he maintain confidentiality while in contact with the obstetrician?

Confidentiality will also be put at risk when billing occurs. Either Ms. Larson will pay for her care directly, or the bill to the insurance company will need to be handled separately from any copy sent to the Larson home, as with the Rosenthal family in Case 1. How can confidentiality be maintained when the billing system works against that process?

Joan Larson may also need special care in the future. If Ms. Larson has delivery troubles or additional medical problems as a result of HSV, the clinician may need to explain the circumstances to her husband. What does Ms. Larson want Dr. Haladay to say then?

Maintaining confidentiality becomes more complicated and complex with each step. Dr. Haladay has friendships with both Larsons and the extra-marital partner, outside of work. Each friendship is important, and their families' frequent interactions as members of the same house of worship extend the difficulty. Again, clinician stress is extenuated by being in a "no-win" position, and with the potential inability to discuss the tension with colleagues or at home. In addition to this, Dr. Haladay faces the potential for more infected patients if all parties are not notified and treated. How can Dr. Haladay achieve the public health goal of reducing the number of the community's sexually transmitted infections, when truth-telling does not occur?

**RESPONDING TO REPRODUCTIVE
HEALTH CARE ETHICS CONFLICTS**

In both cases presented, the solutions to these issues are ideally negotiated within the clinical setting, based on professional guidelines that set clear expectations for care. First, clinicians should provide medical care that is evidence-based, and in accordance with professional standards to ensure the quality of patient care. Secondly, clinicians, within the context of the fiduciary patient-clinician relationship, should provide all the needed information in a confidential manner to foster a shared decision-making process. Thirdly, clinicians and their staff should ensure that they are adhering to the legal requirements, including making written information available for all patients regarding their privacy and confidentiality policies.

BOX 13.7

PROFESSIONAL GUIDELINES FOR REPRODUCTIVE HEALTH CARE

- Appropriate medical care is provided to patients seeking care
- Information exchanged at the office is confidential
- Act in in manner consistent with federal and state laws

CASE 13.1 | Birth control for a minor

Possible responses to the ethics issues presented by Sally Rosenthal's request for birth control and confidentiality depend on the relationship the clinician builds with Sally over the next months. The conflict stemming from the friendship with Sally's parents might be addressed in one of three ways. One possibility would be for Dr. Bennally to agree with Sally's request and to give her the prescription. This would respect Sally's preferences, but might upset her parents greatly in the future, when and if they learn of Sally's activities and the clinician's silence. Another option is to agree with Sally's request and give her the prescription, but encourage her to talk with her parents in the future. The third option would be to agree with Sally's request now, give her the prescription, and at her next appointment offer to play a supportive role in a conversation between her and her parents. In any case, the first option should be honored. Sally should obtain the care requested, and her privacy should be respected. However, Dr. Bennally should also work to achieve option two or three, as they are both clinically and ethically appropriate in this social context. The family and friendship values are secondary to the medical and clinical care needs, but they are important values for the clinician and the community.

Thus, Dr. Bennally should offer Sally the requested birth control and related education, but she should also open the conversation with Sally about talking with her parents. Dr. Bennally should encourage, either at this or a later appointment, discussions about loving relationships, responsible sexual behaviors, and family values. The clinician should also express her willingness to be a part of the discussions because of their importance. The primary relationship between Sally and Dr. Bennally is to obtain the needed birth control while the secondary or larger relationship invites the additional discussion. (In fact, Sally's boyfriend may also be invited to be part of the discussions, depending on how the options unfold.)

The second ethics conflict in Sally's case has to do with billing. Billing is a clinical-systems issue that each clinic needs to address specifically. The clinician does need to be aware of the institution's billing practice, including whether the information included on third-party billing documentation can be controlled. These confidentiality and privacy issues may result in only one alternative—that the patient pays cash for the services rendered and for any medication as well.

The third conflict refers to what the clinician might say if complications were to arise. This issue requires a conversation at this same appointment with Sally. Just as Sally has taken responsibility for her sexual actions with the request for birth control, Dr. Bennally should discuss with Sally the potential consequences of pregnancy or sexually transmitted infections.

CASE 13.2 | Managing and treating sexually transmitted infections

Possible solutions to the conflicts presented in Joan Larson's case depend on how open she becomes to her circumstances in the next months. For the conflict involving a referral to an obstetrician, two options may be possible, depending on the specific circumstances in the rural setting. Ms. Larson has requested that nothing be written in the chart. However this increases the risk of limiting the care Ms. Larson receives from the consultant, both now and in the future. If there is no written recording of the care needed or rendered now, then when Ms. Larson needs additional care in the future, the consultant and her partners will not be able build on previous information, or offer what may be appropriate urgent care at the time of delivery. Thus, it is important to do the proper charting[9] and reassure Ms. Larson that the referral and related paperwork will be protected by the confidentiality of the medical records system. Certainly to do this requires careful and continuing work with the clinic staff. There are civil and criminal penalties for HIPAA violations which can include firing staff who do not maintain the ethical obligation of confidentiality.

In terms of billing, payment will need to be managed by the billing portion of the clinical system (as described previously). Any options for future care require ongoing and evolving conversations with Ms. Larson as the pregnancy develops and her relationships evolve. Dr. Haladay has reason to believe that there may be a need for further interventions because of the HSV, and Ms. Larson is likely to need to explain the circumstances to her husband eventually. Ms. Larson can participate by either having that conversation herself, or by stating what she would like Dr. Haladay to say.

Dr. Haladay's overlapping relationships in this case can lead to clinician stress and require that he find ways to manage the stress while maintaining confidentiality. This stress is amplified by his concern that maintaining confidentiality could risk the community's overall health by increasing sexually transmitted infections. Deciding to pursue the goal of reducing community sexually transmitted infections (STIs) results in the need to confront the community stigmatization of the condition and the behaviors that spread it—in truth-telling at a more extensive level.

To confront this issue at the community level, the clinician can schedule public forums at the clinic, and provide handouts, posters, and clinic Web site information. In addition, the clinician can offer to provide health education classes in the local high school to discuss STIs and related issues. In these ways, the truth-telling is in revealing that the disease(s) are active in the community, while protecting individuals' confidence and privacy.

ANTICIPATING REPRODUCTIVE HEALTH CARE ETHICS CONFLICTS

Relationships between clinicians and patients are complex, and when they occur in rural settings they are not anonymous. In smaller communities, everyone knows one another and there are multiple overlapping relationships.[4] This is the reality within which rural practitioners establish their clinics and work with patients and families. Drawing guidelines is therefore helpful; some suggestions are offered in Box 13.8.

Professional and personal guidelines can be indispensable in creating a practice in which both patients and clinicians know what to expect, particularly when facing the consequences of sexual and reproductive relationships.

Provide Appropriate Medical Care

Two professional health care goals are essential to the structure and function of a clinic in anticipating ethics issues that relate to reproductive

BOX 13.8

PROFESSIONAL AND PERSONAL GUIDELINES
IN THE MANAGEMENT OF REPRODUCTIVE ISSUES

- Provide appropriate medical care
- Assure confidentiality of clinical information
- Maintain clear boundaries in professional relationships
- Be aware of the law and institutional policies and procedures
- Define and examine one's own personal values

health care. First, it is crucial to always extend the best and most appropriate medical care available to all patients.[3] When a patient raises sexual or reproductive health concerns, the patient care available should not be dependent on, nor diminished by, any personal shame or community stigma. Patients may choose not to follow a clinician's recommendation, but state-of-the-art care should always be available and offered. For example, Ms. Larson may never be honest with her husband about her illness, but she still deserves to be given the best available treatments, and her pregnancy needs to be protected.

Assuring Confidentiality of Clinical Information
Information exchanged at the office must be confidential, whether spoken, written, or electronically recorded. Confidentiality must be a prime concern in a rural clinic—and reinforced through hiring, firing, and in-service education. Although confidentiality can be very difficult to maintain in a small community, it is one of the prime ways in which patients (and clinicians) are harmed within the medical setting.[1, 2, 4] As referenced in both cases, charting and billing records are essential in maintaining confidentiality, too.

Maintain Clear Boundaries in Professional Relationships
It is essential for rural clinicians to establish clear boundaries between professional and personal relationships within the community.[1, 4] Personal relationships outside of the office can take many forms, but professional relationships within the clinic need to be strictly defined—and the expectations of confidentiality, responsibilities and obligations may need to be repeatedly stated and discussed with some patients and staff members. Over time, community members will come to know what they can expect and how they will be treated in each relationship setting. For example, if Sally Rosenthal and her parents see Dr. Bennally at a community function,

Sally can feel secure about her health information remaining confidential even though she is not at the clinic.

Recognize and Clarify One's Own Personal Values

A personal guideline is also critical for rural clinicians who care for patients with reproductive health issues. It is important for clinicians to take the time to know themselves and to be reflective about their personal views.[1, 8] Knowing and being able to state personal positions on birth control, abortion, and sexual liaisons, are the provider's first steps to objectivity and integrity in a practice including reproductive health care. They are also essential to truth-telling and managing clinician stress. Personal positions and insights can be supported through local or distant colleagues, and awareness of professional standards of practice. For particular concerns, consultation with local or regional ethics resources can also be helpful. This is especially true in the case of Dr. Haladay, who faces stress due to concerns not only for his patient with HSV, but also for the community. He can help to relieve some of that stress by confiding in a distant colleague or ethics network.

CONCLUSION

For the rural health care professional, it is essential to create a health care practice where community members can expect trust, respect, and safety in their patient-clinician relationships. This goal becomes critical when the practice includes reproductive health care, a specialty where providers may experience heightened ethics concerns regarding the management of clinical information. When health care is needed as a consequence of sexual activity that differs from the majority's culture or norms, the clinician and clinic can be put into a difficult position. Both the medical and social circumstances require appropriate care, confidentiality, truth-telling, and carefully defined boundaries.

To avoid conflicts that often arise in reproductive health care, the clinician may find that adhering to particular professional and personal guidelines can be indispensable. When the clinician establishes professional expectations, the patient will know and trust that he or she will receive appropriate care, whatever the circumstances, and that confidentiality of his or her clinical information will be carefully guarded. Clinician stress and patient-clinician relationships are also easier to manage when clinicians establish and maintain clear boundaries in their clinical relationships, take time to know their own views regarding sexual issues, and maintain supportive professional relationships with colleagues and ethics resources. These professional efforts on the part of the clinician can assure objectivity and integrity in a practice that includes reproductive care.

REFERENCES

1. Roberts LW, Battaglia J, Smithpeter M, Epstein RS. An office on Main Street. Health care dilemmas in small communities. *Hastings Cent Rep.* Jul-Aug 1999;29(4):28-37.

2. Purtilo R, Sorrell J. The ethical dilemmas of a rural physician. *Hastings Cent Rep.* Aug 1986;16(4):24-28.

3. Lo B. *Resolving Ethical Dilemmas: A Guide for Clinicians.* 2nd ed. Philadelphia, PA: Lippincott Williams & Wilkins; 2000.

4. Nelson W, Pomerantz A, Howard K, Bushy A. A proposed rural healthcare ethics agenda. *J Med Ethics.* Mar 2007;33(3):136-139.

5. Cook AF, Hoas H. Ethics and rural healthcare: what really happens? What might help? *Am J Bioeth.* Apr 2008;8(4):52-56.

6. Institute of Medicine. Committee on the Future of Rural Health Care. Board on Health Care Services. *Quality Through Collaboration: The Future of Rural Health* Washington, DC: National Academies Press; 2005.

7. Rudnick CM, Hoekzema GS. Neonatal herpes simplex virus infections. *Am Fam Physician.* Mar 15 2002;65(6):1138-1142.

8. Kaldjian LC, Weir RF, Duffy TP. A clinician's approach to clinical ethical reasoning. *J Gen Intern Med.* Mar 2005;20(3):306-311.

9. ACP Ethics and Human Rights Committee. Documenting sensitive information poses dilemma for physicians. *Am Coll Physicians Obs.* 1996(Dec.). http://www.acpinternist.org/archives/1996/12/sensinfo.htm. Accessed June 27, 2009.

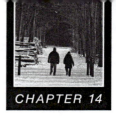

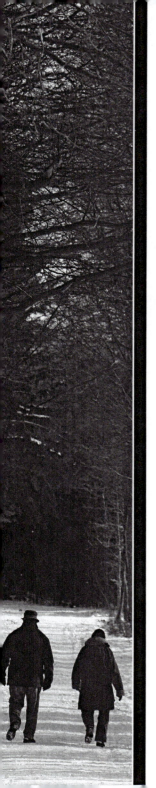

Ethics Conflicts in Rural Communities:
Health Information Technology

David A. Fleming

CHAPTER 14

Ethics Conflicts in Rural Communities: Health Information Technology

David A. Fleming

ABSTRACT

The use of health information technology (HIT) is becoming increasingly important in medical providers' efforts to support decision-making and to promote quality health care delivery and equitable access to services in rural areas. However, technological interventions in remote settings have attracted ethics concern and conflict. Complex patient information processes, service shortages, high demand, and a widening array of medical interventions and treatments constantly challenge health care providers as they struggle to maintain standards of care. For patients in rural areas, barriers to reasonable access for even basic health care services, such as primary care, screenings, and prevention, are also common. Numerous technologies have been introduced in recent years to remote sites, with the intention of enhancing quality and improving access. However, as with any well-meaning and innovative medical advance, these technologies bring both intended and unintended consequences to the lives and welfare of patients. This chapter will address four domains of health information technology: telehealth, electronic medical records, electronic clinical support, and online prescribing services. These technologies bear careful scrutiny when deployed in rural settings, due to both the nature of the setting and the complexity of the technology. When deploying HIT in any setting, rural or urban, health care providers must place patient welfare above all other considerations, protect confidentiality, ensure privacy, promote trust in the healing relationship, and ensure fair and equitable access to quality services.

CASE STUDIES

CASE 14.1 | Privacy and consent issues when
using telehealth in rural areas

Gina Conti is 75 years old, with multiple chronic medical conditions
including severe rheumatoid arthritis. She lives in a rural chronic-
care nursing facility, and requires a wheelchair to get around. Mrs.
Conti was recently seen by her family physician for a persistent rash.
Following several failed diagnoses and treatments, her physician
recommended referral to a dermatologist at a university hospital
60 miles away. Neither Mrs. Conti nor her physician feels that she
can make a trip of this kind due to her fragile condition, but since
the local hospital is part of the university's telehealth network, Mrs.
Conti agrees to have the dermatology consultation done remotely.
Mrs. Conti is not sure what to expect, and has only been informed
that she will, "… be seeing a skin doctor on the TV screen." Upon
arrival at the local hospital, Mrs. Conti is taken to a room near the
emergency room waiting area where the dermatologist appears on a
videoconferencing screen. Mrs. Conti feels a little uneasy while talking
to the dermatologist on the screen, especially when the dermatologist
asks the nurse to disrobe Mrs. Conti so her rash can be examined.
The nurse is instructed to use a special camera for a closer
examination of the rash on Mrs. Conti's buttocks, and scrapings are
taken and sent to the lab. Mrs. Conti notices that the dermatologist
seems to be talking to someone else, but it isn't until the session is
almost over that she realizes that a student and resident have been
present off-camera, without her knowledge or permission having
been requested. When Mrs. Conti is wheeled out of the telehealth
room, she feels as though people in the ER waiting room are staring.
She is grateful to have seen a skin specialist without having to travel
far, but wonders why her physician didn't give her more advance
warning about what to expect in the video consultation.

CASE 14.2 | Availability of, and access to,
electronic medical records (EMR)

Dr. Adams, a rural general internist, is on call for his three-person
group. He is in the ER seeing a patient who normally sees one of

Dr. Adams' partners. Lars Danielson is a 57-year-old male, who was referred to an out-of-town cardiologist last week for evaluation of recurrent chest pain. Mr. Danielson is concerned because he is still having chest pain, and wants to know more about the previous tests, and why he is on so many new medications. He feels dizzy and nauseated and thinks it might be due to one of the new drugs, so he has stopped taking them all. Dr. Adams has Mr. Danielson's medical record, and there is no information from the cardiologist, other than a brief discharge summary stating, "inoperable coronary artery disease," and a list of several new medicines. The letter indicates that the patient's electronic medical record (EMR) provides a full account of his hospital stay. Dr. Adams' group uses a paper record system, and the clinic has only one computer, used only for billing and appointments. Although it would be useful, Dr. Adams' group can't afford an EMR system. If they had the system, however, he still wouldn't be able to access the patient's hospital record because his clinic is not in the same networked health care system as the cardiologist's hospital. Dr. Adams will have to call the referral hospital to get a faxed copy of the patient's record. Meanwhile, Mr. Danielson is complaining of chest pain and becomes short of breath.

CASE 14.3 | Using electronic clinical decision support systems

Robert Taft is a 65-year-old general contractor in a small rural community. He has been unusually tired for several days, and while at a construction site, he becomes very nauseated and fatigued. When symptoms persist for 20 minutes, he agrees to be driven to the emergency department of his 20-bed community hospital. When the physician, Dr. Kimberly Russell, arrives 15 minutes later, Mr. Taft feels much better except for mild fatigue. Dr. Russell examines Mr. Taft and finds no abnormalities other than mild blood pressure elevation and a slightly rapid pulse. Lab work is normal, and an ECG is electronically interpreted as having "nonspecific ST abnormalities." Still concerned, Dr. Russell performs a second ECG using new software that electronically interprets and predicts the probability of cardiac ischemia. The second ECG report estimates an "80% probability of cardiac ischemia." With this information, Mr. Taft agrees to be transferred to a university hospital. There, a cardiac catheterization finds a 95% blockage in one of his coronary arteries, which is then dilated and stented. No cardiac damage is found, and Mr. Taft returns to work the following week.

CASE 14.4 | Addressing patient use of online
treatment and prescribing services

Gwen Thompson lives alone in a remote rural area. She frequently
goes online to get information, and to obtain goods and services
that are not easily accessible due to her isolation. She has recently
been diagnosed with hypertension, but finds it difficult to keep
appointments at the clinic 20 miles away. Ms. Thompson ran out of
one blood pressure medicine several weeks ago and has been feeling
light-headed. She also noticed that her blood pressure has been
running high. It is winter, the roads are bad, and she fears going out,
so she begins taking double the prescribed daily dose of the other
blood pressure medication that she has not run out of. While surfing
the net, she finds *CyberDocs.com* and discovers that a "virtual house
call" can be obtained for a modest fee, so she requests a "house
call...." That same day a physician (in a different state) responds
online and Ms. Thompson describes her symptoms, gives her recent
blood pressure readings, and mentions that she has run out of
medication. The physician offers to provide a one-month prescription,
and even arranges for quick mail delivery of the medication. One
week later, Ms. Thompson is found unconscious by a neighbor. At
the hospital, she is diagnosed with acute kidney failure, possibly a
result of taking two different prescribed diuretics, one from her regular
physician and the other from *CyberDocs*. She ultimately recovers, but
the kidney damage is irreversible, and sadly, she will require chronic
dialysis. Ms. Thompson's attorney contacts *CyberDocs.com*, but
the prescribing physician no longer contracts with them. *CyberDocs*
claims that since no face-to-face contact occurred, no patient-
clinician relationship existed and, therefore, there was no professional
duty to "do no harm." *CyberDocs* also argues that printed warnings
of risk came with the prescription when it was delivered. Arguing that
this was a contracted service with full disclosure of potential risk,
CyberDocs is unwilling to accept any obligation or responsibility for
Ms. Thompson's situation.

OVERVIEW OF ETHICS ISSUES

More than ever, health care is being driven by the need to access and
use health information technology (HIT), regardless of where services
are delivered. Modern technological innovations increasingly influence
standards of care, by allowing patients and providers to be better informed.

This enables more effective diagnosis and treatment of illness, and improves the relief of suffering. Patients are also uniquely empowered, because they are now able to access health information directly, without depending on physicians, clinics, and hospitals to select what they read and hear about health and health care. Although the quality of Web-based health information may be questionable (particularly with regard to meeting standards of evidence-based medical care), and subject to commercial influence, health information is readily available and easily accessible by almost everyone. This means that many patients are better informed, and feel more empowered to participate as partners in the decision-making. Ethically, this is beneficial as long as the information the patient receives is accurate, appropriate, and does not result in greater harm than if the patient had had no information at all. For providers, the day-to-day use of electronic sources of information is unavoidable. In fact, there are few health care interventions today that do not directly or indirectly incorporate health information technology in some fashion. These basic health information technologies (HIT) are summarized below.

- **Telehealth:** Delivery of health-related services and information via telecommunications technologies, including both health care and education
- **Electronic Medical Records:** Computer-based patient records
- **Electronic Clinical Support Systems:** Computer-based knowledge management technologies that support the clinical decision-making process from diagnosis and investigation through treatment and recovery
- **Online Health Care Resources:** Web-based resources that market to health care consumers, as well as providers, linking to information and education about products, medical and dental services, alternative health care, hospitals, providers, employment, publications, and mental health

Traditionally, health care technologies have been developed and introduced predominantly by scientists and physicians for the good of patients. When needed, patients are informed about the technologies or interventions that their clinicians recommend to further their health, and together, patients and physicians decide on a course of treatment. Interventions, such as radiology, surgery, and intravenous therapy, are utilized in the doctor's office or hospital, and are available to patients only through the guiding hand and advice of their provider. Hopefully, patients benefit from the use of these technologies.

In the modern paradigm, however, patients and providers seek health information technology both independently and in partnership. This new paradigm may require adjustment, as multiple individuals and organizations relinquish control over information at some level when it is freely accessible. Even in rural areas where access to technology is often difficult, patients are becoming increasingly empowered and many seek to be partners in the pursuit and use of HIT. The traditional moral precepts, including autonomy, beneficence, nonmaleficence, justice, and confidentiality, that shape our professional behavior while caring for patients, remain the same.[1] However, we must never lose sight of them. These principles are discussed in more detail in Chapter 3 of this *Handbook*.

As information technologies evolve and become available, the skills necessary to access and employ them likewise become increasingly sophisticated. As availability grows, so will the risk that misinformation, missed information, and misused information will potentially lead to poor quality and dissatisfied users. Multiple forms of informational technology, including cell phones, personal digital assistants (PDAs), and laptop computers are now commonplace even in rural settings. The ethical concern for information integrity brings a parallel concern regarding privacy and confidentiality, when electronic devices are used outside the relatively secure confines of homes, cars, and offices. Health information technology may also dramatically impact the relationships between providers and patients, the quality of care, and the clinical outcomes. In response to these external forces, health care providers must remain focused on their primary goal of providing high-quality care. Therefore, a prudent and balanced approach is needed when introducing new health information technologies.

Balancing Ethical Obligations to Patients with Technology Usage

When using health information technology, unintended harms must be considered in pursuit of the intended good.[2] Of utmost concern are patient confidentiality and autonomy. Respecting patient autonomy requires that clinicians do everything in their power to ensure privacy, and to respect the patient's right to make informed decisions.[1] The ethical obligations pertain to actions taken on patients' behalf, to improve their health status and protect their personal information. For example, meeting this obligation may be achieved by clinicians' providing local access to specialty care using telehealth systems, as in the dermatology case, and improving standards of care in the use of electronic decision support. Respect for autonomy, however, requires that information regarding patient encounters be kept private, whether obtained in person or via electronic (virtual) means, unless the patient requests or gives permission to have personal information shared.[3] This task can be especially difficult when the clinical encounter is "broadcast" beyond the privacy of an exam room. When using e-mail, telephone, videoconferencing, or other electronic means, one can never be completely sure who is gleaning information on the other end of the line, or even tapping into such information as it is being sent across the network.

A broader ethics concern is that confidentiality may become less important, or more difficult to enforce, as health information technologies become more universally available and applied, particularly as human curiosity continues to promote behavior that derails even the most secure system.[4] Breaches in confidentiality can be both visual and auditory. Such breeches may be quite innocent, such as when a passer-by inadvertently views or hears a provider's videoconference interactions with patients. Other concerns include unauthorized viewing of patient images or clinic notes in an electronic database that is shared by providers, and/or unauthorized retrieval of patient information from a protected database by staff members for purposes other than billing or quality assurance. Unauthorized viewing of patient information of any kind—intentional or unintentional, whether written, electronic, or auditory—is unethical and, typically, not in compliance with the law or regulatory policies regarding privacy.[5]

Improving access has also become an ethical imperative for HIT. The use of electronic medical records (EMR) and electronic decision support in emergency rooms and other clinical settings is increasingly commonplace. In fact, they are becoming the standard of care in many clinical domains. But significant economic and logistical barriers impede widespread adoption of these tools.[6] Finding cost-effective ways to implement technology where it is most needed may help solve one of the most challenging problems confronting health care today—the uneven distribution and relative shortage of specialty providers in rural areas. Despite concerted efforts by federal and state governments over the past 30 years to address this problem, mal-distribution of skills and provider shortages in rural areas persist.[7] In dermatology, for instance, although the workforce has risen in recent years (presently 3.4 per 100,000 population, compared to 1.8 in 1965 and 2.8 in 1985), there continues to be a major migration of newly trained dermatologists to metropolitan areas. Dermatologists tend to move away from underserved areas (poor urban and rural locations), where they are increasingly needed.[8] Therefore, many patients in remote areas who need treatment don't get it at all, or often delay care until it is too late because they find it difficult or impossible to travel long distances for clinic appointments. This is particularly true for those individuals at greatest risk, including the elderly and chronically ill. These patients are particularly vulnerable to geographic, physical, cognitive, or economic barriers to health care services. Telehealth and other forms of health information technology are important resources in making the lives of these and other rural patients safer, healthier, and more comfortable.

Telehealth: Telehealth is one means by which rural patients can gain access to health care when needed services are a prohibitive distance away. However, the location and accessibility of telehealth may still be a problem for those who find traveling even short distances a challenge, such as debilitated patients and those in nursing homes. Telehealth technology is typically nonportable, and some patients will still have to travel some distance to gain access. Providing telehealth services is primarily an organizational concern with significant fiscal up-front costs, although over time the service pays for itself in savings on travel and in-person visits at the tertiary center. There can be a high cost also in installation and maintenance of the equipment. Rural telehealth units are typically in hospitals or clinics, and may be located hundreds of miles from the tertiary care centers and specialty providers who offer the telehealth services. How these services are financially supported, and subsequently reimbursed, is a fiduciary concern that must be addressed—since both the initiating site and the specialty provider must pay up front for the equipment, and then must dedicate ongoing resources during telehealth "visits." Deploying telehealth requires an additional financial investment that rural hospitals may not have.

Electronic Medical Record: Between 30 and 40% of rural hospitals report using computers to collect basic clinical information that could potentially be used in an electronic medical record (EMR) or computerized provider order entry (CPOE) system.[9] Even though hospitals and clinics have been under great pressure to incorporate HIT for purposes of quality improvement and patient safety, many have been slow to comply, because to do so requires a significant investment of money, time, and human resources. Most clinic and hospital administrators simply feel that they don't have the resources to afford EMR systems. Even if EMR systems were deployed in today's networked health care system, the chance of interoperability among EMR systems is essentially nil for the time being. Electronic records are individually contracted and "firewalled," so outside persons or systems cannot be allowed in. The emerging national and international privacy standards that have created this morass of impenetrability are in response to both legal and ethical requirements that health systems and individual providers must maintain the confidentiality of patient information.[10]

Electronic Clinical Decision Support Systems: Several preliminary studies are encouraging in this arena. One recent study found that physicians using a cardiac ischemia predictive instrument provided an accurate diagnosis to triage patients with chest pain.[11] In another study, an Internet-based antimicrobial prescribing support system improved prescribing behavior in rural Idaho physicians, although organizational and cultural barriers to behavioral change were still evident.[12] These are compelling data, but many physicians still resist the use of electronic triage systems because they feel that experience, knowledge, wisdom, and skill are still the gold standard—as well they should be. Physicians have a professional obligation to hone their skills and utilize knowledge to provide optimal care for their patients. Wisdom, though variably defined, comes with years of experience, instinct, and knowledge of patients with whom physicians have developed long and trusting relationships. Physicians who first rely on their mind, instinct, and senses, and then use technology to confirm their clinical suspicions may be wary lest technology and "informatics" become the driving force in health care, thereby supplanting the "art" of diagnostic and therapeutic excellence. Paradoxically, if electronically derived information about patients becomes the prime focus of attention, the welfare of those same patients may actually become subsidiary to the welfare and integrity of the information itself—even though it is the patient's information to begin with. Decision support and informatics will be an increasingly important means to good health care in the future, but their use and integrity should never be considered the goal of health care.

Use of Online Health Resources: Rural areas have historically trailed urban regions in the use of computers and the Internet; however, this trend is changing. Malecki informs us that Internet access rates for rural households now approximate those of urban areas.[13] There is an expanding and seemingly limitless wealth of information now available to health care consumers everywhere, even in remote areas. However, individuals seeking online information are also often seeking advice, which makes patients vulnerable to misinformation in times of need. As a free society, anyone can publish and offer opinions on the Web, so judging the reliability of scientific and health-related Web sites becomes the responsibility of each individual user. Thus, online research becomes a very challenging—if not precarious—enterprise for those seeking health care. As health information becomes increasingly marketed, commercial influence will be unavoidable in determining what and how information is conveyed. Information may also express unilateral—and therefore biased—opinions of a particular group or organization. Online information of this pedigree is potentially misleading, erroneous, or misinterpreted, and may lead to inappropriate and even harmful decision support for patients.[14]

The laudable incentive for online health information is to provide timely and easily accessible opportunities for patient education and decision support. In *Crossing the Quality Chasm*, the Institute of Medicine (IOM) proposed guidelines for developing an improved health care system.[15] The IOM recommended that health care systems and society improve patients' access to personal medical information and to clinical knowledge. This system they envision would be one in which patients would have unprecedented control of personal health information, and broad access to knowledge. Patients who are better informed will hopefully be encouraged by, and have improved communication with, their physicians and other providers. Evidence-based and reliable online resources, such as those offered by the National Library of Medicine through *MedLine Plus*, offer a tremendous boost to patient understanding. Resources like *MedLine Plus* are particularly effective when used in partnership with, and guided by, health care providers with whom the patient has a close, trusting relationship.

CASE DISCUSSION

The following case analyses were interpreted using a method similar to that presented in Chapter 4.

CASE 14.1 | Privacy and consent issues when using telehealth in rural areas

It would be difficult and perhaps dangerous for Gina Conti to travel a long distance to see a dermatologist. She is thankful that specialty consultation and care can be obtained locally through telehealth. The process is a bit unnerving and uncomfortable for her, though, especially when she is instructed to disrobe on camera. Mrs. Conti also feels exposed due to the proximity of the telehealth room to the emergency waiting room. Most egregiously, Mrs. Conti is disturbed after discovering that other trainees were present with the dermatologist during the telehealth "virtual visit" and examination, about which she was neither notified nor asked to give permission. The ethics concerns involving telehealth are described in brief in Box 14.1.

BOX 14.1

ETHICS CONCERNS IN THE USE OF TELEHEALTH

- Lack of maintaining privacy and confidentiality
- Lack of adequate patient informed consent
- Inadequate disclosure of the possible presence of other clinicians or trainees
- Lack of informed consent for the presence of others, photos being taken and stored, biopsy, or scrapings, or telehealth intervention
- Potential loss of trust between patient and provider

Overall, Mrs. Conti is pleased to be able to see a dermatologist without having to travel a long distance, although she would have appreciated being fully informed about what to expect, including being asked for permission to have others present during the interview and examination. Mrs. Conti was also not told what would become of the photos taken of her skin lesion.

Unquestionably, Mrs. Conti has benefited medically by seeing a specialist via telehealth. But her primary care physician and the dermatologist conducting the telehealth visit should have been more forthcoming about how the visit would be conducted and who, given the patient's permission, would be present. The physical disconnect that occurs with telehealth visits also threatens to undermine clinical relationships and trust, if special attention is not given to the emotional, as well as physical, distance.

CASE 14.2 | Availability of, and access to, electronic medical records (EMR)

The irony in the scenario of the Electronic Medical Record is that one ethical requirement (confidentiality and respect for patient autonomy) impedes the ability to effectively respond to other ethical requirements in the care and safety of patients. In Case 2, it is very difficult for Dr. Adams to effectively treat the patient, Lars Danielson, because the doctor does not have access to important patient information from another hospital. This case exemplifies the frustration that many rural physicians feel when decision-making for a returning patient is hampered by the inability to obtain records from a hospital or provider to which the patient had been referred. Patient harm could be avoided if contingencies were put in place to ensure that critical information is shared, especially when critically needed, such as in this case during an ER visit. Hospital systems and physicians have an obligation to ensure that mutual patient information is shared in a timely fashion—whether or not mutually compatible EMRs exist. Most rural hospitals and physicians don't have electronic systems; therefore, traditional means of communication will need to be used until compatible electronic records allow immediate access to medical information. It is difficult for physicians like Dr. Adams to prevent harm and promote patient autonomy and equitable treatment when information is restricted in this fashion.

This case scenario demonstrates an ethics problem that extends beyond the individual professional concern of two physicians to encompass a greater organizational issue. If health care systems are going to implement information systems like EMRs, and require physicians and staff to use them, as well as firewall them to ensure protection, then parallel mechanisms must be implemented to ensure that important information is made available in a timely fashion. Organizations should ensure that mechanisms are put in place that allow electronic information to be transmitted to referring physicians quickly and effectively. The *prima facie* nature of autonomy dictates that we do everything we can to prevent harm; in this case, by using a "firewall" system to ensure patient privacy and confidentiality. However, autonomy does not dictate that we demand privacy at all costs, if in doing so we compromise patient welfare and the physician's ability to do his or her job. Dr. Adams, the cardiologist, and their respective hospitals should establish policies and practices that communicate patient information in a way that is both secure and efficient, so that patients can receive the best possible care available from both facilities.

CASE 14.3 | Using electronic clinical decision support systems

Rural citizens have a right to expect that their health care needs will be met with certain basic standards of care. Case 3 has a positive outcome on many levels[16] and reflects the potential for moral distress that remote health care providers often feel when trying to ensure access to equitable standards of care. Mr. Taft does well because Dr. Russell is able to meet his acuity needs using decision support technology, thus providing him with a higher standard of care than might normally have been available. More importantly, perhaps, are the warm feelings and renewed trust that Mr. Taft, and perhaps others in the community, now have for Dr. Russell, and the local hospital that employs her. The fact that Mr. Taft returns "well" to his job and community is due, in large part, to the superlative care that she has given him, which is reinforced by the decision support technology deployed by the hospital. Similar stories are playing throughout the world, where access to quality educational and clinical support is being provided electronically in rural and remote regions.[17]

CASE 14.4 | Addressing patient use of online treatment and prescribing services

In Case 4, Gwen Thompson seeks online information, "cyber" advice, and treatment from a doctor she has never met, with whom she has no prior relationship, and who is later unavailable. This *"Cyberdoc"* has only a cursory working knowledge of her situation and, therefore, is unaware of potentially serious complications. Though prescribing guidelines for *CyberDocs.com* only permit giving a one-month prescription, this is enough to result in irreversible harm for Ms. Thompson. No face-to-face contact occurs between this doctor and patient; thus, *Cyberdoc* argues that no "duty" exists beyond a contractual relationship based solely on the buying and selling of goods (in this case, information and a prescription for medication). However, the unique nature of patient-clinician relationships requires accountability through shared trust, an awareness of vulnerability, and a fiduciary response to the patient' needs—regardless of how or where the interaction occurred.[18] Therefore, the *Cyberdoc* is ethically responsible for Ms. Thompson's treatment and the unfortunate resulting complications.

RESPONDING TO HEALTH INFORMATION TECHNOLOGY ETHICS CONFLICTS

CASE 14.1 | Privacy and consent issues when using telehealth in rural areas

Beware of the burden of technology. For patients who suffer from chronic conditions and those who reside in long-term care facilities, the perceived benefit of telehealth may be overshadowed by the foreign experience of videoconferencing. To speak to a doctor via video may be unpleasant or strange for older and chronically ill patients, further adding to their burden of illness. Patients may feel overwhelmed by the technology itself, or by the geographic and emotional distance that they sense between them and their provider when technology is used.[19] Medical staff members may pick up on the patient's discomfort, creating their own internal struggle. Gina Conti is uncomfortable with the situation she finds herself in and, though it isn't discussed directly in the case example, the nurse provider may also

1

1

feel moral discomfort after witnessing Mrs. Conti's distress. Facilitating a discussion about these issues could provide guidance in resolving this case and similar cases in the future. Preparation for telehealth experiences might include some of the suggested tasks listed in Box 14.2.

BOX 14.2

PREPARING FOR TELEHEALTH EXPERIENCES

- Educate nurses and physicians involved in telehealth and related activities about the importance of full disclosure and transparency, as well as what the clinicians may expect of the patient
- When patients become distressed, it is important to provide reassurance, and to further inform the patient and his or her family about the nature, benefits, and risks of the telehealth service being offered
- Patients have the right to refuse, and should be given the information necessary for informed decision-making, including any potential negative aspects of the telehealth experience

Many patients embrace new technologies, once they have become accustomed to them and encouraged by their use. Sometimes patients actually feel more satisfied and closer to their provider(s), knowing that they have more immediate access as a result of telehealth and other forms of HIT.[20] Therefore, at the first sign of discomfort or conflict, it is important for the provider to optimize communication, clarify the issues, and resolve misunderstandings. This requires time and availability. Often, a meeting of all stakeholders can be very helpful, including the patient, family, and care team members. A clinical ethics consultant may also be helpful to facilitate a discussion, including understanding the ethics questions related to HIT, what ethics concepts relate to those questions, what are the value perceptions from all stakeholders, and what possible means exist for conflict resolution.

In the case of Gina Conti, the discomfort and sense of exposure she feels during her tele-dermatology visit would likely be averted if the care team were to ensure a private environment, and effectively communicate with Mrs. Conti about what to expect during the telehealth visit. Improved communication would allow this patient to make a truly informed decision regarding whether or not to be seen via telehealth. The team also should be transparent about who, besides the dermatologist, would be participating.

This could be accomplished by panning the consultant's room with the camera at the beginning of the video visit, and introducing all participants to the patient, while also asking permission for other trainees or clinicians to be there. Virtual visits can be as comfortable and satisfying as face-to-face visits, for all patients, including children, when special attention is given to issues of patient privacy, camera comfort, and specialist comfort.

CASE 14.2 | Availability of, and access to, electronic medical records (EMR)

Case 2 presents a challenging situation because relatively few rural practices, only about one in five, have access to electronic medical record systems.[21] From both an ethical and professional standpoint, this case underscores the obligation of individual physicians and organizations to meet reasonable standards of care, by utilizing available technologies to ensure safe and equitable health care for all patients. The operative word in this claim, however, is "available." In this case Dr. Adams will likely be forced to be much more aggressive in the use of medical resources in treating Lars Danielson, unless outside hospital records are readily available at the time they are needed. Without the information from the cardiologist, Dr. Adams will no doubt treat Mr. Danielson aggressively, as if the other recent hospitalization had not occurred. Dr. Adams is obligated to provide optimal care in response to the information and technologies available. In the interest of good patient care, there is also an obligation to communicate with the referral hospital and to garner as much information as possible, but this will take time. In the meantime, Mr. Danielson must be treated.

The ethics challenge to meet modern standards of care in the use and transmission of health information should be addressed at the organizational level. Modern health care is informatics-driven, and electronic health records have been available in recent years to securely transmit patient data, both between physicians, and among different health care systems. These systems help to coordinate the care of patients with both acute and chronic conditions. Accurate, timely and secure information sharing is critically important for providers when the care of patients is shared between clinicians on different systems. In Box 14.3, three recommendations are offered regarding the implementation of electronic records to enhance care coordination.

To meet the electronic record challenge in future cases like that of Dr. Adams' patient, Mr. Danielson, the medical staff and hospital leadership

BOX 14.3

ENHANCING CARE USING ELECTRONIC MEDICAL RECORDS (EMR)

- Create a common health record to facilitate the exchange of clinical information among health providers
- Create regional governance structures to encourage the exchange of clinical data
- Initiate payment by purchasers of care, both public and private, to physicians for using electronic health records

in both the rural clinic and tertiary hospital should jointly advocate at the organizational and societal level to develop systems that will communicate information, both internally and between systems, when the care and treatment of patients is shared among institutions.[22] Individual physicians, systems, and society must work together to negotiate to make information accessible when and where it is needed. The logistical and ethical challenge of achieving standardization, so that electronic systems will talk to each other, is a major challenge. However, optimal communication and information sharing between providers for the welfare of patients is an ultimate and worthy goal if universal access to quality health care—and sustainability of that care—is to be attained.

CASE 14.3 | Using electronic clinical decision support systems

Case 3 demonstrates both clinical and organizational ethics concerns that relate to meeting new and evolving standards of care resulting from the availability of new technologies. Robert Taft experiences a good outcome, at least in part, because the remote clinic has access to computer-based decision support software that helps providers to make complex clinical decisions where specialty expertise is not available. The ethics challenge is one of ensuring equitable and safe health care that meets modern standards. It has been demonstrated that decision support systems can improve the quality of clinical decisions in the primary care setting.[23] However, the study's authors caution that considerable work is needed to ensure that the introduction of this technology is not detrimental to the quality of the relationship between the doctor and patient. They also advise that providers ensure that systems are adaptable to local needs and practices, and are acceptable to both physicians and patients. A careful analysis is needed in each health care system before introducing new technologies, to ensure that they are a good fit for all parties, including staff and patients who jointly will use them. New technologies should be introduced in a manner that ensures patient safety, through effective training and other quality assurance measures.

Happily, Case 3 has a good outcome, which results from the effective use of decision support technology. The physician makes the correct diagnosis, Mr. Taft does well and is happy with the outcome, and thus no ethics conflict arises. This might not have been the result, however, had the technology not been available when it was needed and wanted, if it had failed to perform as designed, or if the physician had been ill-prepared or unwilling to use it. In each case the patient might have had a bad outcome, due to a delay in appropriate diagnosis and treatment. An ethical analysis of the case again demonstrates that a patient-centered approach, equitable access, and quality health care are necessary precursors for a successful implementation of this technology by providers and systems investing in it. Providers and health care organizations must advocate together to ensure that reasonable and equitable access to evidence-based technologies is made available to patients when need is demonstrated, patients are accepting, and providers are willing and able to use such technologies. Access, quality, and benefit are the defining variables, and should never be subjugated to the economic gain of the physician or the system in which the physician practices.

CASE 14.4 | Addressing patient use of online treatment and prescribing services

The ethics concerns in Case 4 are clear. Gwen Thompson was harmed following inappropriate pharmaceutical treatment by a physician who did not know or examine her, but still responded by prescribing a medication. Because no face-to-face contact between the doctor and patient occurred, it could be argued that no professional duty exists. However, the professional relationship is implied by the fact that medical advice and treatment was requested, and the *Cyberdoc* agreed to provide it; thus the patient-physician relationship was formed. By responding to the call for help, a professional promise was made confluent with the professional oath that defines the practice of medicine. A similar argument of fiduciary responsibility can be made for on-call physicians who prescribe medications sight-unseen for patients of whom they know little; the professional responsibility for safety and quality does not abate after hours or on weekends. Overall, there was a failure in the fiduciary responsibility that physicians, by the nature of their healing profession, traditionally have for patients, by the nature of their vulnerability and need.

Physicians and health care systems play an important role in forewarning and educating patients about dangerous practices, and encouraging state law enforcement and regulatory officials to take action against physicians who engage in illegal and unethical online practices. The FDA also encourages physicians and patients to report potentially illegal Web sites to the FDA or to the National Association of Boards of Pharmacy.[24] Although patients and their families clearly have the right to seek other opinions, and pursue other treatment options beyond what is recommended, physicians still have an indirect responsibility to do all they can to protect their patients from undue harm. In Gwen Thompson's case, her primary physician would probably not be held culpable, from a legal or regulatory perspective, for the harm inflicted by the other doctor's cyber-prescribing. That said, the professional promise to "keep from harm" will always remind the physician to do all he or she can in the future to protect the patient and guide his or her care appropriately.

ANTICIPATING HEALTH INFORMATION TECHNOLOGY ETHICS CONCERNS

Telehealth and other information technologies are still evolving; these technologies promise access and decision support in remote areas for primary care providers as well as specialists. Though health information technologies present unique and ethically challenging opportunities for both patients and clinicians, they tend to be expensive, and should be implemented in direct response to clear and appropriate needs. Health care systems and providers must be cautious against developing excessive reliance on information technologies, such that the traditional patient-clinician relationship is inadvertently weakened.[25] Providers and administrators must also guard against complacency regarding the risks and distractions that accompany the use of such technology. Entrepreneurism and technology-focused programs that grow within health care systems tend to distract from the primary goal of medicine, and may ultimately lead to cost-prohibitive health care for many patients, especially in rural areas.

When using health information technologies, we as providers must never sway from the moral precepts that underscore our obligations as health care professionals: to serve the patient's needs first (beneficence); prevent harm if at all possible (nonmaleficence); provide fair access to reasonable forms of treatment and care (justice); and above all, to respect the patient's right to make informed decisions about his or her health care—including the right to refuse or accept what is offered. Keeping these precepts in mind with each patient will help maintain a balanced and satisfying experience, although conflict is often unavoidable. Suggestions on some ways in which providers may prevent ethics conflicts related to health information technology are given in Box 14.4.

BOX 14.4

PREVENTING ETHICS CONFLICTS IN HEALTH INFORMATIONTECHNOLOGY

Telehealth
Respect privacy and confidentiality; ensure adequate informed consent

Electronic Medical Records
Ensure accuracy, accessibility and accountability by providers; seek information transferability between systems

Electronic Clinical Support Systems
Ensure access and reliability of decision support systems for local sites, with support from tertiary care sites when needed

Online Health Care Resources
Ensure accuracy and reliability of information being accessed; encourage careful scrutiny by those accessing such information

Additional Protections
Establish policies and procedures to ensure consistency, generalization, and quality; develop informational material for providers and patients; provide community-wide education on health information technology

Telehealth

Telehealth will be a unique first-time experience for many patients. Therefore, it is important for clinicians to prepare patients in advance for the "talking head" interaction of videoconferencing. Ensuring that providers who interact with the patient will respect privacy and confidentiality is also very important to the success of a telehealth experience, as shown in Gina Conti's case. Telehealth is a clinical intervention and, therefore, requires verbal or written informed consent from the patient, or his or her representative. There should also be an established hospital policy and procedure regarding the use of telehealth, including patient education materials that clearly describe what one should expect during a telehealth visit.

Electronic Medical Records

Unfortunately, barriers to effectively using electronic medical records in rural areas will not be brought down soon. Individual health care systems will continue to deploy complex and separate firewalls for EMR systems that are inaccessible to outside providers who refer and share patients. Most rural physicians, and many rural hospitals, will not have electronic systems in the foreseeable future, unless such systems become more affordable, and also become standardized to allow critical information to be accessed when needed. Until such time, physicians like Dr. Adams and the cardiologist will need to take responsibility for communicating with each other directly and effectively, sharing important information, and ensuring that redundancy is minimized and safety optimized for their patient(s).

Electronic Decision Support

Electronic decision support for rural physicians is of burgeoning importance and is increasingly available. By enhancing standards of care and implementing improved quality and patient-safety standards, providers and administrators will improve care and promote equitable outcomes everywhere, including in remote and rural outposts. The cautionary plea is for the provider not to rely too heavily on technology, or to allow a false sense of security to extend one's self beyond one's own abilities. Decision support interventions are designed to be just that—supportive. Knowledge, skill, experience, and wisdom are still the mainstay of clinical decision-making, but these important human tools can be enhanced by the amazing technologies now available. When electronic decision support tools are used wisely, as in the case of Mr. Taft, patients, clinicians, and the hospital all benefit.

Online Health Information

Patients will continue to become increasingly computer-savvy and informed about health matters. They will continue to bring their physicians stacks of printouts and questions about information just pulled from the Internet regarding their health concerns. This behavior empowers patients to take personal responsibility, and physicians should support the process as an important component of their decision-making. But, in supporting patients, we must also partner with them by assessing what information is relevant and accurate, and by helping them use all forms of information technology wisely. Given the proper direction, patients might avoid the serious health complications that resulted in the case of Gwen Thompson. It is also very helpful to develop and distribute patient-education materials that enlighten patients about the use of online health care resources, distinguishing fact from fiction.

When advising patients about online health-information sources, consider the questions listed in Box 14.5 as a starting point for evaluating medical Web sites. These questions are found on the U.S. Department of Energy Human Genome Project's information Web site and are adapted from the U.S. Food and Drug Administration.

BOX 14.5

QUESTIONS PATIENTS SHOULD ASK WHEN USING MEDICAL WEB SITES

- Who maintains the site?
- Is there an editorial board or listing of names and credentials of those responsible for preparing and reviewing the site's content?
- Does the site link to other reliable sources of medical information?
- Does the site provide references to reliable sources?
- When was the site last updated?
- Has the site been reviewed for mistakes in grammar or spelling?
- Are informative graphics and multimedia files such as video or audio clips available?

As consumers increasingly use the Internet to obtain information about health, it must be the responsibility of each individual user—whether professional, public or private—to check the accuracy, reliability, and overall trustworthiness of information given on health-related Web sites. The questions offered above provide a good starting point for evaluating medical Web sites, and their use should be encouraged, especially for patients who are inquisitive and computer-savvy.

CONCLUSION

Access to health care in rural areas is a burgeoning concern, especially for the elderly.[26] Our society is responding to this intense need with telehealth and other technological means of decision support. The Federal Communications Commission (FCC) Chair announced a comprehensive proposal that would expand access to health care to rural and underserved communities through the creation of broadband telehealth networks in 42 states and three U.S. Territories.[27] This is a welcome initiative that, if successful, will provide relief to rural areas. More is needed at the state and local levels to ensure that reasonable health information technology interventions are deployed equitably and effectively to meet the health care needs of underserved areas.

In light of this evolution, health care providers and systems must never lose touch with their central purpose, which is driven not by information, science, or technology, but by the clinician's primary responsibility to protect the welfare of individual patients. The need for innovative technologies that can promote access to specialized health care services and enhance decision-making for the growing number of underserved in this country should and will continue to be of paramount concern in years to come. In particular, health care systems and providers who are committed to serving the needs of geographically isolated and otherwise disenfranchised persons in rural America should continue to seek innovative means to support rural health care.

When used ethically in the appropriate setting, health information technology can have a tremendously positive impact on the lives and welfare of patients. But it must be emphasized that information technologies, like any innovation, must be developed and implemented under the rubric of strict clinical and ethical standards to ensure safety and quality. Therefore, the goal of health information technology should be to optimize the balance of risks and benefits to the patient, and to augment, but never replace, the skills, shared trust, comfort, and compassion manifested by the healing presence of physicians, nurses, and other health care providers.

REFERENCES

1. Beauchamp TL, Childress JF. *Principles of Biomedical Ethics.* 5th ed. New York, NY: Oxford University Press; 2001.

2. Fleming DA. Ethical implications in the use of telehealth and teledermatology. In: Pak H, Edison K, Whited J, eds. *Teledermatology: A User's Guide.* Cambridge, England: Cambridge University Press; 2008:97-108.

3. Yadav H, Lin WY. Patient confidentiality, ethics and licensing in telemedicine. *Asia Pac J Public Health.* 2001;13 Suppl:S36-38.

4. Hersh W. Health care information technology: progress and barriers. *JAMA.* Nov 10 2004;292(18):2273-2274.

5. Gostin L. Health care information and the protection of personal privacy: ethical and legal considerations. *Ann Intern Med.* Oct 15 1997;127(8 Pt 2):683-690.

6. Anderson JG. Social, ethical and legal barriers to e-health. *Int J Med Inform.* May-Jun 2007;76(5-6):480-483.

7. Hart LG, Salsberg E, Phillips DM, Lishner DM. Rural health care providers in the United States. *J Rural Health.* 2002;18 Suppl:211-232.

8. Resneck J, Jr. Too few or too many dermatologists? Difficulties in assessing optimal workforce size. *Arch Dermatol.* Oct 2001;137(10):1295-1301.

9. Ward MM, Jaana M, Bahensky JA, Vartak S, Wakefield DS. Clinical information system availability and use in urban and rural hospitals. *J Med Syst.* Dec 2006;30(6):429-438.

10. Nordberg R. EHR in the perspective of security, integrity and ethics. In: Bos L, Roa L, Yogesan K, O'Connell B, Marsh A, Blobel B, eds. *Medical and Care Compunetics 3.* Washington, DC: IOS Press; 2006.

11. Westfall JM, Van Vorst RF, McGloin J, Selker HP. Triage and diagnosis of chest pain in rural hospitals: implementation of the ACI-TIPI in the High Plains Research Network. *Ann Fam Med.* Dec. 13, 2008 2006;4(2):153-158.

12. Stevenson KB, Barbera J, Moore JW, Samore MH, Houck P. Understanding keys to successful implementation of electronic decision support in rural hospitals: analysis of a pilot study for antimicrobial prescribing. *Am J Med Qual.* Nov-Dec 2005;20(6):313-318.

13. Malecki E. Digital development in rural areas: potentials and pitfalls. *J Rural Studies.* 2003;19(2):201-214.

14. Eysenbach G, Powell J, Kuss O, Sa ER. Empirical studies assessing the quality of health information for consumers on the world wide web: a systematic review. *JAMA.* May 22-29 2002;287(20):2691-2700.

15. Institute of Medicine. Committee on Quality of Health Care in America. *Crossing the Quality Chasm: A New Health System for the 21st Century.* Washington, DC: National Academy Press; 2001.

16. Moscovice I, Rosenblatt R. Quality-of-care challenges for rural health. *J Rural Health.* Spring 2000;16(2):168-176.

17. Walker J, Thomson A, Smith P. Maximising the world wide web for high quality educational and clinical support to health and medical professionals in rural areas. *Int J Med Inform.* Jun 1998;50(1-3):287-291.

18. Deady KE. Cyberadvice: the ethical implications of giving professional advice over the Internet. *Georget J Leg Ethics.* Spring 2001;14(3):891-907.

19. Irvine R. Mediating telemedicine: ethics at a distance. *Intern Med J.* Jan 2005;35(1):56-58.

20. Gustke S, Balch D, West V, Rogers L. Patient satisfaction with telemedicine. *Telemed J.* 2000;6(1):5-13.

21. Andrews JE, Pearce KA, Sydney C, Ireson C, Love M. Current state of information technology use in a US primary care practice-based research network. *Inform Prim Care.* 2004;12(1):11-18.

22. Burton LC, Anderson GF, Kues IW. Using electronic health records to help coordinate care. *Milbank Q.* 2004;82(3):457-481, table of contents.

23. Thornett A. Computer decision support systems in general practice. *Int J Inform Manage.* 2001;21(1):39-47.

24. Henney JE, Shuren JE, Nightingale SL, McGinnis TJ. Internet purchase of prescription drugs: buyer beware. *Ann Intern Med.* Dec 7 1999;131(11):861-862.

25. Evans H. High tech vs "high touch": the impact of medical technology on patient care. In: Clair J, Allman R, eds. *Sociomedical Perspectives on Patient Care.* Lexington, KY: University Press of Kentucky; 1993:82-95.

26. Rosenthal TC, Fox C. Access to health care for the rural elderly. *JAMA.* Oct 25 2000;284(16):2034-2036.

27. Kun LG. Telehealth and the global health network in the 21st century. From homecare to public health informatics. *Comput Methods Programs Biomed.* Mar 2001;64(3):155-167.

Rural Ethics Resources

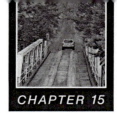

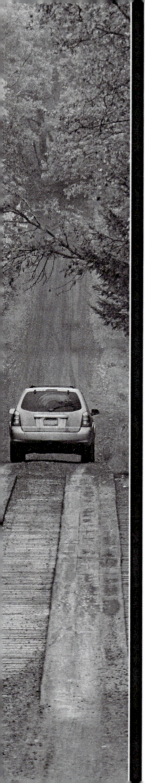

Practical Strategies for
Addressing and
Preventing
Ethics Issues
in Rural Settings

William A. Nelson, Karen E. Schifferdecker

Practical Strategies for Addressing and Preventing Ethics Issues in Rural Settings

William A. Nelson, Karen E. Schifferdecker

ABSTRACT

Ethics questions and conflicts will always be commonplace in rural health care practices. Despite the ethics knowledge and skills that clinicians and administrators may possess, ethics conflicts are stressful and time-consuming because of the inherent uncertainty surrounding such conflicts. To manage the potential negative effect of ethics conflicts, health care professionals and institutions should employ various strategies for anticipating and potentially decreasing the occurrence of such ethics conflicts in the delivery of today's health care. Effective strategies for clinicians and institutions to employ include identifying ethics resources; creating networks with professional colleagues, ethicists, and hospital ethics committees; developing and propagating ethical standards of practice in rural facilities and clinical practices; facilitating community-wide ethics training and discussions, and collaborating with professional organizations. These proactive strategies for anticipating and potentially decreasing ethics conflicts can both enhance the quality of health care, and decrease the negative impact that such conflicts generate, including the stress and time consumed in addressing them. An additional approach for addressing rural ethics issues is for faculty in health care professional schools to implement strategies which focus on rural health care ethics and prepare professionals choosing to practice in rural settings. Ethics faculty should expand their understanding of the rural context's influence on ethics challenges, and use cases focused on rural studies in the ethics curriculum.

INTRODUCTION

Ethics conflicts, such as professional-personal boundary conflicts, end-of-life decision-making, and maintaining patient privacy and confidentiality, are a few of a broad spectrum of ethics challenges occurring in today's rural health care settings. Rural health care professionals respond to the ethics challenges that occur in their clinics or in critical access hospitals based on their personal beliefs and experiences, community values, organizational policy, and/or understanding of ethical guidelines.

The presence of ethics conflicts can create uncertainty and stress for both the involved health care professionals and the patient. For example, a nurse recognizes that a physician in a small, economically struggling rural clinic has written a prescription for an incorrect medication, only to have the physician tell her to "forget it, we are a having a hard enough time paying our overhead, so we do not want to acknowledge that I made a mistake." Even though the patient was not harmed by the error, the nurse feels that she has a moral obligation to inform the patient, who is actually a neighbor. In another situation, a Medicare patient requests that a family physician write a prescription for a hypertension medication, which is actually to be used by his wife, who is not Medicare-eligible. The physician knows the couple well from their contact at a place of worship and other community activities, and is aware that such an action would be fraudulent, with dire consequences if it were ever discovered. But the physician also realizes that without writing the prescription to the man, his wife will go without the necessary medication. In both cases, the ethics conflict creates uncertainty, stress, and questions regarding how the provider should best respond to the situation. The cases can be further contextually complicated due to the frequent overlapping of personal and professional relationships and the "openness" of rural communities.

As these briefly presented cases suggest, ethics conflicts are not a benign event for the involved persons, or for the clinic or hospital. There is a growing understanding that organizational and clinical ethics conflicts have a potential for a detrimental impact on today's health care organizations in many ways.[1-7] Box 15.1 lists potential problems arising from ethics conflicts.

In considering this list of the potential implications of ethics conflicts, it is easy to see that such conflicts are anything but trivial. The reality is that ethics conflicts can have a significant impact on the health care professional's stress, workload, time management, and respect from

BOX 15.1

IMPACT OF ETHICS CONFLICTS IN HEALTH CARE PRACTICES

Staff
| Caregiver stress, deflated morale, weakened professionalism

Patients
| Poor patient satisfaction, loss of self-referrals

Organization's Culture
| Diminished quality of care

Relationship with Community
| Diminished organizational image, decreased trust, poor public relations and lower levels of philanthropic giving

Legal
| Increased litigation and settlements

Regulations
| Negatively influences adherence to Joint Commission standards and other regulatory organizations

Organization's Bottom Line
| Operational, legal, and public relations costs[8]

the community. Similarly, ethics conflicts can impact the overall culture and financial success of critical access hospitals as well as clinics, and can ultimately impact quality of care. The vulnerability of rural health care settings and communities to ethical challenges and the frequency of ethics issues encountered increases the need for clinicians and institutions to develop their knowledge and skills in recognizing and managing ethics conflicts.[9, 10]

An important approach in response to ethics issues is the development of proactive, preventive approaches to ethical uncertainty and conflicts. Because of the significant impact of ethics issues on today's health care organizations and the recurring nature of many ethics challenges, providers should pursue a strategy of moving upstream to prevent or diminish ethics conflicts from occurring. By moving upstream we mean a systematic exploration and analysis of the factors leading to ethics conflicts. After determining the causes fostering the ethics conflict, health care professionals are in a better position to apply quality improvement strategies for addressing the root cause of the conflict. Such an approach is a shift in managing ethics conflicts from the traditional reactive style. Throughout this *Handbook's* chapters, authors not only offered their reasoning in response to ethics cases, but also suggested various approaches for anticipating and decreasing the ethics challenges from arising.

Several constructive basic strategies that rural health hospitals and clinics can implement to assist providers in proactively addressing ethics conflicts and potentially decreasing the frequency of the challenges are listed in Box 15.2.

BOX 15.2

CONSTRUCTIVE STRATEGIES FOR PREVENTING AND COPING WITH ETHICS CONFLICTS

- Understand personal and community values and how they may impact the delivery of health care
- Identify and use ethics resources
- Develop and propagate ethical standards of rural practices in both clinic and hospital settings
- Enhance ethics awareness in rural communities through public forums and discussions
- Collaborate with professional organizations to increase understanding of ethics conflicts
- Expand rural ethics training in professional schools

UNDERSTANDING PERSONAL AND COMMUNITY VALUES

Rural health care professionals should examine their own values and how those values might influence their clinical or administrative thinking, behaviors and decisions. Personal values or beliefs are frequently based on one's own religious, ethnic, and cultural background. Health care professionals need to acknowledge their own values and balance them in relationship to professional standards of care, including the policies and practice of the health care facility and the values of the community.

Related to recognizing one's own values, health care professionals need to recognize and incorporate the values of the community within patient-care relationships. Each rural community is unique; however, rural communities frequently share values of their common dominant culture, such as a Native American culture in the American Southwest. If a provider did not understand a community's values, this could create ethics issues.

"Cultural ethics mistakes may arise when clinicians manifest unawareness of or disregard for indigenous values and behaviors by, for example, interfering with a healing ceremony, failing to work with the natural supports within families and communities... A second kind of ethical mistake may occur when clinicians overemphasize indigenous values to the point of diminishing the clinician's own professional values and ethics...that are the basic guideposts for decision-making in most clinical situations."[11] Avoiding such ethics issues requires a provider to be familiar with community values, and to know the appropriate levels of balancing such values with ethical standards of professionalism.

IDENTIFYING AND USING ETHICS RESOURCES
Rural clinicians often feel isolated from other health care professionals in rural settings. This isolation can increase the stress level of rural practices. Addressing ethics issues can be complex, time-consuming, and challenging for the provider. Therefore, identifying and using expert resources can be beneficial in addressing ethics issues. For the rural health professional, it is not only important to develop one's own ethics knowledge and skills, but also critically important to cultivate and use a network of various resources to provide consultation for patients' medical, mental health issues, and ethics issues. For example, a rural family physician caring for a patient with an acute psychiatric disorder may discuss the patient's care with a distant mental health expert. Similarly, when ethics issues arise regarding a patient-care issue, having a trusted colleague or ethicist with whom to discuss the situation can be beneficial. Potential ethics resources and networks are listed and described in Box 15.3.

BOX 15.3

ETHICS RESOURCES AND PROFESSIONAL NETWORKS

- Ethics literature and Web-based resources
- Professional clinician or administrative colleagues
- Health care ethicists
- Hospital ethics committees
- Academic-based ethics programs

Ethics Literature and Resources
To successfully manage a broad spectrum of ethics challenges in rural practices, clinicians should acquire a basic understanding of health care

ethics, including an awareness of basic ethical standards of practice. Ethical standards are generally-accepted guidelines for providers to use when responding to common ethics conflicts[12, 13] as noted in basic ethics textbooks. Even though these textbook-based guidelines may lack a specific rural focus, they are an important foundation. Ethical standards can also be found in a wide variety of profession–specific sources including the American College of Physicians Ethics Manual,[14] professional codes of ethics, and various position papers on a wide variety of ethics concerns. This *Handbook* provides an expanded bibliography with a useful list of resources. In addition, many ethics centers have created useful Web sites that offer a wide range of resources.

Networking with Professional Colleagues

In addition to developing his or her own ethics-related knowledge and skills, the rural health care professional can develop a network of colleagues, who can be consulted to provide support or advice regarding ethics challenges. Seeking the perspective of clinicians outside the immediate situation can provide the rural provider with insight, clarity, and supportive advice.

The network of colleagues should include professionals from various disciplines, such as dentists and mental health providers. Depending on the particular clinical situation, additional colleagues outside the health care field could also be useful resources, including clergy, school principals, local government leaders, and police officials.

The importance of identifying and using professional colleagues is not limited to ethical challenges—such a network can be beneficial to clinician-care issues, as well as decreasing the stress often associated with working in rural communities.

Networking with Ethicists

Rural health care professionals should also identify health care ethicists to provide them with consultation and training. Despite the general lack of trained ethicists living or working in rural settings, many are available through the telephone, e-mail, Internet, or telehealth programs. Ethicists can assist the rural clinician or administrator in reasoning through an ethically challenging situation. The rural provider's development of contacts with ethicists and clinicians can alleviate the potential sense of isolation which can come when dealing with ethics situations in rural areas.

The American Society of Bioethics and the Humanities (ASBH) is a large professional society that focuses on scholarship and teaching of health care ethics issues. The ASBH Web site offers a directory of members by state that can be accessed to help identify a nearby member.

Identifying Hospital Ethics Committees

Clinicians should identify those health care facilities that have ethics committees with case-consultation services. Many critical access hospitals have ethics committees that can provide a forum in which to discuss ethics issues with a multi-disciplinary group of professionals who have knowledge and skills in applied ethics. The chair of the committee should be able to describe the scope of the committee's activities, including when the committee meets, and how a clinician can access the committee.

In those hospitals where there is no ethics committee or program, clinicians might consider working with others and the hospital's administration to develop such a program.[15]

Accessing Academic-Based Ethics Centers

Rural clinicians should identify and use academic-based ethics centers and Web sites that can provide ethics resources. Ethics centers' Web sites can be valuable sources of information, resources, and material. Many of those Web sites are listed in the *Handbook's* bibliography. In addition to ethics-focused sites, there are several outstanding general rural resources, including the Rural Assistance Center (RAC) and the National Rural Health Association (NRHA).

DEVELOPING AND PROPAGATING ETHICAL STANDARDS OF PRACTICE

Rather than just reacting to ethics questions, rural clinicians can anticipate and proactively address recurring ethics conflicts. For instance, rural health care professionals can collaborate with clinical colleagues, ethicists, and ethics committee members to draft, disseminate and provide training around ethics practice guidelines that pertain to recurring rural ethics conflicts.

One approach is to proactively identify recurring ethics conflicts in a particular clinic or rural health care facility. A recurring clinical ethics case involves different patients, at different times, in different settings, but raises the same basic ethics conflict, such as end-of-life decision-making, or conflicts of interest. Once the recurring ethics conflict is identified, the team could develop an ethical practice protocol that provides guidance for addressing the conflict in the future. The guidance can help reduce the situation's impact, or even prevent it from becoming a conflict. This type of proactive approach has been suggested by several authors.[16-20] The proactive approach to addressing ethics conflicts is based on five basic steps, as listed in Box 15.4.

BOX 15.4

A PROACTIVE APPROACH TO ETHICS CONFLICTS

- Identify the recurring ethics issues that create conflict or uncertainty
- Study the ethics issues in a systematic, system-oriented manner
- Develop ethical practice protocols to guide clinicians and executives on handling the conflict when it arises again
- Propagate the protocols into the organization's culture so that all staff are aware of the guidelines and the rationale driving the guidelines
- Review whether the protocols are adequately addressing the ethics conflict and decreasing its recurrence

This proactive, preventive approach can be used in various settings and situations. For example, in a practice staff meeting the question could be asked, "What are the situations that create uncertainty or conflict, which come up over and over in this practice?" These ethics issues could then be prioritized, and systematically and thoughtfully discussed, to create an ethically-grounded, proactive guideline. Once established, the guidelines could be shared, and theoretically might decrease the uncertainty of how the conflict or question should be addressed.

A preventive approach to ethics conflicts can also be employed with hospital ethics committees. A common activity for almost all ethics committees is to have an ethics consultation service, which can assist staff in addressing ethics conflicts. This approach tends to be reactive, in response to a current conflict. This traditional reactive approach to complex and challenging ethics conflicts can be helpful to involved parties. However, this process has several potential concerns. First, responding to an ethics conflict can be demanding, occasionally necessitating a rapid response. Second, time limitations can affect the availability of ethics consultants and thus preclude a thoughtful review of the conflict. Third, as has been noted, the traditional process accepts the perspective that ethics conflicts are recurring. Additionally, the presence of ethics conflicts can potentially take a toll on the culture of the organization, because of staff's ethical uncertainty or questions.

Despite these concerns, having a competent and available ethics consultation program is essential, because ethics conflicts will arise that need immediate reflection. However, the addition of a preventive approach is also critically important. After an ethics committee or ethics consultation service responds to a conflict, the consultants should facilitate a process to identify the underlying causes for the conflict, and consider corrective actions to decrease its potential occurrence in the future. For example, in applying a Root Cause Analysis process to ethics conflicts, ethicists would seek to determine why the conflict occurred, and what can be done to prevent it from happening again. The process is used to focus on improving systems and processes, and when needed, redesigning them, rather than focusing on the individuals involved in the conflict.

Having a proactive approach to ethics conflicts may be just as important to the rural provider as employing an effective ethics consultation service. Emphasizing the prevention of ethics conflicts by fostering the development of ethical practice protocols or guidelines, which are integrated into the culture of the organization, can enhance the quality of patient care by reducing the frequency of ethics conflicts.

The proactive approach to addressing ethics conflicts within the context of hospital ethics committees' activities would use the same basic five steps as noted above. For example, a member of the ethics committee or consult team could meet with the patient safety officer, the head of Human Resources, or a Vice President of Operations, and ask the question, "What are some of the recurring ethics issues that you or your staff encounter that create uncertainty or conflict?" Those identified ethics issues could then be systematically and thoughtfully discussed by ethics consultants and staff from the particular program or section over a period of time, leading to ethically grounded, proactive guidelines. Once the guidelines were propagated, along with the ethical reasoning underpinning them, the ethics committee could then provide staff with guidance for addressing the conflict when it reoccurred. This proactive ethics approach is similar in reasoning and process to the patient safety movement, with its goal of improving quality of care by reducing medical errors.[21]

Even though a proactive process that leads to the development of ethical practice guidelines may seem arduous, it has the advantage of creating an

environment of increased ethical certainty and staff morale—thus avoiding
emotionally draining and time-consuming ethics conflicts. In the end,
practical, anticipatory approaches can enhance the clinic's or hospital's
overall ethics environment by helping the staff better understand what is the
right thing to do; thus reducing the recurrence of ethics conflicts.

ETHICS AWARENESS AND DISCUSSIONS IN RURAL COMMUNITIES

Rural professionals can develop and implement community-wide education
programs to foster patient awareness. Such programs often address
topics to promote preventive care, such as weight loss/fitness, smoking
cessation, and advance-care planning. However, community forums can
also address ethics-related topics, including privacy and confidentiality,
boundary issues, and end-of-life decision-making. For example, a critical
access hospital can organize two to three community forums a year.
Health care professionals can talk about a particular topic in an informal
open atmosphere. The community forum session can create a dialog
about the selected topic to enhance the understanding of the issue. Some
educational events can be facilitated in collaboration with community
leaders, such as clergy, to gain broad support and interest.

The National Rural Bioethics program, based in Missoula, Montana,
has facilitated community forums using the Readers Theater approach.
A Readers Theater is designed to provide education and to stimulate
informed conversation. The Readers Theater technique was developed
and pioneered at East Carolina School of Medicine, where actors read
a story line that describes problems that develop when providing health
care. The scripts can be based on various common ethics issues
encountered in rural settings, and participants may try on different roles. As
described in the National Rural Bioethics Project's Educational Resources
Web site, "incidents are described in the voices of physicians, nurses,
hospital administrators, patients, families, and clergy. An administrator or
physician may read a nurse's or a patient's lines, a patient may assume the
physician's role. After the reading, the actors and audience engage in a
discussion of the issues and themes."[22] It has been noted that the scripts
have been well accepted by a wide variety of rural audiences and health
care providers, providing a way to talk about the ethics issues. Potential
scripts can be found on the National Rural Bioethics Project's Web site.[22]

In addition to community-wide programs, rural clinicians working in various
settings such as a small clinic should have clearly thought-out ethics
practices. These ethics-grounded practices should be openly shared

with patients and built into the overall culture of the clinic. Clinicians can also develop pamphlets delineating their ethical standards of practice to complement the discussions. Pamphlets on various topics can be available in the clinic waiting room, or given to patients during one-on-one visits.

COLLABORATING WITH PROFESSIONAL ORGANIZATIONS

In addition to collaborating with colleagues and ethicists, rural health care professionals can foster linkages with national and state professional organizations that focus on rural studies for educational opportunities, networking contacts, and as a vehicle for promoting and addressing rural health care concerns.

Even though professional organizations rarely focus on rural issues, rural health care professionals can encourage planners of health care conferences, often held at state or national professional meetings, to include a spotlight or seminar on rural issues. These meetings can provide an opportunity to engage with others concerning rural health care, including the ethics challenges inherent in rural practice. Rural health care professionals can also actively participate in national professional organizations' committees that establish standards of care to ensure that a rural perspective is recognized. They also can work with such organizations in advocating for adequate rural health care resources.

Despite the lack of a rural focus in many professional organizations, there are state- and national-level organizations focused on rural health that provide information and support on rural specific issues. These organizations also serve as strong advocates for rural health care.

EXPANDING PROFESSIONAL TRAINING IN
RURAL HEALTH CARE ETHICS

In addition to strategies employed by rural health care professionals in their practices, health care faculty at professional schools that train future rural health care professionals should implement strategies to address rural health care ethics issues in the curriculum. Such strategies can enhance the knowledge and skills of future rural health care professionals in addressing ethics challenges. In some schools, training could also be inter-disciplinary, that is, training that includes multiple professions, such as nurses and physicians.

The overall goals of rural ethics training, as noted in Box 15.5, should ensure students' ability to perform the skills identified.

BOX 15.5

RURAL ETHICS TRAINING GOALS

- Identify ethics issues present in clinical care
- Recognize how the rural context influences ethics issues and the professionals' responses to them
- Perform an ethical analysis; applying ethical principles and professional standards
- Locate rural ethics resources
- Identify strategies to anticipate and decrease ethics issues in clinical practice

Rural ethics training can be planned and implemented in both the pre-clinical and clinical years of training, involving mentors and preceptors as well as classroom faculty. To achieve the basic goals of rural ethics training, several strategies are suggested in Box 15.6.

BOX 15.6

STRATEGIES TO EXPAND RURAL ETHICS FOCUS IN PROFESSIONAL EDUCATION

- Increase the faculty's understanding of the impact of the rural context on ethics issues
- Build opportunities into the curriculum for students to learn about rural ethics issues
- Have the faculty use rural-based cases in teaching and publications
- Have the faculty share their own ethics challenges or situations for discussion to enhance students' awareness and comfort in identifying and discussing ethics situations
- Evaluate the student's recognition and response to ethics conflicts

Rural ethics education and training should not be just an "add-on" to the current full curriculum. To avoid a silo approach to ethics training, rural ethics should be integrated into the existing curriculum, in both the pre-clinical and clinical training. To achieve this goal, several steps need to be planned and implemented.

Increase Awareness

Educators should increase their own awareness and understanding of rural health care ethics issues, as perceived by rural residents and health care professionals, including the contextual influence on ethics issues, and how the issues are different in rural and non-rural settings. This *Handbook* provides a thorough overview of health care ethics in rural settings, and lists additional resources to assist faculty in raising their understanding of the issues.

Develop Learning Goals

Educators can partner with health care ethicists, or can review the goals for student training listed above (e.g., perform an ethical analysis) to develop a set of learning goals and objectives that can be integrated into the existing curriculum. These goals and objectives should build on any existing ethics curriculum at the school to enhance students' overall understanding and skills related to ethics problems.

Implement Training

Educators should determine the best means to meet the specific learning goals and objectives, and should implement rural ethics training using these strategies. The Rural Ethics Training Manual provides a number of materials (e.g., PowerPoint slides, case studies, small group discussion questions) to facilitate interactive discussions on rural ethics. In addition, faculty can collaborate with rural clinicians, administrators, and policy-makers to help facilitate the training, either at training sites or in classroom settings. For example, a pediatric or family medicine course director might include a session in collaboration with the school's ethicist to present a rural ethics case for student discussion.

Encourage Discourse

Faculty should encourage students to bring up ethics challenges or questions to help them begin to identify ethics situations and to offer a framework for thinking about and addressing these situations, particularly in future practice. One way faculty can encourage this is by relating personal ethical challenges that they have encountered, and strategies (effective or not effective) that they used to address such challenges. Faculty can also share the eight-step method, designed by Nelson[23] for thinking about ethics problems, and can refer students to additional online resources that focus on rural ethics to aid them in their future practices.

Develop Evaluation Methods

Faculty, should develop and implement, in both the preclinical and clinical training, explicit evaluation methods regarding rural ethics. The evaluation should not be limited to whether the student appreciated learning about rural ethics issues—the evaluation should focus on the student's ability to recognize and respond to ethics conflicts.

In addition to those professional schools that have many graduates going into rural settings, schools that are urban-based and -focused should also implement some level of rural ethics training. Ethicists teaching in such settings could include a few cases and provide resource material focusing on rural contexts to foster the students' understanding of how context can influence health care ethics. Either way, rural or urban-based professional training programs have an obligation to expose students to the influence of context on ethics challenges as well as the response to those challenges.

In addition to changes in the formal curriculum to include a focus on rural ethics, course directors can foster special events that emphasize how rural ethics issues are encountered and addressed. For example, they could organize an evening panel discussion with a group of rural clinicians that is focused around these questions. Several professional schools have developed special interests, such as Dartmouth Medical School's Rural Scholars Program. This program brings together medical students planning to practice in rural settings for a regular evening gathering to meet with rural clinicians.

CONCLUSION

Ethics conflicts are a common occurrence in today's rural health care settings. Managing and responding to an ethics conflict can be challenging for the provider, because inherent in all ethics conflicts are feelings of uncertainty and questioning about what is the most appropriate course of action. Ethics conflicts affect not only patients and families; they also affect staff and administrators. Ethics conflicts can be time-consuming and stressful; they can potentially negatively impact the patient's quality of care. Additionally, ethics conflicts that occur in small rural hospitals can affect the health care organization's culture, and, ultimately, its overall financial success.

Traditionally, when an ethics conflict occurs, the involved parties respond to the situation based on their experience(s), training, and personal values. In some situations, health care professionals may seek the support of an ethics committee or other ethics resource. Most often, professionals seek to carefully and thoughtfully respond to ethics conflicts. By using the strategies suggested in this chapter, however, health care professionals can "move upstream" to prospectively seek and prevent conflicts from occurring, or decrease the impact of ethics conflicts that do occur.

REFERENCES

1. Hamric AB, Blackhall LJ. Nurse-physician perspectives on the care of dying patients in intensive care units: collaboration, moral distress, and ethical climate. *Crit Care Med.* Feb 2007;35(2):422-429.

2. Bischoff SJ, DeTienne KB, Quick B. Effects of ethics stress on employee burnout and fatigue: an empirical investigation. *J Health Hum Serv Adm.* Spring 1999;21(4):512-532.

3. Schneiderman LJ, Gilmer T, Teetzel HD, et al. Effect of ethics consultations on nonbeneficial life-sustaining treatments in the intensive care setting: a randomized controlled trial. *JAMA.* Sep 3 2003;290(9):1166-1172.

4. Weeks WB. Quality improvement as an investment. *Qual Manag Health Care.* Spring 2002;10(3):55-64.

5. Nelson WA, Weeks WB, Campfield JM. The organizational costs of ethical conflicts. *J Healthc Manag.* Jan-Feb 2008;53(1):41-52; discussion 52-43.

6. Heilicser BJ, Meltzer D, Siegler M. The effect of clinical medical ethics consultation on healthcare costs. *J Clin Ethics.* Spring 2000;11(1):31-38.

7. Schneiderman LJ, Gilmer T, Teetzel HD. Impact of ethics consultations in the intensive care setting: a randomized, controlled trial. *Crit Care Med.* Dec 2000;28(12):3920-3924.

8. Nelson WA. Ethical uncertainty and staff stress. *Healthc Exec.* 2009;24(4):38-39.

9. Nelson WA. The challenges of rural health care. In: Klugman CM, Dalinis PM, eds. *Ethical Issues in Rural Health Care* Baltimore, MD: Johns Hopkins University Press; 2008:34-59.

10. Nelson WA, Schmidek JM. Rural healthcare ethics. In: Singer PA, Viens AM, eds. *The Cambridge Textbook of Bioethics.* New York, NY: Cambridge University Press; 2008:289-298.

11. Roberts LW, Dyer AR. Caring for people in small communities. In: *Concise Guide to Ethics in Mental Health Care.* Washington, DC: American Psychiatric Publishing; 2004:175.

12. Lo B. *Resolving Ethical Dilemmas: A Guide for Clinicians.* 2nd ed. Philadelphia, PA: Lippincott Williams & Wilkins; 2000.

13. Singer PA, Viens AM, eds. *The Cambridge Textbook of Bioethics.* New York, NY: Cambridge University Press; 2008.

14. Ethics manual. Fourth edition. American College of Physicians. *Ann Intern Med.* Apr 1 1998;128(7):576-594.

15. Nelson WA. Ethics programs in small rural hospitals. Ethics committees are essential all healthcare facilities, not just large ones. *Healthc Exec.* Nov-Dec 2007;22(6):30, 32-33.

16. Nelson WA. Dealing with ethical challenges. How occurrences can be addressed before they happen. *Healthc Exec.* Mar-Apr 2007;22(2):36, 38.

17. McCullough LB. Preventive ethics, managed practice, and the hospital ethics committee as a resource for physician executives. *HEC Forum.* Jun 1998;10(2):136-151.

18. Forrow L, Arnold RM, Parker LS. Preventive ethics: expanding the horizons of clinical ethics. *J Clin Ethics*. Winter 1993;4(4):287-294.

19. McCullough LB. Practicing preventive ethics-the keys to avoiding ethical conflicts in health care. *Physician Exec*. Mar-Apr 2005;31(2):18-21.

20. Chervenak FA, McCullough LB. An ethical framework for identifying, preventing, and managing conflicts confronting leaders of academic health centers. *Acad Med*. Dec. 14, 2008 2004;79(11):1056-1061.

21. Nelson WA, Neily J, Mills P, Weeks WB. Collaboration of ethics and patient safety programs: opportunities to promote quality care. *HEC Forum*. Mar 2008;20(1):15-27.

22. Educational resources. National Rural Bioethics Project, University of Montana. http://www.umt.edu/bioethics/healthcare/resources/educational/default.aspx. Accessed July 2, 2009.

23. Nelson WA. An organizational ethics decision-making process. *Healthc Exec*. Jul-Aug 2005;20(4):8-14.

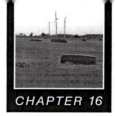

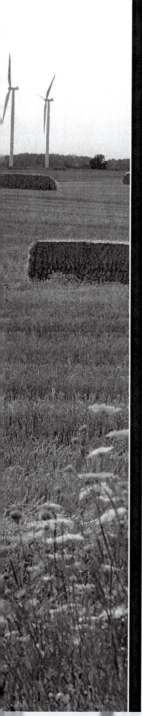

Developing
Rural Ethics
Networks

Lisa Anderson-Shaw, Jacqueline J. Glover

CHAPTER 16

Developing Rural Ethics Networks

Lisa Anderson-Shaw, Jacqueline J. Glover

ABSTRACT

Rural ethics networks are a tool that small, rural health care institutions can join in order to share ideas, explore questions with peers, and gain educational opportunities and support. Because there are few existing rural ethics networks, the development of new networks might help many hospitals or clinics that currently lack health care ethics resources in their workplaces. Health care institutions in rural geographical areas are often challenged with limited finances and overworked staff, which may make it difficult for those working on institutional ethics committees or providing ethics consultation to access ongoing education and development opportunities. This chapter will discuss various ethics network models that are currently available, including academic, government and independently-based networks, as well as informal networks. This chapter will also describe how an interested professional might begin building a new rural ethics network to meet rural health care needs.

INTRODUCTION

There are approximately 5708 registered hospitals in the United States, 1997 of which are community hospitals located in rural areas.[1] This means that approximately 37% of the nation's hospitals are considered rural. The American Hospital Association (AHA) defines a rural hospital, in general, as a large or small hospital that is located outside a metropolitan statistical area. A small hospital is defined as one having less than 150 beds; many rural hospitals have less than 150 beds.[2]

Ethics issues of a clinical and administrative nature cross over all health care environments, including rural and small institutions. Illness, and the ethics conflicts associated with it, occur no matter where we live. Rural areas require supportive professionals who appreciate and understand this context. Rural health care also requires ethics resources that may include networks of rural practitioners who communicate about their struggles with ethical issues, as well as practitioners who sit on the ethics committees and/or provide clinical health care ethics consultation.[2] Networking can be formal or informal. Formal networking might include inviting a trained ethicist to visit a rural institution's ethics committee to hold training sessions for committee members, or contracting an ethicist to provide ongoing training and/or consultation. Informal networking can include phone or e-mail contact with an outlying ethics consultant, or discussing issues with other local institutional ethics committee members.

Limited Ethics Resources

Many small, rural health care institutions (hospitals, nursing homes, and outreach clinics) are not affiliated with colleges or universities, where they might have access to scholarly resources or individuals trained in health care ethics.[3] It might also be true that many small and rural institutions do not need a full-time ethicist on site, but rather would benefit from an ethicist who serves several institutions part-time through some form of health care ethics network. Limited financial and educational resources can be enhanced when several rural institutions work together. An ethics network can provide not only clinical ethicists, but also resources related to health policy, research, legal updates, committee education, and peer feedback.

Benefits of Rural Ethics Networks

There are important reasons for rural institutions to create networks, because rural health care ethics issues are often unique from those experienced by their urban counterparts. Ethics committee members and others interested in rural ethics could benefit from the opportunity to participate in the network, sharing a common rural understanding, perspective, and lived experience. As committee members, we feel more at home when others immediately understand the rural dynamics shaping the presentations of common challenges. The benefits of rural ethics networks are listed in Box 16.1.

BOX 16.1

BENEFITS OF RURAL ETHICS NETWORKS

- Access to health care ethics consultant(s)
- Collegial support
- Ethics committee member interaction and sharing of ideas
- Specific educational programs to meet the needs of small and rural institutions
- Opportunities to share research ideas and activities

A major benefit of rural ethics networks is that members are colleagues and professionals who all live and work in rural settings. Therefore, each has a greater understanding of the unique rural challenges and what kinds of solutions for ethics issues are most fitting for rural care situations. Cook and Hoas wrote, "Merely transplanting urban models, guidelines, standards, and training requirements into resource-limited rural health care scenes appear(s) to be inadequate. Identifying resources, disseminating materials, and developing linkages among similarly sized institutions could be useful interventions."[4] Providers can improve the rural health care experience by recognizing the unique attributes of the rural context, and seeking ethics network support from within as well as without individual health care facilities.[5]

TYPES OF RURAL ETHICS NETWORKS

There are several types of rural health care ethics networks in place throughout the United States and Canada today, listed in Box 16.2.

Again, networks may be formal or informal, depending on the needs of those groups or individuals who make up the general group. Membership also depends on the individuals representing the various institutions, such as physicians, nurses, allied health care providers, and the like. The structures and purpose of the various networks differ, but there are several general types of rural networks.

BOX 16.2

TYPES OF HEALTH CARE ETHICS NETWORKS

- Academic-based networks with academic funding
- Academic-based networks with membership funding
- Government-sponsored networks
- Independent-based networks with independent funding
- Informal rural networks

Academic-Based Ethics Networks with Academic-Based Funding
Academic-based and -funded networks are those that are both facilitated and funded by a sponsoring academic institution. The Illinois Healthcare Ethics Committee Forum, based at the University of Illinois at Chicago Medical Center, is one example of such a network that provides useful resources to small and rural health care institutions. This network was developed in 2003 to assist institutions throughout the state of Illinois. There are 194 hospitals in Illinois, 88 of which are classified as small, rural, or both.[6] The ethics committee membership focuses on members specifically, and not just the ethics consultant, as not all hospitals have an ethics-consulting service or department. However, even small and rural institutions must have some form of ethics committee or mechanism to address medical ethical issues, in order to meet basic patient rights and ethics standards as specified by The Joint Commission.

In order to successfully develop an ethics network of any kind, a dedicated, committed, and institution-supported leader must carefully plan the development of a network with as many rural facility professionals as possible. An early step in the development process includes surveying potential users of the network.

Preparation for the Illinois Healthcare Ethics Committee Forum began with a survey sent to 88 small and rural hospitals, including critical access hospitals, as listed by the Illinois Hospital Association (IHA). The surveys were addressed to the institutional risk manager, because most institutions have a defined person for this role. If the manager was not a member of the hospital's ethics committee, they were asked to pass the survey on to the appropriate contact. The survey described a future health care ethics committee network, in which members would be able to share ideas, experiences, JCAHO insights, and educational topics via a Web-based discussion board. Survey questions asked hospitals about the organization of their institutional ethics committee, how often the committee met, what responsibilities members had, and what kinds of resources were available. Survey participants were asked if they would be interested in joining a statewide network and, if so, if they would be willing to pay a fee for this service. The survey in Figure 16.1 was used to better understand the level of interest in a statewide network.

Of the 88 surveys sent out to small and rural Illinois hospitals, 51 responses were returned, a 58% return rate. All 51 indicated that their committee work included policy review, case review, and/or education. Twelve of the 51 would not be willing or able to pay any fee for membership to an ethics network, but the remaining 39 stated that they would be willing to pay $25-50 for an annual membership. All but two of the respondents said that they would find membership in a statewide ethics network helpful.

After receiving positive feedback from the original surveys, work began with the University of Illinois Information Services support staff to build our virtual online forum discussion board Web site. Within six months following the survey, the University of Illinois at Chicago Medical Center launched the Illinois Healthcare Ethics Committee Forum. The forum was advertised via e-mail and letters sent out again to the Illinois Hospital Association's small and rural hospitals. The forum was also easily accessed via the Medical Center's Clinical Ethics Consult Service home page, where individuals could sign up for the secured discussion site. This forum is now offered free of charge as a service of the University of Illinois Medical Center. Within three months the forum had 23 members, and five years later there are over 175 members representing institutions throughout the state. The University of Illinois is committed to this resource and to the ongoing support of the virtual network.

Membership is not restricted to just members of small and rural institutions. All members have benefited from the varied experiences and expertise that we share online. In June 2004 the Illinois Healthcare Ethics Committee Forum held its first conference in central Illinois, with over 100 participants. The conference has become an annual event, and is an important opportunity for attendees to network face-to-face, to share experiences and ideas, and for those active in ethics committee work to conduct continuing education. The conference topics are member-driven, with most speakers coming from the membership, thus allowing for the forum to meet the specific needs of its members. For example, education might

FIGURE 16.1

SAMPLE ETHICS COMMITTEE SURVEY

1. Does your institution have an Ethics Committee?   Yes   No

2. If no, please explain:_____

3. If yes, what professional classifications make up the committee membership? (Circle all that apply)

   MD   RN   Social Worker   Clergy
   Respiratory Therapy   Administrator   Lawyer
   Other:_____

4. How many members are on your Ethics Committee? _____

5. How often does your committee meet? (Circle one)

   Monthly   Bi-monthly   Quarterly
   Annually   Other:_____

6. What activities does your Ethics Committee do? (Circle all that apply)

   Policy review/revision   Case review
   Education   Other:_____

7. Do your committee members provide clinical ethics case consultations?

   Yes   No   Other: _____

8. What ethics resources are available to your committee?

   _____

9. Would it be helpful to your committee to participate in an informal network of ethics committees to share ideas and educational resources?

   Yes   No

10. Do you think your institution would be willing to pay a nominal fee (annually) to be included as a member of an Ethics Committee Network?

    Yes   No

11. If you answered yes to the question above, what fee range would be acceptable to your institution? (Circle one)

    $25-$50 $50-$100 $150-$200

12. If such an Ethics Committee Network were available, would you be most likely to participate in: (Circle all that apply)

    Virtual Discussion Board (Internet-based)   Annual Conference
    Face-to-Face meetings   Other: _____

be available on the consultative process, for those institutions that may have less than five consultations per year; or a program might be given on home hospice care for rural locations where such services are challenging to obtain.

Academic-Based Ethics Networks with Membership Funding

A second type of health care ethics network is the academic- or university-based network, in which funding is provided directly by members. Here are examples from two well-established networks, both having been in operation for about 20 years.

The first network is the West Virginia Network of Ethics Committees (WVNEC), which began in 1988 as the West Virginia Network of Hospital Ethics Committees. There were 12 original members, and they raised start-up monies through conference registrations with the kind support of West Virginia University Health Sciences Center. The West Virginia Network of Ethics Committees expanded to include nursing homes, home care agencies, and hospices, in addition to hospitals. It currently has an institutional membership of 44 hospitals, 22 nursing homes, 5 home care agencies, 9 hospices, and 12 individual members. The network is governed by a Network Advisory Committee which represents the diversity of membership. The mission of the West Virginia Network of Ethics Committees is to promote ethical decision-making in both daily patient care and during quality end-of-life care, by educating patients, families, professionals, and institutions about ethical and legal issues. In addition to serving as a resource for ethical decision-making for all West Virginians, the West Virginia Network assists hospitals, nursing homes, hospices, and home health agencies to start or strengthen ethics committees and to develop knowledge and skills in palliative care. The services that this ethics network provides are summarized in Box 16.3.

These services keep network members connected, even when they are separated by significant distance.

The yearly membership dues are $150 for institutions with annual gross revenues of less than $500,000 per year; $250 for those institutions with revenues from $600,000 to $5,000,000 per year; and $350 for those institutions with revenues in excess of $5,000,000. Individual membership is $25 annually.

Another example of an academic-based network that has membership

BOX 16.3

EXAMPLE OF NETWORK SERVICES
(WEST VIRGINIA NETWORK OF ETHICS COMMITTEES)

- Web site, wvethics.org, with a complete toolkit for ethics committees
- E-mail newsletters with information about ethical and legal issues
- Telephone consultations
- List-serve to keep members current on pending health care legislation
- Assistance in drafting policies on ethics-related issues
- Quarterly newsletter containing articles on current topics and other help as needed

fees is the Midwest Ethics Committee Network. This network was started in 1987 for hospital ethics committees in Wisconsin as a way to meet, discuss policies, and discuss other health care ethics topics of interest, including topics relevant to the rural settings in which many institutions in Wisconsin are located. The Center for the Study of Bioethics at the Medical College of Wisconsin provided leadership for this network, and sent the original membership invitations. There are currently 120 hospital members of the Midwest Ethics Committee Network, representing 1500 individuals. Institutional membership is available on a sliding scale membership fee based on institution size. Institutions with over 500 beds pay an annual membership fee of $1,200, while those with less than 150 beds pay $300 annually. Individual membership is $75 per year. The Medical College of Wisconsin funds the Midwest Ethics Committee Network on a partial basis. A variety of network activities are available to members, including an online discussion board, a member newsletter, and frequent educational programs at locations throughout the state, including regional meetings.[7]

Government-Sponsored and -Funded Ethics Networks

Ethics Networks that are government-based and government-funded include those networks that are financed and run by some type of state-sponsored organization.

There is evidence that having some type of system-wide or location-driven network successfully helps provide needed ethics resources to practitioners and ethics committee members in small and rural locations.[5,6] The Provincial Health Ethics Network from Alberta, Canada is an example of a government-based ethics network that serves the entire province of Alberta, including both urban and rural health care institutions. Most of this geographical area remains very rural, despite the large landmass it occupies. Activities sponsored by the network include an annual conference, distance-education offerings, and Web seminars and workshops.[7]

The Department of Veterans Affairs (VA), the largest integrated health care system in the United States, includes many rural hospitals and outpatient clinics across the country. All VA medical centers have ethics committees or programs to assist clinicians and administrators in addressing ethics issues. Local VA medical center ethics committees are linked to the VA's National Center for Health Care Ethics, based at the VA's national headquarters in Washington, DC. The Ethics Center provides many educational and consultation activities and resources to assist local VA ethics programs. The Center drafts position papers regarding a wide range of clinical and organizational ethics issues that are relevant for all health care facilities. The wide variety of National Center for Health Care Ethics resources can be accessed through their Web site. The resources are useful for both VA and non-VA health care organizations.

Independently Based Ethics Networks with Independent Funding
Independently based networks are those which are organized by private institutions or groups that receive funding from various sources, in addition to providing resources to institutions on a fee-for-service basis.

The Kansas City Area Ethics Committee Consortium is an example of an independent network that provides support to ethics committees throughout the Kansas City region, which includes a large rural constituent. This consortium was formed in 1986, and provides ethics committee education, research, policy development assistance, and bi-monthly meetings. The consortium is a service of the Center for Practical Bioethics, which is a nonprofit, independent health care ethics center that is funded by a combination of membership dues and community and foundational support. Consortium membership is a benefit of organizational membership to the Center for Practical Bioethics. Two representatives of each member hospital's ethics committee attend consortium meetings, which are hosted by various institutions during the year. Consortium meetings are supplemented by Center staff assistance to member institutions with on-site visits, phone consultations, and consultation on any difficult health care ethics issues that may arise. The Center staff also provides support by chairing the ethics committees of member hospitals.

The Consortium hosts an online discussion forum that is moderated and administered by Center staff. Members may subscribe to this forum by request only. The forum provides members with a means of communicating about bioethical issues in real time without travel. Forum members also receive monthly "Ethics E-Alert" messages to provide links to news and events at the Center and elsewhere in the Kansas City area. In addition, the Center sponsors a long-term-care ethics committee consortium to assist institutions that may not have access to ethics consultation and educational resources.[8]

Informal Rural Ethics Networks

In addition to the more formal ethics networks, there are informal ways that rural health care institutions can interact in order to meet their individual needs. Ethics committee members can contact the ethics committees of other small and rural health care institutions by obtaining membership lists from state hospital associations. For a small fee, state hospital associations often offer membership lists with contact information that can be used to locate institutions of a similar size. Sending a letter to the ethics committee chairperson of an identified similar institution can start informal networking that may lead to valuable interactions.

Informal networks can also be started by looking into various rural health care resources available via the Internet. For example, The University of Montana in Missoula is host to the National Rural Bioethics Initiative (NRBI), which was established to "create a formal mechanism for sustained health care ethics-related research and program development in rural communities and rural health care settings."[9] NRBI research is funded by federal grants and foundations. This initiative is not a membership network, however. The initiative works with rural hospitals and other health agencies in the West through its research projects. Health care providers can contact the NRBI for resources and assistance.

Established organizations, such as state medical societies and regional health care organizations, may also assist in the ethics networking process. Such organizations may be able to provide financial support to get a network started, or technical support to develop a Web-based or online network for rural institutions. In states with large rural populations, there are often local and state rural organizations related to health care, such as public health departments. Additionally, state universities may have important departments and research initiatives in place, related to rural health care, that could be helpful in organizing a specific network. It only takes one person with an interest to get a network started.

Many rural health care ethics networks are successful, allowing members from small and rural institutions to ask questions, share information, and communicate with resource members from both academic and non-academic institutions. However, we must now go the next step and produce research through organizing scholarly work on the issues that small and rural institutions find interesting or challenging in their unique settings.

BUILDING A RURAL ETHICS NETWORK

Careful planning is important when building a rural ethics network. Important planning steps are suggested in Box 16.4.

BOX 16.4

GETTING AN ETHICS NETWORK STARTED

- Determine a sponsoring institution that is willing to house and support the initial efforts (state hospital, long-term home care and/ or hospice association, medical or nursing society, major hospital in the area, university, etc.)
- Enlist a dedicated network leader and organizer
- Organize focus groups to brainstorm a network outline or plan
- Conduct a needs assessment of your state or region
- Host an initial planning meeting (either via conference call, an in-person meeting, or video conference)
- Prioritize the meeting based on initial planning meeting data
- Utilize resources from existing rural networks and resources
- Provide ongoing network assessment and evaluation
- Update the network as needed based on assessment andevaluations

It is very important to research the resources available in one's area, if any, and what resources are important and needed for all potential network members. Focus groups including individuals from sample rural institutions may be useful for brainstorming ideas about how a potential network could, or should operate in the particular rural area. From the brainstorming session(s), a network outline describing its purpose and activities can be established to further guide development. Then, a network model can be used to decide what type of funding, as well as other resources, will be needed to get the network running. E-mail is an efficient way to communicate with various potential network members. Preliminary Internet searches are also very useful as prospective members do background research regarding the rural ethics resources currently available in the area.

These steps are vital to the success of a rural ethics network. A well-thought-out plan, supported by feedback from focus groups and needs assessments, will reduce the likelihood for unnecessary spending, and will increase the likelihood for efficient and helpful network resources. Similarly, ongoing review and updating of the network will ensure the continual improvement of its programs.

Implementation of the Network

Once professionals have established an overall network outline and plan of action, implementation will begin. This process will take time and dedication, as members begin to interact and the network grows. Ongoing assessment and evaluation of network operations, goals, member interactions, and possible network projects are extremely important. Reviewing assessments and evaluations will allow the network to continuously evolve to meet the needs of the network membership.

CONCLUSION

Ethics issues in health care cut across all types of health care institutions, including those located in small and/or rural areas throughout the country. It is often the case that both the financial and professional resources that would assist small and rural institutions in solving problems relating to health care ethics are limited. Rural ethics networks can be a useful way to share health care ethics resources—both financial and professional—to optimally serve network members.

With the use of the Internet and Web-based discussion boards, small and rural institutions can network in ways that were impossible in past years. The exchange of information among network members can be extremely useful, as many of the ethics issues that rural institutions face are often similar in nature.

This chapter has described several types of networks, and given examples of how such networks can be developed and built into a useful resource for members. Health care providers in rural areas have an opportunity to improve ethics management by employing similar networks within and without their own institutions.

REFERENCES

1. American Hospital Association. Fast facts on US hospitals. American Hospital Association. 2009. Accessed March 16, 2009.

2. Anderson-Shaw L. Rural health care ethics: what assumptions and attitudes should drive the research? *Am J Bioeth.* Mar-Apr 2006;6(2):61-62.

3. Nelson W, Weeks WB. Rural and non-rural differences in membership of the American Society of Bioethics and Humanities. *J Med Ethics.* Jul 2006;32(7):411-413.

4. Cook AF, Hoas H, Guttmannova K. Bioethics activities in rural hospitals. *Camb Q Healthc Ethics.* Spring 2000;9(2):230-238.

5. Niemira DA. Grassroots grappling: ethics committees at rural hospitals. *Ann Intern Med.* Dec 15 1988;109(12):981-983.

6. Rauh JR, Bushy A. Biomedical conflicts in the heartland. A systemwide ethics committee serves rural facilities. *Health Prog.* Mar 1990;71(2):80-83.

7. Provincial Health Ethics Network. Ethics committees. http://phen.ab.ca/ecommittees/forum.asp. Accessed March 17, 2009.

8. Center for Practical Bioethics. Welcome to the Center. http://practicalbioethics.org/. Accessed March 17, 2009.

9. National Rural Bioethics Project. Goals and intent of the project. University of Montana - Missoula. 2003; http://www.umt.edu/bioethics/goals_and_intent.htm. Accessed March 17, 2009.

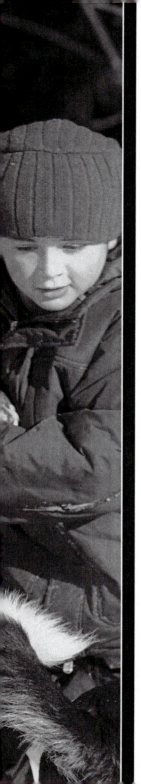

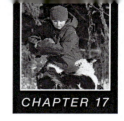

Rural Health Care Ethics:
A Selected Bibliography

Mary Ann Greene

Rural Health Care Ethics:
A Selected Bibliography

Mary Ann Greene

This bibliography is intended to guide the reader in both the theory and practice of ethics in rural health care. It is organized from the general to more specific: sources in health care ethics are introduced first, followed by those publications that provide discussion of rural health care issues and more specifically, rural ethics. Next are sections that are not limited to rural health but are related to the various common ethics issues discussed in the *Handbook*: patient/provider relationships, boundary issues, confidentiality, ethics committees, end-of-life issues, mental health issues, medical errors and patient safety, health information technology, informed consent, and allocation of resources. Unless they inform the discussion of ethics, sources that are of a legal or statistical nature, or those that generally describe the characteristics of rural life, are not included. If the reader is interested in those topics, specific chapters in the Handbook should be consulted.

In addition, a list of pertinent journals and informative Web sites follows the bibliography.

HEALTH CARE ETHICS

Beauchamp TL, Childress JF. *Principles of Biomedical Ethics*. 5th ed. New York, NY: Oxford University Press; 2001.

Beauchamp TL, Walters L. *Contemporary Issues in Bioethics*. 7th ed. Belmont, CA: Wadsworth Pub; 1999.

Bell J, Breslin JM. Healthcare provider moral distress as a leadership challenge. *JONAS Healthc Law Ethics Regul*. Oct-Dec 2008;10(4):94-97; quiz 98-99.

Boyle PJ, DuBose ER, Ellingson SJ, Guinn DE, McCurdy DB. *Organizational Ethics in Health Care: Principles, Cases, and Practical Solutions*. San Francisco, CA: Jossey-Bass; 2001.

Chervenak FA, McCullough LB. An ethical framework for identifying, preventing, and managing conflicts confronting leaders of academic health centers. *Acad Med*. Dec. 14, 2008 2004;79(11):1056-1061.

Collier J, Rorty M, Sandborg C. Rafting the ethical rapids. *HEC Forum*. Dec 2006;18(4):332-341.

Culver CM, Gert B. *Philosophy in Medicine: Conceptual and Ethical Issues in Medicine and Psychiatry*. New York, NY: Oxford University Press; 1982.

Drane JF. *Clinical Bioethics: Theory and Practice in Medical Ethical Decision-Making*. Kansas City, MO: Sheed & Ward; 1994.

Edelstein L. *The Hippocratic Oath: Text, Translation and Interpretation*. Baltimore, MD: Johns Hopkins Press; 1943.

Emanuel EJ, Wendler D, Grady C. What makes clinical research ethical? *JAMA*. May 24-31 2000;283(20):2701-2711.

Engelhardt HT. *The Foundations of Bioethics*. New York, NY: Oxford University Press; 1986.

Ethics manual. Fourth edition. American College of Physicians. *Ann Intern Med*. Apr 1 1998;128(7):576-594.

Fletcher JC, Lombardo PA, Marshall MF, Miller FG, eds. *Introduction to Clinical Ethics*. Frederick, MD: University Publishing Group; 1997.

Forrow L, Arnold RM, Parker LS. Preventive ethics: expanding the horizons of clinical ethics. *J Clin Ethics*. Winter 1993;4(4):287-294.

Friedman E, ed. *Choices and Conflict: Explorations in Health Care Ethics*. Chicago, Il: American Hospital Publishers; 1992.

Gallagher E, Alcock D, Diem E, Angus D, Medves J. Ethical dilemmas in home care case management. *J Healthc Manag*. Mar-Apr 2002;47(2):85-96; discussion 96-87.

Gert B. *Common Morality: Deciding What to Do*. New York, NY: Oxford University Press; 2004.

Gert B, Nelson WA, Culver CM. Moral theory and neurology. *Neurol Clin*. Nov 1989;7(4):681-696.

Gilbert JA. *Strengthening Ethical Wisdom: Tools for Transforming Your Health Care Organization*. Chicago, IL: Health Forum, Inc.; 2007.

HEALTH CARE ETHICS (CONTINUED)

Glover JJ. Ethical decision-making guidelines and tools. In: Harman LB, ed. *Ethical Challenges in the Management of Health Information.* 2nd ed. Sudbury, MA: Jones and Bartlett; 2006.

Hall RT. *An Introduction to Healthcare Organizational Ethics.* New York, NY: Oxford University Press; 2000.

Hofmann PB, Nelson WA, eds. *Managing Ethically: An Executive's Guide.* Chicago, IL: Health Administration Press; 2001.

Hosford B. *Bioethics Committees: The Health Care Provider's Guide.* Rockville, MD: Aspen Systems Corp; 1986.

Joint Commission on Accreditation of Healthcare Organizations JCAHO. Ethics, rights, and responsibilities. In: *Standards for Long Term Care: 2005-2006 Accreditation Policies, Standards Elements of Performance.* Oak Brook, Il: Joint Commission Resources; 2005:MC-14.

Jonsen AR, Siegler M, Winslade WJ. *Clinical Ethics: A Practical Approach to Ethical Decisions in Clinical Medicine.* New York, NY: McGraw Hill, Medical Pub. Division; 2002.

Jonsen JR. *The Birth of Bioethics.* New York, NY: Oxford University Press; 1998.

Junkerman C, Schiedermayer D. *Practical Ethics for Students, Interns, and Residents: A Short Reference Manual.* Frederick, MD: University Publishing Group; 1998.

Kaldjian LC, Weir RF, Duffy TP. A clinician's approach to clinical ethical reasoning. *J Gen Intern Med.* Mar 2005;20(3):306-311.

Lo B. *Resolving Ethical Dilemmas: A Guide for Clinicians.* 4th ed. Philadelphia, PA: Lippincott Williams & Wilkins; 2008.

Markel H. "I swear by Apollo"—on taking the Hippocratic oath. *N Engl J Med.* May 13 2004;350(20):2026-2029.

McCruden P, Kuczewski M. Is organizational ethics the remedy for failure to thrive? Toward an understanding of mission leadership. *HEC Forum.* Dec 2006;18(4):342-348.

McCullough LB. Practicing preventive ethics-the keys to avoiding ethical conflicts in health care. *Physician Exec.* Mar-Apr 2005;31(2):18-21.

Nelson W. Must I maintain another person's promise? Weighing how decisions affect stakeholders in the hospital. *Healthc Exec.* Jan-Feb 2006;21(1):34-35.

Nelson WA. The ethics of patient preferences. Autonomy has limitations when contrary to medical judgment, illegal or unethical. *Healthc Exec.* Sep-Oct 2007;22(5):34, 36-37.

Nelson WA. Ethical uncertainty and staff stress. *Healthc Exec.* 2009;24(4):38-39.

Nelson WA, Gardent PB. Ethics and quality improvement. Quality care and ethical principles cannot be separated when considering quality improvement activities. *Healthc Exec.* Jul-Aug 2008;23(4):40-41.

Nelson WA, Weeks WB, Campfield JM. The organizational costs of ethical conflicts. *J Healthc Manag.* Jan-Feb 2008;53(1):41-52; discussion 52-43.

HEALTH CARE ETHICS (CONTINUED)

Oosterhoff DD, Cand SJ, Rowell M. Shared leadership: the freedom to do bioethics. *HEC Forum*. Dec 2004;16(4):297-316.

Ozar D, Berg J, Werhane PH, Emanuel L. Organizational ethics in healthcare: toward a model of ethical decision-making by provider organizations. 2000. American Medical Assocation website. http://www. ama-assn.org/ama/upload/mm/369/ organizationalethics.pdf Accessed April 11, 2009.

Pence GE. *Classic Cases in Medical Ethics: Accounts of Cases That Have Shaped Medical Ethics, With Philosophical, Legal, and Historical Backgrounds*. Boston, MA: McGraw-Hill; 2004.

Perry F. *The Tracks We Leave: Ethics in Healthcare Management*. Chicago, IL: Health Administration Press; 2002.

Purtilo R. *Ethical Dimensions in the Health Professions*. 4th ed. Philadelphia, PA: Saunders; 2005.

Purtilo R. New respect for respect in ethics education. In: Purtilo R, Jensen GM, Royeen CB, eds. *Educating for Moral Action: A Sourcebook in Health and Rehabilitation Ethics*. Philadelphia, PA: F.A. Davis; 2005:1-10.

Reich WT, ed. *Encyclopedia of Bioethics*. New York: Macmillan; 1995.

Roberts LW, Dyer AR. *Concise Guide to Ethics in Mental Health Care*. Washington, DC: American Psychiatric Publishing; 2004.

Siegler M. Sounding Boards. Confidentiality in medicine--a decrepit concept. *N Engl J Med*. Dec 9 1982;307(24):1518-1521.

Siegler M. The progression of medicine. From physician paternalism to patient autonomy to bureaucratic parsimony. *Arch Intern Med*. Apr 1985;145(4):713-715.

Singer PA, Viens AM, eds. *The Cambridge Textbook of Bioethics*. New York, NY: Cambridge University Press; 2008.

Spencer EM, Mills AE, Rorty MV, Werhane PH. *Organization Ethics in Health Care*. New York, NY: Oxford University Press; 2000.

Weber LJ. *Business Ethics in Healthcare: Beyond Compliance*. Bloomington, IN: Indiana University Press; 2001.

Werhane PH. Business ethics, stakeholder theory, and the ethics of healthcare organizations. *Camb Q Healthc Ethics*. Spring 2000;9(2):169-181.

Werhane PH, Rorty MV. Organization ethics in healthcare. *Camb Q Healthc Ethics*. Spring 2000;9(2):145-146.

Worthley JA. *Organizational Ethics in the Compliance Context*. Chicago, IL: Health Administration Press; 1999.

RURAL HEALTH CARE

Anderson DG, Hatton DC. Accessing vulnerable populations for research. *West J Nurs Res*. Mar 2000;22(2):244-251.

Annual update of the HHS poverty guidelines. *Federal Register*. June 2, 2009;74(Jan. 23, 2009):4199-4200.

Baer LD, Johnson-Webb KD, Gesler WM. What is rural? A focus on urban influence codes. *J Rural Health*. Fall 1997;13(4):329-333.

Bailey J. Health care in rural America: a series of features from the Center for Rural Affairs Newsletter. 2004. http://www.cfra.org/pdf/Health_Care_in_Rural_America.pdf. Accessed Feb. 23, 2009.

Baldwin LM, MacLehose RF, Hart LG, Beaver SK, Every N, Chan L. Quality of care for acute myocardial infarction in rural and urban US hospitals. *J Rural Health*. Spring 2004;20(2):99-108.

Baldwin LM, Patanian MM, Larson EH, et al. Modeling the mental health workforce in Washington State: using state licensing data to examine provider supply in rural and urban areas. *J Rural Health*. Winter 2006;22(1):50-58.

Bennett KJ, Olatosi B, Probst JC. *Health Disparities: A Rural-Urban Chartbook*. Columbia, SC: South Carolina Rural Health Research Center; 2008.

Berger J, Mohr J. *A Fortunate Man: The Story of a Country Doctor*. 1st ed. New York, NY: Holt, Rinehart and Winston; 1967.

Bigbee JL, Lind B. Methodological challenges in rural and frontier nursing research. *Appl Nurs Res*. May 2007;20(2):104-106.

Bird DC, Dempsey P, Hartley D. Addressing mental health workforce needs in underserved rural areas: accomplishments and challenges. Working Paper # 23. 2001. http://muskie.usm.maine.edu/Publications/rural/wp23.pdf. Accessed Dec. 7, 2008.

Blackhall LJ, Murphy ST, Frank G, Michel V, Azen S. Ethnicity and attitudes toward patient autonomy. *JAMA*. Sep 13 1995;274(10):820-825.

Blalock SJ, Byrd JE, Hansen RA, et al. Factors associated with potentially inappropriate drug utilization in a sample of rural community-dwelling older adults. *Am J Geriatr Pharmacother*. Sep 2005;3(3):168-179.

Boffa J. Is there a doctor in the house? *Aust N Z J Public Health*. Aug 2002;26(4):301-304.

Braden J, Beauregard K. Health status and access to care of rural and urban populations. In: *National Medical Expenditure Survey Research Findings 18*. Rockville, MD: AHCPR; 1994.

Brasure M, Stensland J, Wellever A. Quality oversight: why are rural hospitals less likely to be JCAHO accredited? *J Rural Health*. Fall 2000;16(4):324-336.

Burchum JL. Cultural competence: an evolutionary perspective. *Nurs Forum*. Oct-Dec 2002;37(4):5-15.

Bushy A, ed. *Rural Nursing*. Newbury Park, CA: Sage Publications; 1991.

_____. When your client lives in a rural area. Part I: Rural health care delivery issues. Issues *Ment Health Nurs*. May-Jun 1994;15(3):253-266.

RURAL HEALTH CARE (CONTINUED)

____. Women in rural environments: considerations for holistic nurses. *Holist Nurs Pract*. Jul 1994;8(4):67-73.

____. *Rural Minority Health Resource Book*. Kansas City, MO: National Rural Health Association; 2002.

____. Creating nursing research opportunities in rural healthcare facilities. *J Nurs Care Qual*. Apr-Jun 2004;19(2):162-168.

____. Defining 'rural' before tackling access issues. *Am Nurse*. Sep 1993;25(8):20.

____. Nursing in rural and frontier areas: issues, challenges and opportunities. *Harvard Health Policy Review*. 2006;7(1):17-27.

____. Rural nursing: practice and issues. ANA Continuing Education website. http://nursingworld.org/mods/mod700/rurlfull.htm. Accessed July 2, 2009.

Bushy A, Baird-Crooks K. *Orientation to Nursing in the Rural Community*. Thousand Oaks, CA: Sage; 2000.

Canadian Rural Partnership. Canadian rural population trends. *Rural Research Notes*. 2002. http://www.rural.gc.ca/research/note/note1_e.pdf. Accessed Dec. 13, 2008.

Chan L, Hart LG, Goodman DC. Geographic access to health care for rural Medicare beneficiaries. *J Rural Health*. Spring 2006;22(2):140-146.

Christianson J. Potential effects of managed care organizations in rural communities: a framework. *J Rural Health*. Summer 1998;14(3):169-179.

Coburn AF, Wakefield M, Casey M, Moscovice I, Payne S, Loux S. Assuring rural hospital patient safety: what should be the priorities? *J Rural Health*. Fall 2004;20(4):314-326.

Commission on the Future of Health Care in Canada. Rural and remote communities. *Building on values: The future of health care in Canada – final report*. Ottawa2007: http://www.hc-sc.gc.ca/hcs-sss/alt_formats/hpb-dgps/pdf/hhr/romanow-eng.pdf. Accessed October 20, 2008.

Conesa C, Rios A, Ramirez P, et al. Rural primary care centers as a source of information about organ donation. *Transplant Proc*. Nov 2005;37(9):3609-3613.

Cox J. Rural general practice: a personal view of current key issues. *Health Bull* (Edinb). Sep 1997;55(5):309-315.

Davis DJ, Droes NS. Community health nursing in rural and frontier counties. *Nurs Clin North Am*. Mar 1993;28(1):159-169.

Eberhardt MS, Pamuk ER. The importance of place of residence: examining health in rural and nonrural areas. *Am J Public Health*. Oct 2004;94(10):1682-1686.

Gamm LD, Hutchison LL, Dabney BJ, Dorsey AM, eds. *Rural Healthy People 2010: A Companion Document to Healthy People 2010. Volume 1*. College Station, TX: The Texas A&M University System Health Science Center, School of Rural Public Health, Southwest Rural Health Research Center; 2003.

RURAL HEALTH CARE (CONTINUED)

Gamm LD, Hutchison LL, Dabney BJ, Dorsey AM, eds. *Rural Healthy People 2010: A Companion Document to Health People 2010. Volume 2*. College Station, TX: Texas A&M University System Health Science Center, School of Rural Public Health, Southwest Rural Health Research Center; 2003.

Gamm LD, Hutchison LL, eds. *Rural Healthy People 2010: A Companion Document to Healthy People 2010. Volume 3*. College Station, TX: Texas A&M Univerity System Health Science Center, School of Rural Public Health, Southwest Rural Health Research Center; 2004.

Gazewood JD, Rollins LK, Galazka SS. Beyond the horizon: the role of academic health centers in improving the health of rural communities. *Acad Med*. Sep 2006;81(9):793-797.

Gessert CE, Haller IV, Kane RL, Degenholtz H. Rural-urban differences in medical care for nursing home residents with severe dementia at the end of life. *J Am Geriatr Soc*. Aug 2006;54(8):1199-1205.

Geyman JP, Norris TE, Hart LG, eds. *Textbook of Rural Medicine*. New York, NY: McGraw-Hill; 2001.

Goldsmith HF, Wagenfeld MO, Manderscheid RW, Stiles D. Specialty mental health services in metropolitan and nonmetropolitan areas: 1983 and 1990. *Adm Policy Ment Health*. Jul 1997;24(6):475-488.

Guo G, Phillips L. Key informants' perceptions of health care for elders at the U.S.-Mexico border. *Public Health Nurs*. May-Jun 2006;23(3):224-233.

Hart LG, Larson EH, Lishner DM. Rural definitions for health policy and research. *Am J Public Health*. Jul 2005;95(7):1149-1155.

Hart LG, Salsberg E, Phillips DM, Lishner DM. Rural health care providers in the United States. *J Rural Health*. 2002;18 Suppl:211-232.

Hassinger EW, Hicks LL, Godino V. A literature review of health issues of the rural elderly. *J Rural Health*. Winter 1993;9(1):68-75.Henderson CB. Small-town psychiatry. *Psychiatr Serv*. Feb 2000;51(2):253-254.

Helling TS. The challenges of trauma care in the rural setting. *Mo Med*. Sep-Oct 2003;100(5):510-514.

Humphreys JS, Jones JA, Jones MP, et al. The influence of geographical location on the complexity of rural general practice activities. *Med J Aust*. Oct 20 2003;179(8):416-420.

Huttlinger K, Schaller-Ayers J, Lawson T. Health care in Appalachia: a population-based approach. *Public Health Nurs*. Mar-Apr 2004;21(2):103-110

Institute of Medicine. Committee on Quality of Health Care in America. *Crossing the Quality Chasm: A New Health System for the 21st Century*. Washington, DC: National Academy Press; 2001.

Institute of Medicine. Committee on the Future of Rural Health Care. Board on Health Care Services. *Quality Through Collaboration: The Future of Rural Health* Washington, DC: National Academies Press; 2005.

RURAL HEALTH CARE (CONTINUED)

Johnson-Webb KD, Baer LD, Gesler WM. What is rural? Issues and considerations. *J Rural Health.* Summer 1997;13(3):253-256.

Kaiser Commission on Medicaid and the Uninsured. The uninsured in rural America. 2003. http://www.kff.org/uninsured/upload/The-Uninsured-in-Rural-America-Update-PDF.pdf. Accessed April 5, 2009.

Larson O. Values and beliefs of rural people. In: Ford TR, ed. *Rural U.S.A.: Persistence and Change.* Ames, IA: Iowa State University Press; 1978.

Larson SL, Machlin SR, Nixon A, Zodet M. Health care in urban and rural areas, combined years 1998-2000. *MEPS Chartbook No.13.* AHRQ Pub. No. 04-0050. 2004. Agency for Healthcare Research and Quality website. http://www.meps.ahrq.gov/mepsweb/data_files/publications/cb13/cb13.shtml. Accessed Dec. 13, 2008.

Lee GR, Cassidy ML. Family and kin relations of the rural elderly. In: Coward RT, Lee GR, eds. *The Elderly in Rural Society: Every Fourth Elder.* New York, NY: Springer; 1985.

Long KA, Weinert C. Rural nursing: developing the theory base. *Sch Inq Nurs Pract.* Summer 1989;3(2):113-127.

Loue S, Quill BE, eds. *Handbook of Rural Health.* New York, NY: Kluwer Academic; 2001

Marshall CA. American Indian and Hispanic populations have cultural values and issues similar to those of Appalachian populations. *Prev Chronic Dis.* Jul 2007;4(3):A77.

McConnel CE, Zetzman MR. Urban/rural differences in health service utilization by elderly persons in the United States. *J Rural Health.* Fall 1993;9(4):270-280.

Minkler M, Blackwell AG, Thompson M, Tamir H. Community-based participatory research: implications for public health funding. *Am J Public Health.* Aug 2003;93(8):1210-1213.

Mohatt DF, Bradley MM, Adams SJ, Morris CD. Mental health and rural America: 1994-2005. An overview and annotated bibliography. Rockville, MD: Office of Rural Health Policy, US Dept of Health and Human Services; 2007: ftp://ftp.hrsa.gov/ruralhealth/RuralMentalHealth.pdf. Accessed Dec. 13, 2008.

Moscovice I, Rosenblatt R. Quality-of-care challenges for rural health. *J Rural Health.* Spring 2000;16(2):168-176.

Moscovice I, Wholey DR, Klingner J, Knott A. Measuring rural hospital quality. *J Rural Health.* Fall 2004;20(4):383-393.

Nyman JA, Sen A, Chan BY, Commins PP. Urban/rural differences in home health patients and services. *Gerontologist.* Aug 1991;31(4):457-466.

Payer L. *Medicine and Culture: Varieties of Treatment in the United States, England, West Germany, and France.* New York, NY: Henry Holt & Co.; 1996.

Reynnells L. What is rural? USDA National Agriculture Library website. http://www.nal.usda.gov/ric/ricpubs/what_is_rural.shtml. Accessed April 5, 2009.

RURAL HEALTH CARE (CONTINUED)

Ricketts TC. The changing nature of rural health care. *Annu Rev Public Health*. 2000;21:639-657.

Ricketts TC, ed. *Rural Health in the United States*. New York, NY: Oxford University Press; 1999.

Ricketts TC. Workforce issues in rural areas: a focus on policy equity. *Am J Public Health*. 2005;95(1):42-48.

Rogers CC. Rural children at a glance. *Economic Information Bulletin*. 2005(No. 1). USDA website. http://www.ers.usda.gov/publications/eib1/eib1.pdf. Accessed Dec. 7, 2008.

Romanow R. *Building on Values: The Future of Health Care in Canada*. Saskatoon, SK: Commission on the Future of Health Care in Canada; 2002.

Rosenblatt RA, Andrilla CH, Curtin T, Hart LG. Shortages of medical personnel at community health centers: implications for planned expansion. *JAMA*. Mar 1 2006;295(9):1042-1049.

Rosenblatt RA, Hart LG. Physicians and rural America. In: Ricketts III TC, ed. *Rural Health in the United States*. New York, NY: Oxford University Press; 1999:38-51.

Rosenthal TC, Fox C. Access to health care for the rural elderly. *JAMA*. Oct 25 2000;284(16):2034-2036.

Rost K, Owen RR, Smith J, Smith RJ. Rural-urban differences in service use and course of illness in bipolar disorder. *J Rural Health*. 1998;14(1):36-43.

Rowley T. The rural uninsured: highlights from recent research. Health Resources and Services Administration website. http://ruralhealth.hrsa.gov/policy/UninsuredSummary.htm. Accessed Aug. 8, 2009.

Rudman WJ, Bailey JH, Garrett PK, Peden A, Thomas EJ, Brown CA. Teamwork and safety culture in small rural hospitals in Mississippi. *Patient Safety & Quality Healthcare*. 2006(Nov/Dec).

Schoenman JA, Mueller CD. Rural implications of Medicare's post-acute-care transfer payment policy. *J Rural Health*. Spring 2005;21(2):122-130.

Schultz CG, Neighbors C. Perceived norms and alcohol consumption: differences between college students from rural and urban high schools. *J Am Coll Health*. Nov-Dec 2007;56(3):261-265.

Seshamani M, Van Nostrand J, Kennedy J, Cochran C. *Hard Times In the Heartland: Health Care in Rural America*. Washington, DC: US Dept of Health and Human Services;2009.

Shreffler MJ. Culturally sensitive research methods of surveying rural/frontier residents. *West J Nurs Res*. Jun 1999;21(3):426-435.

Simpson JL, Carter K. Muslim women's experiences with health care providers in a rural area of the United States. *J Transcult Nurs*. Jan 2008;19(1):16-23.

Smith MH, Anderson RT, Bradham DD, Longino CF, Jr. Rural and urban differences in mortality among Americans 55 years and older: analysis of the National Longitudinal Mortality Study. *J Rural Health*. Fall 1995;11(4):274-285.

RURAL HEALTH CARE (CONTINUED)

US Department of Health and Human Services. *Tracking Health People 2010*. Washington, DC: US Dept of Health and Human Services; 2000.

Virnig BA, Kind S, McBean M, Fisher E. Geographic variation in hospice use prior to death. *J Am Geriatr Soc*. Sep 2000;48(9):1117-1125.

Wallace AE, Weeks WB, Wang S, Lee AF, Kazis LE. Rural and urban disparities in health-related quality of life among veterans with psychiatric disorders. *Psychiatr Serv*. Jun 2006;57(6):851-856.

Ward MM, Jaana M, Wakefield DS, et al. What would be the effect of referral to high-volume hospitals in a largely rural state? *J Rural Health*. 2004;20(4):344-354.

Weeks WB, Kazis LE, Shen Y, et al. Differences in health-related quality of life in rural and urban veterans. *Am J Public Health*. 2004;94(10):1762-1767.

Weeks WB, Lushkov G, Nelson WA, Wallace AE. Characteristics of rural and urban cadaveric organ transplant donors and recipients. *J Rural Health*. Summer 2006;22(3):264-268.

Westfall JM, Van Vorst RF, McGloin J, Selker HP. Triage and diagnosis of chest pain in rural hospitals: implementation of the ACI-TIPI in the High Plains Research Network. *Ann Fam Med*. Dec. 13, 2008 2006;4(2):153-158.

White MA. Values of elderly differ in rural setting. *Generations*. 1977;1(4):6-7.

Willging CE, Salvador M, Kano M. Brief reports: Unequal treatment: mental health care for sexual and gender minority groups in a rural state. *Psychiatr Serv*. 2006;57(6):867-870.

Winterstein AG, Hartzema AG, Johns TE, et al. Medication safety infrastructure in critical-access hospitals in Florida. *Am J Health Syst Pharm*. Mar 1 2006;63(5):442-450.

Ziller EC, Coburn AF, Loux SL, Hoffmah C, McBride T. Health Insurance Coverage in Rural America: Chartbook. Kaiser Commission on Medicaid and the Uninsured; 2003: http://www.kff.org/uninsured/upload/Health-Insurance-Coverage-in-Rural-America-PDF.pdf. Accessed Dec. 7, 2008.

RURAL HEALTH CARE ETHICS

Anderson-Shaw L. Rural health care ethics: what assumptions and attitudes should drive the research? Am J Bioeth. Mar-Apr 2006;6(2):61-62.

Aultman JM. A foreigner in my own country: forgetting the heterogeneity of our national community. Am J Bioeth. Mar-Apr 2006;6(2):56-59.

Cook AF, Hoas H. Where the rubber hits the road: implications for organizational and clinical ethics in rural healthcare settings. HEC Forum. Dec 2000;12(4):331-340.

____. Voices from the margins: a context for developing bioethics-related resources in rural areas. Am J Bioeth. Fall 2001;1(4):W12.

____. Re-framing the question: what do we really want to know about rural healthcare ethics? Am J Bioeth. Mar-Apr 2006;6(2):51-53.

____. Ethics and rural healthcare: what really happens? What might help? Am J Bioeth. Apr 2008;8(4):52-56.

Cook AF, Hoas H, Guttmannova K. Ethical issues faced by rural physicians. S D J Med. Jun 2002;55(6):221-224.

Cook AF, Hoas H, Joyner JC. Ethics and the rural nurse: a research study of problems, values, and needs. J Nurs Law. May 2000;7(1):41-53.

Cook AF, Joyner JC. No secrets on Main Street. Am J Nurs. Aug 2001;101(8):67, 69-71.

D'Agincourt-Canning L. Genetic testing for hereditary cancer: challenges to ethical care in rural and remote communities. HEC Forum. Dec 2004;16(4):222-233.

Flannery MA. Simple living and hard choices. Hastings Cent Rep. Aug 1982;12(4):9-12.

Fraser J, Alexander C. Publish and perish: a case study of publication ethics in a rural community. J Med Ethics. Sep 2006;32(9):526-529.

Fryer-Edwards K. On cattle and casseroles. Am J Bioeth. Mar-Apr 2006;6(2):55-56.

Glover JJ. Rural bioethical issues of the elderly: how do they differ from urban ones? J Rural Health. Fall 2001;17(4):332-335.

Hardwig J. Rural health care ethics: what assumptions and attitudes should drive the research? Am J Bioeth. Mar-Apr 2006;6(2):53-54.

Jennings FL. Ethics of rural practice. Psychother Priv Pract. 1992;10(3):85-104.

Johnson ME, Brems C, Warner TD, Roberts LW. Rural-urban health care provider disparities in Alaska and New Mexico. Adm Policy Ment Health. Jul 2006;33(4):504-507.

Kelly SE. Bioethics and rural health: theorizing place, space, and subjects. Soc Sci Med. Jun 2003;56(11):2277-2288.

Klugman CM. Haves and have nots. Am J Bioeth. Mar-Apr 2006;6(2):63-64.

Klugman CM, Dalinis PM, eds. Ethical Issues in Rural Health Care. Baltimore, MD: Johns Hopkins University Press; 2008.

RURAL HEALTH CARE ETHICS (CONTINUED)

Merwin E, Snyder A, Katz E. Differential access to quality rural healthcare: professional and policy challenges. *Fam Community Health*. Jul-Sep 2006;29(3):186-194.

Mitchell GW. Rural hospitals: a different take on conflict of interest. *Trustee*. Mar 2008;61(3):30.

Nelson W. Addressing rural ethics issues. The characteristics of rural healthcare settings pose unique ethical challenges. *Healthc Exec*. Jul-Aug 2004;19(4):36-37.

Nelson W, Lushkov G, Pomerantz A, Weeks WB. Rural health care ethics: is there a literature? *Am J Bioeth*. Mar-Apr 2006;6(2):44-50.

Nelson W, Pomerantz A, Howard K, Bushy A. A proposed rural healthcare ethics agenda. *J Med Ethics*. Mar 2007;33(3):136-139.

Nelson W, Weeks WB. Rural and non-rural differences in membership of the American Society of Bioethics and Humanities. *J Med Ethics*. Jul 2006;32(7):411-413.

Nelson WA. The challenges of rural health care. In: Klugman CM, Dalinis PM, eds. *Ethical Issues in Rural Health Care* Baltimore, MD: Johns Hopkins University Press; 2008:34-59.

Nelson WA, Neily J, Mills P, Weeks WB. Collaboration of ethics and patient safety programs: opportunities to promote quality care. *HEC Forum*. Mar 2008;20(1):15-27.

Nelson WA, Pomerantz AS. Ethics issues in rural health and hospitals. In: Friedman E, ed. *Choices and Conflict: Explorations in Health Care Ethics*. Chicago, Il: American Hospital Publishers; 1992.

____. Ethics issues in rural health care. *Trustee*. Aug 1992;45(8):14-15.

Nelson WA, Pomerantz AS, Weeks WB. Response to commentaries on "is there a rural ethics literature?". *Am J Bioeth*. Jul-Aug 2006;6(4):W46-47.

Nelson WA, Schmidek JM. Rural healthcare ethics. In: Singer PA, Viens AM, eds. *The Cambridge Textbook of Bioethics*. New York, NY: Cambridge University Press; 2008:289-298.

Perkins DV, Hudson BL, Gray DM, Stewart M. Decisions and justifications by community mental health providers about hypothetical ethical dilemmas. *Psychiatr Serv*. Oct 1998;49(10):1317-1322.

Purtilo R, Sorrell J. The ethical dilemmas of a rural physician. *Hastings Cent Rep*. Aug 1986;16(4):24-28.

Purtilo RB. Rural health care: the forgotten quarter of medical ethics. *Second Opin*. Nov 1987(6):10-33.

Roberts LW, Battaglia J, Epstein RS. Frontier ethics: mental health care needs and ethical dilemmas in rural communities. *Psychiatr Serv*. Apr 1999;50(4):497-503.

Roberts LW, Battaglia J, Smithpeter M, Epstein RS. An office on Main Street. Health care dilemmas in small communities. *Hastings Cent Rep*. Jul-Aug 1999;29(4):28-37.

RURAL HEALTH CARE ETHICS (CONTINUED)

Roberts LW, Dyer AR. Caring for people in small communities. In: *Concise Guide to Ethics in Mental Health Care*. Washington, DC: American Psychiatric Publishing; 2004:175.

Roberts LW, Johnson ME, Brems C, Warner TD. Ethical disparities: challenges encountered by multidisciplinary providers in fulfilling ethical standards in the care of rural and minority people. *J Rural Health*. Fall 2007;23 Suppl:89-97.

Roberts LW, Warner TD, Hammond KG. Ethical challenges of mental health clinicians in rural and frontier areas. *Psychiatr Serv*. Mar 2005;56(3):358-359.

Robillard HM, High DM, Sebastian JG, Pisaneschi JI, Perritt LJ, Mahler DM. Ethical issues in primary health care: a survey of practitioners' perceptions. *J Community Health*. Spring 1989;14(1):9-17.

Schank JA. Ethical issues in rural counseling practice. *Can J Counselling*. 1998;32(4):270-283.

Simpson C, Kirby J. Organizational ethics and social justice in practice: choices and challenges in a rural-urban health region. *HEC Forum*. Dec 2004;16(4):274-283.

Sriram TG, Radhika MR, Shanmugham V, Murthy RS. Comparison of urban and rural respondents' experience and opinion of ethical issues in medical care. *Int J Soc Psychiatry*. Autumn 1990;36(3):200-206.

Turner LN, Marquis K, Burman ME. Rural nurse practitioners: perceptions of ethical dilemmas. *J Am Acad Nurse Pract*. Jun 1996;8(6):269-274.

Vernillo A. Preventive ethics and rural healthcare: addressing issues on a systems level. *Am J Bioeth*. Apr 2008;8(4):61-62; author reply W63-64.

Warner TD, Monaghan-Geernaert P, Battaglia J, Brems C, Johnson ME, Roberts LW. Ethical considerations in rural health care: a pilot study of clinicians in Alaska and New Mexico. *Community Ment Health J*. 2005;41(1):21-33.

PATIENT-PROVIDER RELATIONSHIPS

ABIM Foundation, American Board of Internal Medicine, ACP-ASIM Foundation, American College of Physicians-American Society of Internal Medicine, European Federation of Internal Medicine. Medical professionalism in the new millennium: a physician charter. *Ann Intern Med.* Dec. 6, 2008 2002;136(3):243-246.

American Medical Association, Council on Ethical and Judicial Affairs. Opinions on the patient-physician relationship. *Code of Medical Ethics*: http://www.ama-assn.org/ama/pub/physician-resources/medical-ethics/code-medical-ethics/opinion1001.shtml. Accessed April 5, 2009.

Andrews MM, Boyle JS. Transcultural concepts in nursing care. *J Transcult Nurs.* Jul 2002;13(3):178-180.

Balint J, Shelton W. Regaining the initiative. Forging a new model of the patient-physician relationship. *JAMA.* Mar 20 1996;275(11):887-891.

Bendapudi NM, Berry LL, Frey KA, Parish JT, Rayburn WL. Patients' perspectives on ideal physician behaviors. *Mayo Clin Proc.* Mar 2006;81(3):338-344.

Bischoff SJ, DeTienne KB, Quick B. Effects of ethics stress on employee burnout and fatigue: an empirical investigation. *J Health Hum Serv Adm.* Spring 1999;21(4):512-532.

Cassel CK. The patient-physician covenant: an affirmation of Asklepios. *Conn Med.* May 1996;60(5):291-293.

Cooper-Patrick L, Gallo JJ, Gonzales JJ, et al. Race, gender, and partnership in the patient-physician relationship. *JAMA.* Aug 11 1999;282(6):583-589.

Crocker J, Major B, Steele C. Social stigma. In: Gilbert DT, Fiske ST, Lindzey G, eds. *The Handbook of Social Psychology.* Vol 2. Boston, MA: McGraw-Hill; 1998:504-553.

Dycus D. On being a doctor...where I'm from. *Tenn Med.* Aug 2005;98(8):382-383.

Forster HP, Schwartz J, DeRenzo E. Reducing legal risk by practicing patient-centered medicine. *Arch Intern Med.* Jun 10 2002;162(11):1217-1219.

Han GS, Humphreys JS. Overseas-trained doctors in Australia: community integration and their intention to stay in a rural community. *Aust J Rural Health.* Aug 2005;13(4):236-241.

Henry MS. Uncertainty, responsibility, and the evolution of the physician/patient relationship. *J Med Ethics.* Jun 2006;32(6):321-323.

Kiser K. Doctoring the old-fashioned way. *Minn Med.* Jan 2006;89(1):8-10.

Larson L. How many hats are too many? *Trustee.* Feb 2001;54(2):6-10, 11.

Levin A. Stress of practicing in rural area takes toll on psychiatrist Psychiatric News. Dec. 13, 2008 2006;41(9):4.

Link BG, Phelan JC. Conceptualizing stigma. *Annu Rev Sociol.* 2001;27:363-385.

Loxterkamp D. Hearing voices. How should doctors respond to their calling? *N Engl J Med.* Dec 26 1996;335(26):1991-1993.

PATIENT-PROVIDER RELATIONSHIPS (CONTINUED)

Martinez R. Professional role in health care institutions: towards an ethics of authenticity. In: Wear D, Bickel J, eds. *Educating for Professionalism: Creating a Culture of Humanism in Medical Education.* Iowa City, IA: University of Iowa Press; 2000:35-48.

Maslach C, Jackson SE, Leiter MP. *Maslach Burnout Inventory Manual.* Palo Alto, CA: Consulting Psychologists Press; 1996.

Morath J, Hart LG. Partnering with families: disclosure and trust. Paper presented at: National Patient Safety Foundation/ JCAHO Patient Safety Initiative 2000: Spotlighting Strategies, Sharing Solutions; October 6, 2000; Chicago, IL. http://www.npsf.org/download/Morath.pdf. Accessed Dec. 13, 2008.

Moszczynski AB, Haney CJ. Stress and coping of Canadian rural nurses caring for trauma patients who are transferred out. *J Emerg Nurs.* Dec 2002;28(6):496-504.

Nassar ME. Racial and ethnic disparities in health care. *Ann Intern Med.* Jan 18 2005;142(2):153; author reply 153-154.

Phelan JC, Bromet EJ, Link BG. Psychiatric illness and family stigma. *Schizophr Bull.* 1998;24(1):115-126.

President's Commission for the Study of Ethical Problems in Medicine and Biomedical and Behavioral Research. Making health care decisions: the ethical and legal implications of informed consent in the patient-practioner relationship. 1982;Volume 1: Report. http://www.bioethics.gov/reports/past_commissions/making_health_care_decisions.pdf. Accessed March 19, 2009.

Roberts LW, Johnson ME, Brems C, Warner TD. Preferences of Alaska and New Mexico psychiatrists regarding professionalism and ethics training. *Acad Psychiatry.* May-Jun 2006;30(3):200-204.

Rourke LL, Rourke JT. Close friends as patients in rural practice. *Can Fam Physician.* Jun 1998;44:1208-1210, 1219-1222.

Schneck SA. "Doctoring" doctors and their families. *JAMA.* Dec 16 1998;280(23):2039-2042.

Shanafelt TD, Bradley KA, Wipf JE, Back AL. Burnout and self-reported patient care in an internal medicine residency program. *Ann Intern Med.* Mar 5 2002;136(5):358-367.

Woods D. The rural doctor: among friends on the Canada-US border. *Can Med Assoc J.* 1977;117(7):809, 812-804.

Boundary Issues

Campbell CC, Gordon MC.
Acknowledging the inevitable:
Understanding multiple relationships in
rural practice. *Prof Psychol Res Pract.*
2003;34(4):430-434.

Endacott R, Wood A, Judd F, Hulbert
C, Thomas B, Grigg M. Impact and
management of dual relationships in
metropolitan, regional and rural mental
health practice. *Aust N Z J Psychiatry.*
Nov-Dec 2006;40(11-12):987-994.

Fiske ST. Controlling other people. The
impact of power on stereotyping. *Am
Psychol.* Jun 1993;48(6):621-628.

Kullnat MW. A piece of my mind.
Boundaries. *JAMA.* Jan 24
2007;297(4):343-344.

Martinez R. A model for boundary
dilemmas: ethical decision-making in
the patient-professional relationship.
Ethical Hum Sci Serv. Spring
2000;2(1):43-61.

Miller PJ. Dual relationships in rural
practice: a dilemma of ethics and
culture. *Hum Serv Rural Environ.*
1994;18(2):4-7.

Nadelson C, Notman MT. Boundaries in
the doctor-patient relationship. *Theor
Med Bioeth.* 2002;23(3):191-201.

Scopelliti J, Judd F, Grigg M, et al. Dual
relationships in mental health practice:
issues for clinicians in rural settings.
Aust N Z J Psychiatry. Nov-Dec
2004;38(11-12):953-959.

Simon RI, Williams IC. Maintaining
treatment boundaries in small
communities and rural areas. *Psychiatr
Serv.* Nov 1999;50(11):1440-1446.

Sobel SB. Small town practice of
psychotherapy: ethical and personal
dilemmas. *Psychother Priv Pract.*
1992;10(3):61-69.

Stockman AF. Dual relationships in rural
mental health practice: An ethical
dilemma. *J Rural Comm Psych.*
1990;11(2):31-45.

CONFIDENTIALITY

American Medical Association, Council on Ethical and Judicial Affairs. Confidentiality. Opinion 5.05 - *Code of Medical Ethics*: http://www.ama-assn.org/ama/pub/physician-resources/medical-ethics/code-medical-ethics/opinion505.shtml. Accessed July 2, 2009.

Annas GJ. HIPAA regulations - a new era of medical-record privacy? *N Engl J Med*. Apr 10 2003;348(15):1486-1490.

Burnum JF. Secrets about patients. *N Engl J Med*. Apr 18 1991;324(16):1130-1133.

Centers for Disease Control and Prevention (CDC). HIPAA privacy rule and public health. Guidance from CDC and the U.S. Department of Health and Human Services. *MMWR Morb Mortal Wkly Rep*. May 2 2003;52 Suppl:1-17, 19-20.

Confidentiality of mental health information: ethical, legal, and policy issues. In: *Mental Health: A Report of the Surgeon General*. Rockville, MD: US Dept of Health and Human Services,Substance Abuse and Mental Health Services Administration, Center for Mental Health Services, National Institutes of Health, National Institute of Mental Health; 1999.

Gostin LO, Turek-Brezina J, Powers M, Kozloff R, Faden R, Steinauer DD. Privacy and security of personal information in a new health care system. *JAMA*. Nov 24 1993;270(20):2487-2493.

Slowther A, Kleinman I. Confidentiality. In: Singer PA, Viens AM, eds. *The Cambridge Textbook of Bioethics*. New York, NY: Cambridge University Press; 2008:43-48.

Spiegel PB. Confidentiality endangered under some circumstances without special management. *Psychotherapy*. Winter 1990;27(4):636-643.

Ullom-Minnich PD, Kallail KJ. Physicians' strategies for safeguarding confidentiality: the influence of community and practice characteristics. *J Fam Pract*. Nov 1993;37(5):445-448.

Yadav H, Lin WY. Patient confidentiality, ethics and licensing in telemedicine. *Asia Pac J Public Health*. 2001;13 Suppl:S36-38.

ETHICS COMMITTEES

Arnold RM, Youngner SJ, Aulisio MP. Core Competencies for Health Care Ethics Consultation: The Report of the American Society for Bioethics and Humanities. Glennview, IL: American Society for Bioethics and Humanities; 1998.

Aulisio MP, Arnold RM, Youngner SJ. Health care ethics consultation: nature, goals, and competencies. A position paper from the Society for Health and Human Values-Society for Bioethics Consultation Task Force on Standards for Bioethics Consultation. Ann Intern Med. Jul 4 2000;133(1):59-69.

Bayley C. Ethics committee DX: failure to thrive. HEC Forum. Dec 2006;18(4):357-367.

Blake DC. Reinventing the Healthcare Ethics Committee. HEC Forum. Mar 2000;12(1):8-32.

Bushy A, Rauh JR. Implementing an ethics committee in rural institutions. J Nurs Adm. Dec 1991;21(12):18-25.

Cook A, Hoas H. Are healthcare ethics committees necessary in rural hospitals? HEC Forum. Jun 1999;11(2):134-139.

Cook AF, Hoas H, Guttmannova K. Bioethics activities in rural hospitals. Camb Q Healthc Ethics. Spring 2000;9(2):230-238.

Cranford RE, Doudera AE, eds. Institutional Ethics Committees and Health Care Decision Making. Ann Arbor, MI: Health Administration Press; 1984.

Davis W. Failure to thrive or refusal to adapt? Missing links in the evolution from ethics committee to ethics program. HEC Forum. Dec 2006;18(4):291-297.

Derenzo EG, Mokwunye N, Lynch JJ. Rounding: how everyday ethics can invigorate a hospital's ethics committee. HEC Forum. Dec 2006;18(4):319-331.

Foglia MB, Pearlman RA. Integrating clinical and organizational ethics. A systems perspective can provide an antidote to the "silo" problem in clinical ethics consultations. Health Prog. Mar-Apr 2006;87(2):31-35.

Fox E, Myers S, Pearlman RA. Ethics consultation in United States hospitals: a national survey. Am J Bioeth. Feb 2007;7(2):13-25.

Having KM, Hale D, Lautar CJ. Ethics committees in the rural Midwest: exploring the impact of HIPAA. J Rural Health. Summer 2008;24(3):316-320.

Heilicser BJ, Meltzer D, Siegler M. The effect of clinical medical ethics consultation on healthcare costs. J Clin Ethics. Spring 2000;11(1):31-38.

Hinderer DE, Hinderer SR. A Multidisciplinary Approach to Health Care Ethics. Mountain View, CA: Mayfield; 2001.

Jiwani B. A mandate for regional health ethics resources. HEC Forum. Dec 2004;16(4):247-260.

La Puma J, Schiedermayer D, Siegler M. How ethics consultation can help resolve dilemmas about dying patients. West J Med. Sep 1995;163(3):263-267.

Maddalena V, Sherwin S. Vulnerable populations in rural areas: challenges for ethics committees. HEC Forum. Dec 2004;16(4):234-246.

Ethics Committees (continued)

McCullough LB. Preventive ethics, managed practice, and the hospital ethics committee as a resource for *physician exec*utives. *HEC Forum*. Jun 1998;10(2):136-151.

McCullough LB. Practicing preventive ethics-the keys to avoiding ethical conflicts in health care. *Physician Exec*. Mar-Apr 2005;31(2):18-21.

Mills AE, Rorty MV, Spencer EM, eds. Introduction: Ethics Committees and Failure to Thrive. *HEC Forum*. 2006;18(4, theme issue):270-376.

Mills AE, Rorty MV, Spencer EM. Introduction: ethics committees and failure to thrive. *HEC Forum*. Dec 2006;18(4):279-286.

Milmore D. Hospital ethics committees: a survey in Upstate New York. *HEC Forum*. Sep 2006;18(3):222-244.

Moreno JD. Consensus, contracts, and committees. *J Med Philos*. Aug 1991;16(4):393-408.

Moreno JD. Ethics committees: beyond benign neglect. *HEC Forum*. Dec 2006;18(4):368-369.

Nelson W. Where is the evidence: a need to assess rural ethics committee models. *J Rural Health*. Summer 2006;22(3):193-195.

Nelson WA. Using ethics advisory committees to cope with ethical issues. *Mo Med*. Dec 1992;89(12):827-830.

____.Evaluating your ethics committees. *Healthc Exec*. Jan-Feb 2000;15(1):48-49.

____.An organizational ethics decision-making process. *Healthc Exec*. Jul-Aug 2005;20(4):8-14.

____.Defining ethics. How to determine whether a conflict falls under your ethics committee's purview. *Healthc Exec*. Jul-Aug 2006;21(4):38-39.

____.Dealing with ethical challenges. How occurrences can be addressed before they happen. *Healthc Exec*. Mar-Apr 2007;22(2):36, 38.

____.Ethics programs in small rural hospitals. Ethics committees are essential all healthcare facilities, not just large ones. *Healthc Exec*. Nov-Dec 2007;22(6):30, 32-33.

____.Addressing organizational ethics. How to expand the scope of a clinical ethics committee to include organizational issues. *Healthc Exec*. Mar-Apr 2008;23(2):43, 46.

Nelson WA, Wlody GS. The evolving role of ethics advisory committees in VHA. *HEC Forum*. Jun 1997;9(2):129-146.

Niemira DA. Grassroots grappling: ethics committees at rural hospitals. *Ann Intern Med*. Dec 15 1988;109(12):981-983.

Niemira DA, Meece KS, Reiquam CW. Multi-institutional ethics committees. *HEC Forum*. 1989;1(2):77-81.

Niemira DA, Orr RD, Culver CM. Ethics committees in small hospitals. *J Rural Health*. Jan 1989;5(1):19-32.

Nilson EG, Fins JJ. Reinvigorating ethics consultations: an impetus from the "quality" debate. *HEC Forum*. Dec 2006;18(4):298-304.

Pape D, Manning S. The educational ladder model for ethics committees: confidence and change flourishing through core competency development. *HEC Forum*. Dec 2006;18(4):305-318.

ETHICS COMMITTEES (CONTINUED)

Post LF, Blustein J, Dubler NN. *Handbook for Health Care Ethics Committees.* Baltimore, MD: Johns Hopkins Press; 2006.

Potter RL. On our way to integrated bioethics: clinical/organizational/communal. *J Clin Ethics.* Fall 1999;10(3):171-177.

Rauh JR, Bushy A. Biomedical conflicts in the heartland. A systemwide ethics committee serves rural facilities. *Health Prog.* Mar 1990;71(2):80-83.

Research Notes: Ethics Practices and Beliefs. *Healthc Exec.* Nov/Dec 2006;21(6):74-75.

Ross JW, Glaser JW, Rasinski-Gregory D, Gibson JM, Bayley C. *Health Care Ethics Committees: The Next Generation.* Chicago, IL: American Hospital Publisher; 1993.

Schneiderman LJ, Gilmer T, Teetzel HD. Impact of ethics consultations in the intensive care setting: a randomized, controlled trial. *Crit Care Med.* Dec 2000;28(12):3920-3924.

Schneiderman LJ, Gilmer T, Teetzel HD, et al. Effect of ethics consultations on nonbeneficial life-sustaining treatments in the intensive care setting: a randomized controlled trial. *JAMA.* Sep 3 2003;290(9):1166-1172.

White ED, 2nd. Reflections on the success of hospital ethics committees in my health system. *HEC Forum.* Dec 2006;18(4):349-356.

END-OF-LIFE ISSUES

Cantor MD, Braddock CH, 3rd, Derse AR, et al. Do-not-resuscitate orders and medical futility. *Arch Intern Med*. Dec 8-22 2003;163(22):2689-2694.

Conrad E. Terminal success. *HEC Forum*. Dec 2006;18(4):287-290.

Covinsky KE, Goldman L, Cook EF, et al. The impact of serious illness on patients' families. SUPPORT Investigators. Study to Understand Prognoses and Preferences for Outcomes and Risks of Treatment. *JAMA*. Dec 21 1994;272(23):1839-1844.

Doukas DJ, McCullough LB. The values history. The evaluation of the patient's values and advance directives. *J Fam Pract*. Feb 1991;32(2):145-153.

Field MJ, Cassel CK, eds. *Approaching Death: Improving Care at the End of Life*. Washington, DC: National Academy Press; 1997.

Gazelle G. The slow code--should anyone rush to its defense? *N Engl J Med*. Feb 12 1998;338(7):467-469.

Gessert CE, Calkins DR. Rural-urban differences in end-of-life care: the use of feeding tubes. *J Rural Health*. Winter 2001;17(1):16-24.

Gessert CE, Elliott BA, Peden-McAlpine C. Family decision-making for nursing home residents with dementia: rural-urban differences. *J Rural Health*. Winter 2006;22(1):1-8.

Halevy A, Brody BA. A multi-institution collaborative policy on medical futility. *JAMA*. Aug 21 1996;276(7):571-574.

Hamric AB, Blackhall LJ. Nurse-physician perspectives on the care of dying patients in intensive care units: collaboration, moral distress, and ethical climate. *Crit Care Med*. Feb 2007;35(2):422-429.

Hastings Center. Making treatment decisions: guidelines on the decision-making process. In: *Guidelines on the Termination of Life-Sustaining Treatment and the Care of the Dying*: A Report. Briarcliff Manor, NY: Hastings Center; 1987.

_____.Prospective planning: guidelines on advance directives. In: *Guidelines on the Termination of Life-Sustaining Treatment and the Care of the Dying*. Briarcliff Manor, NY: Hastings Center; 1987.

Hern HE, Jr., Koenig BA, Moore LJ, Marshall PA. The difference that culture can make in end-of-life decisionmaking. *Camb Q Healthc Ethics*. Winter 1998;7(1):27-40.

JAMA Patient Page: advance directives. *JAMA*. Mar 15 2000;283(11):1518.

Jennings B, Kaebnick GE, Murray TH. Improving end of life care: why has it been so difficult?. . Garrison, NY: Hastings Center; 2005: http://www.thehastingscenter.org/pdf/improving_eol_care_why_has_it_been_so_difficult.pdf. Accessed Dec. 13, 2008.

Lo B. *Resolving Ethical Dilemmas: A Guide for Clinicians*. 4th ed. Philadelphia, PA: Lippincott Williams & Wilkins; 2008.

Lorenz KA, Lynn J, Dy SM, et al. Evidence for improving palliative care at the end of life: a systematic review. *Ann Intern Med*. Jan 15 2008;148(2):147-159.

End-of-Life Issues (continued)

Lynn J. Perspectives on care at the close of life. Serving patients who may die soon and their families: the role of hospice and other services. *JAMA*. Feb 21 2001;285(7):925-932.

Lynn J. Why I don't have a living will. *Law Med Health Care*. Spring-Summer 1991;19(1-2):101-104.

Meisel A, Snyder L, Quill T, American College of Physicians--American Society of Internal Medicine End-of-Life Care Consensus P. Seven legal barriers to end-of-life care: myths, realities, and grains of truth. *JAMA*. Nov 15 2000;284(19):2495-2501.

National Rural Health Association. Providing Hospice and Palliative Care in Rural and Frontier Areas. Kansas City: National Rural Health Association; 2005: Available from: http://www.capc.org/palliative-care-across-the-continuum/hospital-hospice/Rural-Toolkit-READER.pdf/view?searchterm=Providing%20hospice%20and%20palliative%20care%20in%20rural%20and%20frontier%20areas. Accessed Dec. 13, 2008.

Ostertag SG, Forman WB. End-of-life care in Hancock County, Maine: a community snapshot. *Am J Hosp Palliat Care*. Apr-May 2008;25(2):132-138.

Patrick DL, Curtis JR, Engelberg RA, Nielsen E, McCown E. Measuring and improving the quality of dying and death. *Ann Intern Med*. Sep 2 2003;139(5 Pt 2):410-415.

Perkins HS. Controlling death: the false promise of advance directives. *Ann Intern Med*. Jul 3 2007;147(1):51-57.

Qaseem A, Snow V, Shekelle P, et al. Evidence-based interventions to improve the palliative care of pain, dyspnea, and depression at the end of life: a clinical practice guideline from the American College of Physicians. *Ann Intern Med*. Jan 15 2008;148(2):141-146.

Quill TE. Perspectives on care at the close of life. Initiating end-of-life discussions with seriously ill patients: addressing the "elephant in the room". *JAMA*. Nov 15 2000;284(19):2502-2507.

Rhodes R. Futility and the goals of medicine. *J Clin Ethics*. Summer 1998;9(2):194-205

Rogers FB, Shackford SR, Hoyt DB, et al. Trauma deaths in a mature urban vs rural trauma system. A comparison. *Arch Surg*. Apr 1997;132(4):376-381; discussion 381-372.

Schneiderman LJ, Jecker N. Futility in practice. *Arch Intern Med*. Feb 22 1993;153(4):437-441.

Schneiderman LJ, Jecker NS, Jonsen AR. Medical futility: response to critiques. *Ann Intern Med*. Oct 15 1996;125(8):669-674.Schrader SL, Nelson ML, Eidsness LM. Palliative care teams on the prairie: composition, perceived challenges & opportunities. *S D Med*. Apr 2007;60(4):147-149, 151-143.

Summaries for patients. Treatment of seriously ill patients who are near the end of life: recommendations from the American College of Physicians. *Ann Intern Med*. Jan 15 2008;148(2):I42.

END-OF-LIFE ISSUES (CONTINUED)

Teno JM, Hakim RB, Knaus WA, et al. Preferences for cardiopulmonary resuscitation: physician-patient agreement and hospital resource use. The SUPPORT Investigators. *J Gen Intern Med*. Apr 1995;10(4):179-186.

Van Vorst RF, Crane LA, Barton PL, Kutner JS, Kallail KJ, Westfall JM. Barriers to quality care for dying patients in rural communities. *J Rural Health*. Summer 2006;22(3):248-253.

MEDICAL ERRORS AND PATIENT SAFETY

ACP Ethics and Human Rights
Committee. Documenting sensitive
information poses dilemma for
physicians. *Am Coll Physicians Obs.*
June 27, 2009 1996(Dec.).

American Medical Association, Council on
Ethical and Judicial Affairs. Reporting
impaired, incompetent, and unethical
colleagues, Opinion 9.031. *Code of
Medical Ethics*: http://www.ama-assn.
org/ama/pub/physician-resources/
medical-ethics/code-medical-ethics/
opinion9031.shtml. Accessed April 5,
2009.

Banja JD. *Medical Errors and Medical
Narcissism.* Sudbury, MA: Jones and
Bartlett; 2005.

Berlinger N, Wu AW. Subtracting insult
from injury: addressing cultural
expectations in the disclosure of
medical error. *J Med Ethics.* Feb
2005;31(2):106-108.

Boyle D, O'Connell D, Platt FW, Albert
RK. Disclosing errors and adverse
events in the intensive care unit. *Crit
Care Med.* May 2006;34(5):1532-1537.

Calvert JF, Jr., Hollander-Rodriguez
J, Atlas M, Johnson KE. Clinical
inquiries. What are the repercussions
of disclosing a medical error? *J Fam
Pract.* Feb 2008;57(2):124-125.

Clark PA. Medication errors in family
practice, in hospitals and after
discharge from the hospital: an ethical
analysis. *J Law Med Ethics.* Summer
2004;32(2):349-357, 192.

Cook A, Hoas H. You have to see errors
to fix them (letter). *Mod Healthc.*
2004(Dec. 6, 2004):21.

Cook AF, Hoas H, Guttmannova K. Not
by technology alone .... Project seeks
to assess and aid patient safety in rural
areas. *Biomed Instrum Technol.* Mar-
Apr 2003;37(2):128-130.

____. From here to there: lessons from
an integrative patient safety project in
rural health care settings. In: *Advances
in Patient Safety: From Research to
Implementation.* Rockville, MD: Agency
for Healthcare Research and Quality;
2005. Available at: http://www.ncbi.
nlm.nih.gov/books/bv.fcgi?rid=aps.
section.1290. Accessed Dec. 6, 2008.

Cook AF, Hoas H, Guttmannova K,
Joyner JC. An error by any other name.
Am J Nurs. Jun 2004;104(6):32-43;
quiz 44.

Cook AF, Hoas H, Kennedy J. R.Ph.s'
take on patient safety: they're caught
in the middle. *Drug Topics.* 2005;July
25:6-8.

Devers KJ, Pham HH, Liu G. What
is driving hospitals' patient-safety
efforts? *Health Aff (Millwood).* Mar-Apr
2004;23(2):103-115.

Emmons K. Commentary: The
transtheoretical model of behavior
change: Application to clinical practice.
Adv Mind Body Med. 2006;1:221-223.

Gallagher TH, Waterman AD, Ebers AG,
Fraser VJ, Levinson W. Patients' and
physicians' attitudes regarding the
disclosure of medical errors. *JAMA.*
Feb 26 2003;289(8):1001-1007.

Jeffe DB, Dunagan WC, Garbutt
J, et al. Using focus groups to
understand physicians' and nurses'
perspectives on error reporting in
hospitals. *Jt Comm J Qual Saf.* Sep
2004;30(9):471-479.

Medical Errors and Patient Safety (continued)

Kohn LT, Corrigan JM, Donaldson MS, eds. *To Err is Human: Building a Safer Health System*. Washington, DC: National Academy Press; 2000.

Lamb RM, Studdert DM, Bohmer RM, Berwick DM, Brennan TA. Hospital disclosure practices: results of a national survey. *Health Aff (Millwood)*. Mar-Apr 2003;22(2):73-83.Lindblad B, Chilcott J, Rolls L. Mary Lanning Memorial Hospital: communication is key. *Jt Comm J Qual Saf*. Oct 2004;30(10):551-558.

Liang BA. A system of medical error disclosure. *Qual Saf Health Care*. Mar 2002;11(1):64-68.

Loux SL, Payne SM, Knott A. Comparing patient safety in rural hospitals by bed count. *Advances in Patient Safety: from Research to Implementation*. Rockville, MD: Agency for Healthcare Research and Quality; 2005. http://www.ncbi.nlm.nih.gov/books/bv.fcgi?rid=aps.section.1319. Accessed Dec. 6, 2008.

Mazor KM, Simon SR, Gurwitz JH. Communicating with patients about medical errors: a review of the literature. *Arch Intern Med*. Aug 9-23 2004;164(15):1690-1697.

Morgan DG, Crossley MF, Stewart NJ, et al. Taking the hit: focusing on caregiver "error" masks organizational-level risk factors for nursing aide assault. *Qual Health Res*. Mar 2008;18(3):334-346.

Rubin SB, Zoloth L, eds. *Margin of Error: The Ethics of Mistakes in the Practice of Medicine*. Hagerstown, MD: University Publishing Group; 2000.

Sharpe VA. Promoting patient safety. An ethical basis for policy deliberation. *Hastings Cent Rep*. Sep-Oct 2003;33(5):S3-18.

Schade CP, Hannah K, Ruddick P, Starling C, Brehm J. Improving self-reporting of adverse drug events in a West Virginia hospital. *Am J Med Qual*. Sep-Oct 2006;21(5):335-341.

Smith ML, Forster HP. Morally managing medical mistakes. *Camb Q Healthc Ethics*. Winter 2000;9(1):38-53.

Wachter RM, Shojania KG. *Internal Bleeding: The Truth Behind America's Terrifying Epidemic of Medical Mistakes*. New York, NY: Rugged Land; 2005.

Weeks WB. Quality improvement as an investment. *Qual Manag Health Care*. Spring 2002;10(3):55-64.

Wu AW, Cavanaugh TA, McPhee SJ, Lo B, Micco GP. To tell the truth: ethical and practical issues in disclosing medical mistakes to patients. *J Gen Intern Med*. Dec 1997;12(12):770-775.

HEALTH INFORMATION TECHNOLOGY

Anderson JG. Social, ethical and legal barriers to e-health. *Int J Med Inform.* May-Jun 2007;76(5-6):480-483.

Anderson JG, Goodman KW. *Ethics and Information Technology: A Case-Based Approach to a Health Care System in Transition.* New York, NY: Springer; 2002.

Andrews JE, Pearce KA, Sydney C, Ireson C, Love M. Current state of information technology use in a US primary care practice-based research network. *Inform Prim Care.* 2004;12(1):11-18.

Bauer JC. Rural America and the digital transformation of health care. New perspectives on the future. *J Leg Med.* Mar 2002;23(1):73-83.

Berner ES. Ethical and legal issues in the use of health information technology to improve patient safety. *HEC Forum.* Sep 2008;20(3):243-258.

Black L, Anderson EE. Physicians, patients and confidentiality: the role of physicians in electronic health records. *Am J Bioeth.* Mar 2007;7(3):50-51.

Brooks RG, Menachemi N, Burke D, Clawson A. Patient safety-related information technology utilization in urban and rural hospitals. *J Med Syst.* Apr 2005;29(2):103-109.

Burton LC, Anderson GF, Kues IW. Using electronic health records to help coordinate care. *Milbank Q.* 2004;82(3):457-481, table of contents.

Culler SD, Atherly A, Walczak S, et al. Urban-rural differences in the availability of hospital information technology applications: a survey of Georgia hospitals. *J Rural Health.* Summer 2006;22(3):242-247.

D'Alessandro DM, D'Alessandro MP, Galvin JR, Kash JB, Wakefield DS, Erkonen WE. Barriers to rural physician use of a digital health sciences library. *Bull Med Libr Assoc.* Oct 1998;86(4):583-593.

Deady KE. Cyberadvice: the ethical implications of giving professional advice over the internet. *Georget J Leg Ethics.* Spring 2001;14(3):891-907.

Derse AR, Miller TE. Net effect: professional and ethical challenges of medicine online. *Camb Q Healthc Ethics.* Fall 2008;17(4):453-464.

Dick PT, Filler R, Pavan A. Participant satisfaction and comfort with multidisciplinary pediatric telemedicine consultations. *J Pediatr Surg.* Jan 1999;34(1):137-141; discussion 141-132.

Evans H. High tech vs "high touch": the impact of medical technology on patient care. In: Clair J, Allman R, eds. *Sociomedical Perspectives on Patient Care.* Lexington, KY: University Press of Kentucky; 1993:82-95.

Eysenbach G, Powell J, Kuss O, Sa ER. Empirical studies assessing the quality of health information for consumers on the world wide web: a systematic review. *JAMA.* May 22-29 2002;287(20):2691-2700.

Fleming DA. Ethical implications in the use of telehealth and teledermatology. In: Pak H, Edison K, Whited J, eds. *Teledermatology: A User's Guide.* Cambridge, England: Cambridge University Press; 2008:97-108.

HEALTH INFORMATION TECHNOLOGY (CONTINUED)

Gostin L. Health care information and the protection of personal privacy: ethical and legal considerations. *Ann Intern Med*. Oct 15 1997;127(8 Pt 2):683-690.

Gustke S, Balch D, West V, Rogers L. Patient satisfaction with telemedicine. *Telemed J*. 2000;6(1):5-13.

Harman LB, ed. *Ethical Challenges in the Management of Health Information*. 2nd ed. Sudbury, MA: Jones and Bartlett 2006.

Henney JE, Shuren JE, Nightingale SL, McGinnis TJ. Internet purchase of prescription drugs: buyer beware. *Ann Intern Med*. Dec 7 1999;131(11):861-862.

Hersh W. Health care information technology: progress and barriers. *JAMA*. Nov 10 2004;292(18):2273-2274.

Irvine R. Mediating telemedicine: ethics at a distance. *Intern Med J*. Jan 2005;35(1):56-58.

Jennett PA, Affleck Hall L, Hailey D, et al. The socio-economic impact of telehealth: a systematic review. *J Telemed Telecare*. 2003;9(6):311-320.

Kaplan B, Litewka S. Ethical challenges of telemedicine and telehealth. *Camb Q Healthc Ethics*. Fall 2008;17(4):401-416.

Kon AA, Rich B, Sadorra C, Marcin JP. Complex bioethics consultation in rural hospitals: using telemedicine to bring academic bioethicists into outlying communities. *J Telemed Telecare*. 2009;15(5):264-267.

Kun LG. Telehealth and the global health network in the 21st century. From homecare to public health informatics. *Comput Methods Programs Biomed*. Mar 2001;64(3):155-167.

Malecki E. Digital development in rural areas: potentials and pitfalls. *J Rural Studies*. 2003;19(2):201-214.

Nordberg R. EHR in the perspective of security, integrity and ethics. In: Bos L, Roa L, Yogesan K, O'Connell B, Marsh A, Blobel B, eds. *Medical and Care Compunetics 3*. Washington, DC: IOS Press; 2006.

Norris AC. *Essentials of Telemedicine and Telecare*. New York, NY: J. Wiley; 2002.

Ohsfeldt RL, Ward MM, Schneider JE, et al. Implementation of hospital computerized physician order entry systems in a rural state: feasibility and financial impact. *J Am Med Inform Assoc*. Jan-Feb 2005;12(1):20-27.

Sachs GA. A piece of my mind: sometimes dying still stings. *JAMA*. Nov 15 2000;284(19):2423.

Singer PA, Martin DK, Kelner M. Quality end-of-life care: patients' perspectives. *JAMA*. Jan 13 1999;281(2):163-168.

Stanberry B. *The Legal and Ethical Aspects of Telemedicine*. London, England: Royal Society of Medicine Press; 1998.

Steinhauser KE, Christakis NA, Clipp EC, McNeilly M, McIntyre L, Tulsky JA. Factors considered important at the end of life by patients, family, physicians, and other care providers. *JAMA*. Nov 15 2000;284(19):2476-2482.

HEALTH INFORMATION TECHNOLOGY (CONTINUED)

Stevenson KB, Barbera J, Moore JW, Samore MH, Houck P. Understanding keys to successful implementation of electronic decision support in rural hospitals: analysis of a pilot study for antimicrobial prescribing. *Am J Med Qual*. Nov-Dec 2005;20(6):313-318.

Thornett A. Computer decision support systems in general practice. *Int J Inform Manage*. 2001;21(1):39-47.

Tulsky JA. Beyond advance directives: importance of communication skills at the end of life. *JAMA*. Jul 20 2005;294(3):359-365.

Walker J, Thomson A, Smith P. Maximising the world wide web for high quality educational and clinical support to health and medical professionals in rural areas. *Int J Med Inform*. Jun 1998;50(1-3):287-291.

Ward MM, Jaana M, Bahensky JA, Vartak S, Wakefield DS. Clinical information system availability and use in urban and rural hospitals. *J Med Syst*. Dec 2006;30(6):429-438.

Woodward B. The computer-based patient record and confidentiality. *N Engl J Med*. 1995;333(21):1419-1422.

INFORMED CONSENT AND SHARED DECISION-MAKING

Cassell EJ. Consent or obedience? Power and authority in medicine. *N Engl J Med*. Jan 27 2005;352(4):328-330.

Ganzini L, Volicer L, Nelson WA, Fox E, Derse AR. Ten myths about decision-making capacity. *J Am Med Dir Assoc*. Jul-Aug 2004;5(4):263-267.

Roberts LW. Informed consent and the capacity for voluntarism. *Am J Psychiatry*. May 2002;159(5):705-712.

Towle A, Godolphin W. Framework for teaching and learning informed shared decision making. *BMJ*. Sep 18 1999;319(7212):766-771.

Whitney SN, McGuire AL, McCullough LB. A typology of shared decision making, informed consent, and simple consent. *Ann Intern Med*. Jan 6 2004;140(1):54-59.

ALLOCATION OF RESOURCES

Asthana S, Gibson A, Moon G, Brigham P. Allocating resources for health and social care: the significance of rurality. *Health Soc Care Community*. Nov 2003;11(6):486-493.

Daniels N. *Just Health Care*. Cambridge, MA: Cambridge University Press; 1985.

Danis M. The ethics of allocating resources toward rural health and health care. In: Klugman CM, Dalinis PM, eds. *Ethical Issues in Rural Health Care*. Baltimore, MD: Johns Hopkins University Press; 2008

Daniels N, Sabin JE. *Setting Limits Fairly: Learning to Share Resources for Health*. New York, NY: Oxford University Press; 2008.

Emanuel EJ. Justice and managed care. Four principles for the just allocation of health care resources. *Hastings Cent Rep*. May-Jun 2000;30(3):8-16.

Fordyce MA, Chen FM, Doescher MP, Hart LG. *2005 Physician supply and distribution in rural areas of the United States*. Seattle, WA: WWAMI Rural Health Research & Policy Centers; 2007.

Repenshek M. Stewardship and organizational ethics. How can hospitals and physicians balance scarce resources with their duty to serve the poor? *Health Prog*. May-Jun 2004;85(3):31-35, 56.

Ubel PA, Goold S. Recognizing bedside rationing: clear cases and tough calls. *Ann Intern Med*. Jan 1 1997;126(1):74-80.

HEALTH CARE ETHICS JOURNALS

The American Journal of Bioethics
Quarterly.
ISSN: 1526-5161 (Print); 1536-0075 (Electronic).
MIT Press.
http://bioethics.net/journal/

Cambridge Quarterly of Healthcare Ethics
Quarterly.
ISSN: 0963-1801 (Print); 1469-2147(Electronic).
Cambridge University Press.
http://journals.cambridge.org/action/displayJournal?jid=CQH

Hastings Center Report
Bimonthly.
ISSN: 0093-0334(Print); 1552-146X (Electronic).
The Hastings Center.
http://www.thehastingscenter.org/Publications/HCR/Default.aspx

HEC Forum
Quarterly.
ISSN: 0956-2737 (Print); 1572-8498 (Electronic).
Kluwer Academic Publishers.
http://www.springerlink.com/content/102899

Journal of Business Ethics
20 issues/year.
ISSN: 0167-4544 (Print); 1573-0697 (Electronic).
Kluwer Academic Publishers.
http://www.springer.com/philosophy/ethics/journal/10551

Journal of Clinical Ethics
Quarterly.
ISSN: 1046-7890 (Print).
University Publishing Group.
http://www.clinicalethics.com/

The Journal of Law, Medicine & Ethics
Quarterly.
ISSN: 1073-1105 (Print); 1748-720X (Electronic)
American Society of Law, Medicine & Ethics.
http://www3.interscience.wiley.com/journal/118497548/home

Journal of Medical Ethics
Quarterly.
ISSN: 0306-6800 (Print); 1473-4257 (Electronic).
BMJ Publishing Group.
http://jme.bmj.com/

HEALTH CARE ETHICS JOURNALS (CONTINUED)

Kennedy Institute of Ethics Journal
Quarterly.
ISSN: 1054-6863 (Print); 1086-3249 (Electronic).
Johns Hopkins University Press.
http://www.press.jhu.edu/journals/kennedy_institute_of_ethics_journal/

SELECTED HEALTH CARE ETHICS-RELATED WEB SITE RESOURCES

American College of Healthcare Executives
http://www.ache.org/

American Medical Association Ethics Group
http://www.ama-assn.org/ama/pub/physician-resources/medical-ethics.shtml

American Society of Bioethics and Humanities
http://www.asbh.org/

American Society of Law, Medicine & Ethics
http://www.aslme.org/

Center for Bioethics, University of Pennsylvania
http://www.bioethics.upenn.edu/

The Hastings Center
http://www.thehastingscenter.org/

National Center for Ethics in Health Care
http://www.ethics.va.gov/

The President's Council on Bioethics
http://www.bioethics.gov/

University of Washington Ethics Website
http://depts.washington.edu/bioethx/toc.html

Breinigsville, PA USA
15 July 2010
241798BV00003BA/1/P

9 781584 659587